Neonatal Malignant Disorders

Editor

DANIEL S. WECHSLER

CLINICS IN PERINATOLOGY

www.perinatology.theclinics.com

Consulting Editor
LUCKY JAIN

March 2021 • Volume 48 • Number 1

ELSEVIER

1600 John F. Kennedy Boulevard • Suite 1800 • Philadelphia, Pennsylvania, 19103-2899

http://www.theclinics.com

CLINICS IN PERINATOLOGY Volume 48, Number 1
March 2021 ISSN 0095-5108, ISBN-13: 978-0-323-76166-6

Editor: Kerry Holland
Developmental Editor: Karen Solomon

Clinics in Perinatology (ISSN 0095-5108) is published quarterly by Elsevier Inc., 360 Park Avenue South, New York, NY 10010-1710. Months of issue are March, June, September, and December. Business and Editorial Offices: 1600 John F. Kennedy Blvd., Ste. 1800, Philadelphia, PA 19103-2899. Customer Service Office: 3251 Riverport Lane, Maryland Heights, MO 63043. Periodicals postage paid at New York, NY and additional mailing offices. Subscription prices are $321.00 per year (US individuals), $788.00 per year (US institutions), $365.00 per year (Canadian individuals), $835.00 per year (Canadian institutions), $435.00 per year (international individuals), $835.00 per year (international institutions), $100.00 per year (US and Canadian students), and $195.00 per year (International students). International air speed delivery is included in all Clinics subscription prices. All prices are subject to change without notice. **POSTMASTER:** Send address changes to *Clinics in Perinatology*, Elsevier Health Sciences Division, Subscription Customer Service, 3251 Riverport Lane, Maryland Heights, MO 63043. **Customer Service: Telephone: 1-800-654-2452** (U.S. and Canada); **1-314-447-8871** (outside U.S. and Canada). **Fax: 1-314-447-8029. E-mail: journalscustomerservice-usa@elsevier.com** (for print support); **journalsonlinesupport-usa@elsevier.com** (for online support).

Reprints. For copies of 100 or more, of articles in this publication, please contact the Commercial Reprints Department, Elsevier Inc., 360 Park Avenue South, New York, NY 10010-1710. Tel. 212-633-3874; Fax: 212-633-3820; E-mail: reprints@elsevier.com.

Clinics in Perinatology is also published in Spanish by McGraw-Hill Interamericana Editores S.A., P.O. Box 5-237, 06500 Mexico D.F., Mexico.

Clinics in Perinatology is covered in *MEDLINE/PubMed (Index Medicus) Current Contents, Excepta Medica, BIOSIS and ISI/BIOMED.*

Contributors

CONSULTING EDITOR

LUCKY JAIN, MD, MBA
George W. Brumley Jr Professor and Chairman, Department of Pediatrics, Emory School
of Medicine, Chief Academic Officer, Children's Healthcare of Atlanta, Atlanta, Georgia,
Executive Director, Emory + Children's Pediatric Institute, Atlanta, Georgia

EDITOR

DANIEL S. WECHSLER, MD, PhD
Professor of Pediatrics, Director of Pediatric Oncology, Aflac Cancer and Blood Disorders
Center, Children's Healthcare of Atlanta, Department of Pediatrics, Emory School of
Medicine, Atlanta, Georgia

AUTHORS

DENISE ADAMS, MD
Professor, Medical Director, Complex Vascular Anomalies Frontier Program, Children's
Hospital of Philadelphia, Philadelphia, Pennsylvania

ALLISON AGUADO, MD
Interventional Radiology, Nemours/Alfred I. duPont Hospital for Children, Wilmington,
Delaware

JAMES F. AMATRUDA, MD, PhD
Division of Oncology, Department of Pediatrics, Cancer and Blood Disease Institute,
Children's Hospital Los Angeles, University of Southern California, Keck School of
Medicine of USC, Los Angeles, California

MICHAEL BRIONES, DO
Associate Professor, Clinical Director, Pediatric Hematology and Oncology, Aflac Cancer
and Blood Disorders Center, Emory School of Medicine, Atlanta, Georgia

PATRICK A. BROWN, MD
Director, Pediatric Leukemia Program, Professor, Departments of Oncology and
Pediatrics, Sidney Kimmel Comprehensive Cancer Center, Johns Hopkins School of
Medicine, Baltimore, Maryland

BRADLEY CHEEK, MD
Chief of Pediatric Pathology, Wolfson Children's Hospital, Southeastern Pathology
Associates, Jacksonville, Florida

MURALI M. CHINTAGUMPALA, MD
Texas Children's Cancer Center, Baylor College of Medicine, Houston, Texas

ANDREW M. DAVIDOFF, MD
Full Member and Chairman, Department of Surgery, St. Jude Children's Research Hospital, Memphis, Tennessee

JOSEPH T. DAVIS, MD
Assistant Professor, Department of Radiology, Duke University School of Medicine, Durham, North Carolina

MICHAEL D. DEEL, MD
Assistant Professor, Department of Pediatrics, Division of Hematology/Oncology, Duke University School of Medicine, Durham, North Carolina

KAREN E. EFFINGER, MD, MS
Assistant Professor, Division of Hematology/Oncology/BMT, Department of Pediatrics, Emory University, Medical Director of Cancer Survivor Program, Aflac Cancer and Blood Disorders Center, Children's Healthcare of Atlanta, Atlanta, Georgia

JASON FANGUSARO, MD
Director of Developmental Therapeutics, Medical Director of Clinical Research Office, Carter S. Martin Endowed Chair, Aflac Cancer and Blood Disorders Center, Children's Healthcare of Atlanta, Associate Professor, Department of Pediatrics, Emory School of Medicine, Atlanta, Georgia

A. LINDSAY FRAZIER, MD, ScM
Department of Pediatric Oncology, Children's Cancer and Blood Disorders Center, Children's Hospital Dana-Farber Cancer Center, Harvard Medical School, Boston, Massachusetts

RENEE GRESH, DO
Pediatric Hematology/Oncology, Nemours/Al DuPont Hospital for Children, Assistant Professor of Pediatrics, Sidney Kimmel Medical College at Thomas Jefferson University, Wilmington, Delaware

NATASHA IRANZAD, MD
Department of Pathology, Duke University School of Medicine, Durham, North Carolina

SANYUKTA K. JANARDAN, MD
Division of Hematology/Oncology/BMT, Department of Pediatrics, Emory University, Aflac Cancer and Blood Disorders Center, Children's Healthcare of Atlanta, Atlanta, Georgia

HOWARD M. KATZENSTEIN, MD
Division Director, Pediatric Hematology/Oncology and Bone Marrow Transplantation, Nemours Children's Specialty Care, Wolfson Children's Hospital, Professor of Pediatrics, Mayo Clinic College of Medicine and Science, Jacksonville, Florida

FRANK Y. LIN, MD
Texas Children's Cancer Center, Baylor College of Medicine, Houston, Texas

KENNETH L. McCLAIN, MD, PhD
Professor of Pediatrics, Baylor College of Medicine, Texas Children's Cancer/Hematology Centers, Houston, Texas

SARAH G. MITCHELL, MD
Department of Pediatrics, Aflac Cancer and Blood Disorders Center, Children's Healthcare of Atlanta, Emory School of Medicine, Atlanta, Georgia

DAVID H. NOYD, MD, MPH
Department of Pediatrics, Division of Hematology/Oncology, Duke University School of Medicine, Durham, North Carolina

BOJANA PENCHEVA, MMSc, CGC
Department of Pediatrics, Aflac Cancer and Blood Disorders Center, Children's Healthcare of Atlanta, Emory School of Medicine, Atlanta, Georgia

CHRISTOPHER C. PORTER, MD
Department of Pediatrics, Aflac Cancer and Blood Disorders Center, Children's Healthcare of Atlanta, Emory School of Medicine, Atlanta, Georgia

TOOBA RASHID, BSc
Department of Pediatrics, Division of Hematology/Oncology, Duke University School of Medicine, Durham, North Carolina

RACHANA SHAH, MD, MS
Division of Oncology, Department of Pediatrics, Cancer and Blood Disease Institute, Children's Hospital Los Angeles, University of Southern California, Keck School of Medicine of USC, Los Angeles, California

SHUBIN SHAHAB, MD, PhD
Pediatric Neuro-oncology Fellow, Aflac Cancer and Blood Disorders Center, Children's Healthcare of Atlanta, Instructor, Department of Pediatrics, Emory School of Medicine, Atlanta, Georgia

SEI-GYUNG K. SZE, MD
Maine Children's Cancer Program, Assistant Professor, Department of Pediatrics, Maine Medical Center, Tufts School of Medicine, Scarborough, Maine

BRENT R. WEIL, MD, MPH
Department of Surgery, Boston Children's Hospital, Department of Pediatric Oncology, Children's Cancer and Blood Disorders Center, Children's Hospital Dana-Farber Cancer Center, Harvard Medical School, Boston, Massachusetts

CHRISTOPHER B. WELDON, MD, PhD
Department of Surgery, Boston Children's Hospital, Department of Pediatric Oncology, Children's Cancer and Blood Disorders Center, Children's Hospital Dana-Farber Cancer Center, Harvard Medical School, Boston, Massachusetts

ELLIE WESTFALL, MMSc, CGC
Department of Pediatrics, Aflac Cancer and Blood Disorders Center, Children's Healthcare of Atlanta, Emory School of Medicine, Atlanta, Georgia

Contents

Pediatric cancer is rare, and malignancy during the neonatal period even rarer. However, several malignancies can present in infancy, most commonly in the form of solid tumors. Specific cancer types, bilateral or multifocal disease, associated congenital malformations, and/or cancers in close relatives may herald a diagnosis of an underlying cancer predisposition syndrome. For many patients, surveillance protocols are recommended beginning at birth or during the course of maternal prenatal care. Advantages and disadvantages of genetic testing and surveillance should be discussed with families using a multidisciplinary approach, with input from a genetic counselor with expertise in pediatric cancer predisposition.

Neonates are at risk for 3 major forms of leukemia in the first year of life: acute leukemia, juvenile myelomonocytic leukemia, and transient abnormal myelopoiesis associated with Down syndrome. These disorders are rare but generate interest due to aggressive clinical presentation, suboptimal response to current therapies, and fascinating biology. Each can arise as a result of unique constitutional and acquired genetic events. Genetic insights are pointing the way toward novel therapeutic approaches. This article reviews key epidemiologic, clinical, and molecular features of neonatal leukemias, focusing on risk stratification, treatment, and strategies for developing novel molecularly targeted approaches to improve future outcomes.

Central nervous system (CNS) tumors, including brain and spinal cord tumors, are the most common solid tumors of childhood. Within the neonatal population, however, CNS tumors are relatively rare. These often carry a dismal prognosis in part due to the limited therapeutic options available for newborns and the unique biology of these tumors compared with those seen in older infants and children. This article reviews neonatal CNS tumors, specifically their clinical presentation, imaging findings, treatment, prognosis, and associated genetic syndromes. The unique psychosocial and emotional challenges facing clinicians and families are discussed as well.

Retinoblastoma is the most common ocular malignancy of childhood. With an estimated 300 cases annually in the United States, retinoblastoma is nevertheless considered a rare tumor. Although retinoblastoma primarily affects younger children, diagnosis during the neonatal age range is less common. However, an understanding of patients at risk is critical for appropriate screening. Early detection and treatment by a multidisciplinary specialty team maximizes the chance for survival and ocular/vision salvage while minimizing treatment-related toxicity. Testing for alterations in the RB1 gene has become standard practice, and informs screening and genetic counseling recommendations for patients and their families.

Renal tumors are rare in the neonatal period. Although some may be detected prenatally, a greater proportion present after birth, most often with a palpable abdominal mass with or without other associated symptoms. Cross-sectional imaging is typically followed by radical nephrectomy to make a specific histologic diagnosis to determine the need for additional therapy. This article reviews the clinical presentation, workup, treatment, and outcomes for neonates with some of the more common renal tumors seen in this population.

Malignant liver lesions are uncommon and make up approximately 1% of all pediatric malignancies, comprising approximately 150 new diagnoses each year in the United States. The most common malignancy involving the liver is metastatic disease from neuroblastoma, leukemia, Langerhans cell histiocytosis, or hemophagocytic syndromes. Benign livers lesions often can be well characterized radiographically. Infectious processes are even more rare. The differential diagnosis of both malignant and benign lesions is age dependent. This article first provides a general approach to evaluating and managing liver tumors in infancy, and then discusses specific features of the most common types of liver tumor.

Neuroblastoma accounts for approximately 8% of all pediatric cancers, with 5% diagnosed during the neonatal period. Despite the disproportionate contribution of neuroblastoma to childhood cancer deaths, neonatal neuroblastoma has a favorable prognosis, often with little or no therapy required. Therefore, minimizing therapy and mitigating complications/toxicities are emphasized, including using a watch-and-wait approach for patients at low risk for disease progression/relapse. However, stage MS neuroblastoma exhibits a unique pattern of disseminated disease, can be challenging to manage, and may require early intervention with systemic chemotherapy. In this review, the epidemiology, treatment options, and anticipated outcomes for neonatal neuroblastoma are discussed.

Neonatal sarcomas comprise a heterogeneous group of rare soft tissue neoplasms that present unique diagnostic and therapeutic challenges. Recent advances in molecular profiling have improved diagnostic capabilities and reveal novel therapeutic targets. Clinical trials demonstrate differences in behavior between sarcoma subtypes that allow for better clinical management. Surgical resection has been replaced with a multimodal approach that includes chemotherapy and radiotherapy. Despite these advances, neonates with sarcoma continue to fare worse than histologically similar sarcomas in older children, likely reflecting differences in tumor biology and the complexities of neonatal medicine. This review focuses on recent advances in managing neonatal sarcomas.

Germ cell tumors (GCTs) comprise a wide spectrum of benign and malignant tumors. Neonatal GCTs are predominantly teratomas (mature or immature), which are typically cured with surgery alone. Relapses are infrequent even in the setting of microscopic residual disease; therefore, negative surgical margins at the cost of significant morbidity are not recommended. In neonates with metastatic malignant disease or malignant disease for which upfront surgical resection is not feasible without significant morbidity, an initial biopsy followed by neoadjuvant chemotherapy and delayed surgical resection is recommended. Carboplatin-based regimens should be considered when chemotherapy is indicated.

Langerhans cell histiocytosis, Rosai-Dorfman disease, and juvenile xanthogranuloma may present at birth or any time afterward. Some patients have minimal skin or lymph node involvement, but others present with life-threatening pulmonary, hepatic, bone marrow, or central nervous system lesions. There is often a delay in diagnosis because of confusing overlap with more common neonatal diseases. Many treatment regimens have been applied to these diseases, but those directed at myeloid cells, such as cytarabine and clofarabine or mutation-targeting inhibitors, are gaining favor. This article provides information on the pathophysiology, clinical

PROGRAM OBJECTIVE

The goal of *Clinics in Perinatology* is to keep practicing perinatologists, neonatologists, obstetricians, practicing physicians and residents up to date with current clinical practice in perinatology by providing timely articles reviewing the state of the art in patient care.

TARGET AUDIENCE

Perinatologists, neonatologists, obstetricians, practicing physicians, residents and healthcare professionals who provide patient care utilizing findings from *Clinics in Perinatology*.

LEARNING OBJECTIVES

Upon completion of this activity, participants will be able to:
1. Review cancer predisposition and the most common tumors seen in the neonatal period.
2. Discuss the rapidly changing physiology of infants that places them at high risk for long-term late effects of cancer therapy.
3. Recognize the critical importance of multidisciplinary collaborative efforts in managing neonatal malignant tumors.

ACCREDITATION

The Elsevier Office of Continuing Medical Education (EOCME) is accredited by the Accreditation Council for Continuing Medical Education (ACCME) to provide continuing medical education for physicians.

The EOCME designates this journal-based CME activity for a maximum of 12 *AMA PRA Category 1 Credit*(s)™. Physicians should claim only the credit commensurate with the extent of their participation in the activity.

All other health care professionals requesting continuing education credit for this enduring material will be issued a certificate of participation.

DISCLOSURE OF CONFLICTS OF INTEREST

The EOCME assesses conflict of interest with its instructors, faculty, planners, and other individuals who are in a position to control the content of CME activities. All relevant conflicts of interest that are identified are thoroughly vetted by EOCME for fair balance, scientific objectivity, and patient care recommendations. EOCME is committed to providing its learners with CME activities that promote improvements or quality in healthcare and not a specific proprietary business or a commercial interest.

The planning committee, staff, authors and editors listed below have identified no financial relationships or relationships to products or devices they or their spouse/life partner have with commercial interest related to the content of this CME activity:

Allison Aguado, MD; James F. Amatruda, MD, PhD; Michael Briones, DO; Patrick A. Brown, MD; Regina Chavous-Gibson, MSN, RN; Bradley J. Cheek, MD; Murali M. Chintagumpala, MD; Andrew M. Davidoff, MD; Joseph T. Davis, MD; Michael D. Deel, MD; Karen E. Effinger, MD, MS; Jason Fangusaro, MD; Renee Gresh, DO; Kerry Holland; Natasha Iranzad, MD; Lucky Jain; Sanyukta Janardan, MD; Howard Katzenstein, MD; Frank Y. Lin, MD; Sarah G. Mitchell, MD; Swaminathan Nagarajan; David H. Noyd, MD, MPH; Bojana Pencheva, MMSc, CGC; Christopher C. Porter, MD; Tooba Rashid; Rachana Shah, MD, MS; Shubin Shahab, MD, PhD; Sei-Gyung Sze, MD; Daniel Steven Wechsler, MD, PhD; Brent R. Weil, MD, MPH; Christopher B. Weldon, MD, PhD; Ellie Westfall, MMSc

The planning committee, staff, authors and editors listed below have identified financial relationships or relationships to products or devices they or their spouse/life partner have with commercial interest related to the content of this CME activity:

Denise Adams, MD: consultant/advisor for Novartis AG and Ventura

A. Lindsay Frazier, MD, ScM: consultant/advisor for Decibel Therapeutics, Inc

Kenneth L. McClain, MD, PhD: consultant/advisor for Sobi, Inc

UNAPPROVED/OFF-LABEL USE DISCLOSURE

The EOCME requires CME faculty to disclose to the participants:
1. When products or procedures being discussed are off-label, unlabelled, experimental, and/or investigational (not US Food and Drug Administration [FDA] approved); and
2. Any limitations on the information presented, such as data that are preliminary or that represent ongoing research, interim analyses, and/or unsupported opinions. Faculty may discuss information about pharmaceutical agents that is outside of FDA-approved labelling. This information is intended solely for CME

and is not intended to promote off-label use of these medications. If you have any questions, contact the medical affairs department of the manufacturer for the most recent prescribing information.

TO ENROLL
To enroll in the *Clinics in Perinatology* Continuing Medical Education program, call customer service at 1-800-654-2452 or sign up online at http://www.theclinics.com/home/cme. The CME program is available to subscribers for an additional annual fee of USD 265.00.

METHOD OF PARTICIPATION
In order to claim credit, participants must complete the following:
1. Complete enrolment as indicated above.
2. Read the activity.
3. Complete the CME Test and Evaluation. Participants must achieve a score of 70% on the test. All CME Tests and Evaluations must be completed online.

CME INQUIRIES/SPECIAL NEEDS
For all CME inquiries or special needs, please contact elsevierCME@elsevier.com.

CLINICS IN PERINATOLOGY

Foreword

Can New Frontiers in Cancer Treatment Tame This Malady?

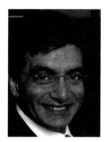

Lucky Jain, MD, MBA
Consulting Editor

In his bestselling book, "The Emperor of All Maladies,"[1] the author digs deep into the "mind" of cancer and asks "Is cancer's end conceivable in the future? Is it possible to eradicate cancer from our bodies and societies forever?"[1] Recent scientific advances in cancer immunobiology and immunotherapy give hope as do genetics and precision medicine. However, the goal can only be viewed from afar: Cancer continues to be a menace and has surpassed all other biologic causes of death in many nations!

Neonatal cancer is uncommon. Yet, when it happens, it brings with it the same level of dread as in older patients. Indeed, outcomes can be quite variable, and few definitive therapies are universally successful. As new knowledge unfolds about predisposition, early diagnosis, and definitive treatment, we remain hopeful that there will be more cures and better outcomes.

After all, spurred by the amazing work done by cancer consortiums, pediatric oncologists have changed the face of pediatric leukemias and many other malignancies.

Immunotherapy is one such approach that holds great promise. It harnesses one's own immune system to target malignant cells and includes use of cytokines, monoclonal antibodies, vaccines, and adaptive-cell transfer therapy.[2] The biology behind these approaches is fascinating. Cells in the body display on their surface endogenous peptides derived from intracellular proteins. In the event the cell undergoes malignant transformation or is infected with a pathogen, peptides derived from the mutant protein or the foreign organism are expressed on the surface, exposing it to T cells carrying highly sensitive and specific T-cell receptor looking for non-self-signals.[3] Chimeric antigen receptors (CARs) are genetic constructs consisting of an antigen-recognizing antibody molecule linked to a T-lymphocyte signaling domain used in ex vivo engineering of tumor reactive lymphocytes (**Fig. 1**).[4] Oncology literature is replete with novel bioengineering approaches being used to refine immunotherapy, including programming of T cells with genetic modules to increase their potency and specificity.

Clin Perinatol 48 (2021) xv–xvii
https://doi.org/10.1016/j.clp.2020.12.003
0095-5108/21/© 2020 Published by Elsevier Inc.

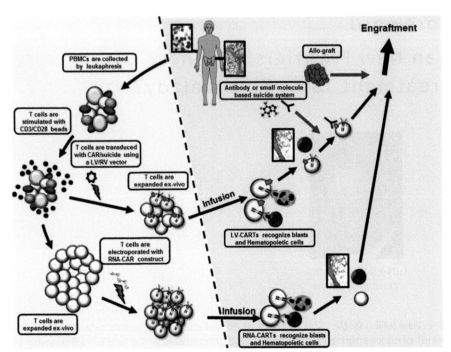

Fig. 1. How myeloid chimeric antigen receptor T-cell therapy can be used in a novel conditioning regimen as a way to induce antileukemic activity and myeloablation. CAR, chimeric antigen receptor; LV-CARTs, left ventricular chimeric antigen receptor T cells; LV/RV, left ventricular/right ventricular; PBMC, peripheral blood mononuclear cell. (With permission from Kenderian SS, Porter DL, Gill S. Chimeric Antigen Receptor Cell Transplantation: How not to put the CART before the horse. Biol Blood Marrow Transplant. 2017;23:235-246.)

Indeed, the successful development of messenger RNA (mRNA)-based vaccines for COVID-19 in record time points to the tantalizing possibility of personalized tumor vaccination using mRNA constructs from the cancer.[5] High-risk individuals could even have preventive immunization if the genetic predisposition and specific cancer type it leads to is known. However, significant challenges remain in broader application of these modalities, including toxicity associated with the treatment and cancer relapse with antigen-negative tumors.[3]

In this issue of the *Clinics in Perinatology*, Dr Wechsler has brought together authors to cover advances in malignant disorders in neonates. The authors point to the need for a uniform approach to tackling these rare but often lethal cancers. As always, I am grateful to the publishing staff at Elsevier, including Kerry Holland and Karen Justine Solomon, for their support in bringing this important publication to you.

Lucky Jain, MD, MBA
Department of Pediatrics
Emory University School of Medicine
Children's Healthcare of Atlanta
Emory + Children's Pediatric Institute
2015 Uppergate Drive NE
Atlanta, GA 30322, USA

E-mail address:
ljain@emory.edu

REFERENCES

1. Mukherjee S. The emperor of all maladies. A biography of cancer. New York: Scribner; 2010.
2. Baxevanis CN, Perez SA, Papamichail M. Cancer immunotherapy. Crit Rev Clin Lab Sci 2009;46:167–89.
3. Labanieh L, Majzner RG, Mackall CL. Programming CAR-T cells to kill cancer. Nat Biomed Eng 2018;2:377–91.
4. Kenderian SS, Porter DL, Gill S. Chimeric antigen receptor cell transplantation: how not to put the CART before the horse. Biol Blood Marrow Transplant 2017; 23:235–46.
5. Corey L, Mascola JR, Fauci AS, Collins FS. A strategic approach to COVID-19 vaccine R&D. Science 2020;368:948–50.

Preface

Neonatal Malignant Tumors

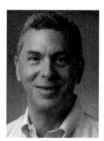

Daniel S. Wechsler, MD, PhD
Editor

Pediatric cancers comprise a large group of heterogeneous tumors that are anatomically and histologically diverse. Over the past few decades, great strides have been made in pediatric oncology, with current overall survival rates in the range of 80%. This issue of *Clinics in Perinatology* focuses on the diagnosis and management of tumors that are commonly seen in neonates within the first months of life.

The incidence of tumors in the neonatal period is estimated to be 1:12,500 to 1:27,500 and to account for approximately 2% of all pediatric cancers.[1] Neonatal cancers differ from those in older patients in incidence, anatomical location, and clinical behavior.[2–5] From an etiologic standpoint, neonates, by definition, will have had minimal environmental exposures that might contribute to the development of cancer. It is therefore particularly important to consider the possibility of a genetic predisposition in an infant diagnosed with cancer in the perinatal period. Therapeutically, it is critical to recognize that surgical management of neonatal tumors, whether benign or malignant, may not be straightforward because of their size and location relative to vital structures. Moreover, the use of chemotherapy in babies can be challenging as a result of rapidly occurring developmental physiological changes.[6,7] The early involvement of a multidisciplinary team that includes pediatric oncologists, pediatric surgeons, and other pediatric subspecialists is essential for the effective management of tumors in neonates.

I am grateful to the expert pediatric hematologists and oncologists who have contributed to this issue of *Clinics in Perinatology*. After first addressing the critical importance of cancer predisposition in neonates and infants (Mitchell and colleagues), we specifically consider the most common tumors that are seen in the neonatal period, including leukemia (Brown), brain tumors (Shahab and Fangusaro), retinoblastoma (Lin and Chintagumpala), tumors of the kidney (Sze) and liver (Katzenstein and colleagues), neuroblastoma (Davidoff), sarcomas (Rashid and colleagues), and germ cell tumors (Shah and colleagues). Although not technically tumors per se, it is important for

Clin Perinatol 48 (2021) xix–xx
https://doi.org/10.1016/j.clp.2020.12.002
0095-5108/21/© 2020 Published by Elsevier Inc.

perinatology.theclinics.com

neonatologists and pediatricians to be familiar with the neonatal presentation and management of histiocytic disorders (McClain) and vascular malformations (Briones and Adams). Finally, the unique and rapidly changing physiology of infants places them at particularly high risk for long-term late effects of therapy, which are discussed in the article by Janardan and Effinger. In summary, this issue provides an overview of tumors that are likely to be encountered in neonates and emphasizes the critical importance of multidisciplinary collaborative efforts in managing these rare conditions.

Daniel S. Wechsler, MD, PhD
Aflac Cancer & Blood Disorders Center
Children's Healthcare of Atlanta
Department of Pediatrics
Emory University School of Medicine
HSRB-W344
1760 Haygood Drive NE
Atlanta, GA 30322, USA

E-mail address:
dan.wechsler@emory.edu

REFERENCES

1. Moore SW, Satgé D, Sasco AJ, et al. The epidemiology of neonatal tumours. Report of an international working group. Pediatr Surg Int 2003;19:509–19.
2. Chandrasekaran A. Neonatal solid tumors. Pediatr Neonatol 2018;59:65–70.
3. Moore SW. Neonatal tumours. Pediatr Surg Int 2013;29:1217–29.
4. Orbach D, Sarnacki S, Brisse HJ, et al. Neonatal cancer. Lancet Oncol 2013;14: e609–20.
5. Shekdar KV, Schwartz ES. Brain tumors in the neonate. Neuroimaging Clin N Am 2017;27:69–83.
6. Veal GJ, Boddy AV. Chemotherapy in newborns and preterm babies. Semin Fetal Neonatal Med 2012;17:243–8.
7. Veal GJ, Errington J, Sastry J, et al. Adaptive dosing of anticancer drugs in neonates: facilitating evidence-based dosing regimens. Cancer Chemother Pharmacol 2016;77:685–92.

Cancer Predisposition in Neonates and Infants
Recognition, Tumor Types, and Surveillance

Sarah G. Mitchell, MD, Bojana Pencheva, MMSc, CGC,
Ellie Westfall, MMSc, CGC, Christopher C. Porter, MD*

KEYWORDS

- Infant malignancy • Neonatal malignancy • Cancer predisposition
- Cancer surveillance

KEY POINTS

- Neonatal malignancies are rare diagnoses, accounting for 1% to 2% of all childhood cancers.
- Neonatal malignancies may be caused by an underlying cancer predisposition syndrome with profound implications for patients and families.
- For neonates with a known cancer predisposition syndrome, recommended biochemical and imaging surveillance often begins at birth if not prenatally.
- Pediatric oncologists and genetic counselors play a significant role in recognition of patients at risk for cancer predisposition syndromes.

INTRODUCTION

Childhood cancer is rare, and malignancy during the neonatal period is even rarer, comprising only approximately 1% to 2% of all childhood cancers.[1,2] Although the cause of pediatric cancer is multifactorial, it is estimated that at least 10% may be related to an underlying genetic predisposition syndrome.[3,4] The age at which patients with cancer predisposition syndromes develop malignancy is variable, although several syndromes are associated with risk for cancer in the neonate, most commonly in the form of solid tumors.[5] Main features that lead to suspicion of a cancer predisposition syndrome include specific types of cancer, bilateral or multifocal disease, associated congenital malformations, and a diagnosis of cancer in close relatives.[6] We discuss here several tumors of neonates and infants associated with cancer predisposition syndromes. We also include current recommendations for imaging and

Department of Pediatrics, Aflac Cancer and Blood Disorders Center, Children's Healthcare of Atlanta, Emory University School of Medicine, 1760 Haygood Drive, Atlanta, GA 30322, USA
* Corresponding author. 1760 Haygood Drive, Atlanta, GA 30322.
E-mail address: chris.porter@emory.edu

Clin Perinatol 48 (2021) 1–14
https://doi.org/10.1016/j.clp.2020.11.001
0095-5108/21/© 2020 Elsevier Inc. All rights reserved.

biochemical surveillance to be initiated perinatally (**Table 1**), because several consensus guidelines were systematically developed and published.[4]

NEUROBLASTOMA

Neuroblastoma is the most commonly diagnosed neonatal malignancy, but tumors in this age group account for less than 5% of all neuroblastoma cases. In light of increasing use of ultrasound during pregnancy, the disease is most often identified as an incidentally detected suprarenal mass on routine prenatal imaging, with a differential diagnosis that includes nonmalignant conditions, such as adrenal hemorrhage, extrapulmonary sequestration, upper pole renal cysts, and bronchogenic cysts.[6] Neonatal neuroblastoma typically carries a favorable prognosis, with most patients classified as having low- or intermediate-risk group disease.[7] Close monitoring with ultrasound imaging and urine catecholamines may be the only intervention, because it is estimated that nearly 50% of neuroblastomas spontaneously regress.[8] If surgery is indicated, minimally invasive procedures are often feasible for well-defined adrenal tumors. Chemotherapy is typically only indicated for localized neuroblastoma if symptomatic, such as for patients with respiratory distress because of large thoracic tumors or neurologic compromise because of dumbbell tumors causing spinal cord compression.[9]

Although neuroblastoma is the most common neonatal cancer diagnosis, it is rarely detected within the context of its known cancer predisposition syndromes at such a young age. Approximately 1% to 2% of neuroblastomas are thought to be hereditary, most of which are related to highly penetrant, autosomal-dominant germline mutations in *PHOX2B* (associated with neural crest disorders including congenital central hypoventilation syndrome and Hirschsprung disease) and *ALK*.[10,11] Neuroblastomas that develop because of these syndromes typically occur earlier than sporadic ones, with one study identifying a mean age of diagnosis of 9 months versus 2 to 3 years, respectively.[12] Additional predisposition syndromes that carry a risk for neuroblastoma development include Li-Fraumeni syndrome (LFS; especially the R337H pathogenic variant of *TP53*), Beckwith-Wiedemann syndrome with a germline *CDKN1C* mutation, germline *RAS* pathway gene mutations (most frequently Costello syndrome and Noonan syndrome), Simpson-Golabi-Behmel syndrome, and germline variants in more newly discovered genes *KIF1B* and *GALNT14*.[13]

Despite most predisposed patients developing neuroblastoma after the neonatal period, malignancy can be present at birth. Most tumors arise in the abdomen, specifically the adrenal gland, but approximately 20% of primary neonatal neuroblastomas may arise in the chest. As a result, neuroblastoma surveillance recommendations offer guidance to begin monitoring neonates at birth, or as soon as a neuroblastoma predisposition syndrome diagnosis is made, with abdominal ultrasound, urine catecholamines (homovanillic acid and vanillylmandelic acid), and chest radiograph every 3 months through the age of 6 years.[10] The exception to these studies is a general recommendation to avoid even the minimal radiation exposure associated with a chest radiograph in patients with pathogenic *TP53* mutations, pursuing solely ultrasound and biochemical laboratory surveillance.

RETINOBLASTOMA

Retinoblastoma is the most common pediatric intraocular malignancy, with 250 to 500 new diagnoses in the United States annually.[14,15] Its well-known association with a pathogenic germline *RB1* mutation, first proposed in 1971 by Alfred Knudson in his "two-hit" hypothesis and validated with the cloning of the *RB1* gene (chromosome

Table 1
Tumors, associated gene and/or syndrome, and surveillance recommendations from birth to 12 months

Malignancy	Associated Gene	Associated Syndrome	Surveillance Recommendations (0–12 mo of Age)
Neuroblastoma	PHOX2B	Congenital Central Hypoventilation Syndrome	Abdomen US, urine HVA/VMA, chest x-ray Q3 months[10]
	ALK	Hereditary Neuroblastoma Syndrome	Abdomen US, urine HVA/VMA, chest x-ray Q3 months[10]
Retinoblastoma	RB1	Hereditary Retinoblastoma Syndrome	Birth: Baseline non-sedated eye exam Age 1 wk – 8 wk: Q2-4 wk non-sedated eye exams Age 8 wk – 12 mo: EUA monthly[10]
Adrenocortical Carcinoma	TP53	Li-Fraumeni Syndrome	Abdomen US, total testosterone, DHEA, androstenedione Q3 months Annual whole-body MRI and annual brain MRI[21]
Rhabdoid Tumor	SMARCB1	Rhaboid Tumor Predisposition Syndrome, Type 1	Brain MRI and abdomen US Q3 months[31]
Pleuropulmonary Blastoma	DICER1	DICER1 Syndrome	Third trimester prenatal US Chest x-ray at birth Chest CT and abdomen US at age 3-6 mo[34]
Medullary Thyroid Carcinoma	RET (p.M918T variant)	Multiple Endocrine Neoplasia, Type 2B	Total thyroidectomy in infancy Thyroid US, serum calcitonin, CEA level Q6 months[38]
Hepatoblastoma	APC (11p15.5 abnormality)	Familial Adenomatous Polyposis	Consideration of abdomen US with AFP level Q4-6 mo[44]
		Beckwith-Wiedemann Syndrome, Isolated Hemihypertrophy, etc	Abdomen US with AFP level Q3 months[47]

(continued on next page)

Table 1
(continued)

Malignancy	Associated Gene	Associated Syndrome	Surveillance Recommendations (0–12 mo of Age)
Wilms Tumor	WT1 (11p15.5 abnormality)	WT1-related disorders (WAGR, Denys-Drash) Beckwith-Wiedemann Syndrome, Isolated Hemihypertrophy, etc	Abdomen US Q3 months[47] Abdomen US Q3 months[26]
Hematologic Neoplasms			
Transient Abnormal Myelopoiesis (benign)	(Trisomy 21)	Down Syndrome	Birth: Complete blood count with differential[50,60]
Myeloproliferative Disorder in Noonan Syndrome (benign)	PTPN11, KRAS	Noonan Syndrome	Birth: Complete blood count with differential
Juvenile Myelomonocytic Leukemia (malignant)			Q6 month complete blood count with differential[57]
Acute Myeloid Leukemia (malignant)	RUNX1, CEBPA, FANCA, etc.	Multiple	At diagnosis: Complete blood count with differential, consider bone marrow evaluation Q 6-12 mo complete blood count with differential[62]
Acute Lymphoblastic Leukemia (malignant)	ETV6, IKZF1, others	Multiple	At diagnosis: Complete blood count with differential, consider bone marrow evaluation Q 6-12 mo complete blood count with differential[62]

13q14.1-q14.2) in 1986, has made hereditary retinoblastoma the standard model for the study of tumor suppressor genes and autosomal-dominant hereditary cancer syndromes.[16,17] Approximately 40% of retinoblastoma diagnoses are hereditary, 80% of which occur as a result of a de novo mutation, without any family history of the disease.[10] Most of these hereditary cases are bilateral and/or multifocal in nature. However, approximately 10% to 15% of children with unilateral, unifocal disease also carry a germline RB1 mutation. In addition to retinoblastoma, patients with a germline RB1 mutation are at an increased risk for second malignancies later in life including sarcoma, thyroid carcinoma, and melanoma.[13] This risk is higher if radiation therapy was a component of treatment of the patient's retinoblastoma. The average age at diagnosis for children with an RB1 germline mutation is 10 to 12 months, often identified by the presence of leukocoria on a routine well-baby examination. Identification of tumors in the neonatal age group is becoming more common, however, in an era of rapid, reliable genetic testing.[18]

Surveillance for known carriers of a germline RB1 pathogenic mutation begins at birth, and perhaps even before. If a fetus is known to harbor the gene defect, prenatal surveillance is undertaken, although this is not uniformly recommended in the United States. Fetal ultrasound has been used with particular attention paid to the ocular structures, evaluating for the presence of calcification or increased echogenicity that could signify a more advanced retinoblastoma. Prenatal MRI protocols have been developed at some centers, although the risks of such a study to the developing fetus are not definitively clear.[18] In Canada, experts have advocated for induction of labor at 36 weeks to allow affected neonates to undergo early diagnosis and management when retinoblastomas could be treated with focal modalities including cryotherapy and laser ablation.[19] One small study of 20 prenatally diagnosed infants with pathogenic RB1 mutations demonstrated an increased likelihood of being born without detectable tumors, improved vision outcomes, and less need for invasive therapies with early term delivery at 36 to 38 weeks' gestation. In the United States, however, the focus has been on delivery at term with an intensive retinal surveillance protocol initiated postnatally.[20] Typical intraocular screening recommendations include a nonsedated ophthalmic examination by a pediatric ophthalmologist or retinal specialist shortly after or within 1 week of birth. Follow-up, nonsedated examinations then take place every 2 to 4 weeks through the age of approximately 2 to 3 months, at which point monthly dilated examinations under anesthesia for full retinal visualization become the standard through the age of 1 year. For those infants who develop an intraocular tumor, a brain MRI is recommended to evaluate for pineoblastoma, a diagnosis designated as trilateral retinoblastoma. However, considering the 2% to 5% risk of pineoblastoma in hereditary retinoblastoma patients along with potential risks of anesthesia on the developing brain, routine surveillance sedated brain MRI protocols have been called into question. Current recommendations range from one baseline brain imaging study at the time of intraocular tumor diagnosis to every 6 month screening brain MRI scans from birth to 5 years of age.[10]

ADRENOCORTICAL CARCINOMA

Adrenocortical carcinoma (ACC) is one of the "core cancers" associated with LFS, an aggressive cancer predisposition syndrome with a high risk for early onset malignancies first described in 1969 by Frederick Li and Joseph Fraumeni Jr.[21] It is estimated that 50% to 70% of children with ACC have a germline pathogenic variant in TP53 (chromosome 17p13.1), identified in 1990 as the genetic link to LFS.[22,23] Furthermore, per National Comprehensive Cancer Network guidelines, all individuals with

ACC meet criteria for germline analysis of *TP53*.[13] Neonatal ACC may be diagnosed as an incidental finding on prenatal ultrasound or palpated as an abdominal mass on routine infant examination. However, ACC is known to secrete cortisol and androgens, and as a result may more commonly present as neonatal Cushing syndrome and/or virilization with clinical manifestations including obesity/weight gain, rounded facies, easy bruising, acne, hirsutism, hypertrophy of the clitoris or penis, hypertension, proximal muscle weakness, increased infection risk, hyperglycemia, hypokalemia, and hyperlipidemia.[24] Two-thirds of patients with ACC have resectable tumors at diagnosis, and overall survival for this cohort is excellent. Management in these cases includes a curative, en bloc resection of the tumor and the peritumoral/periadrenal fat, either in a laparoscopic or open fashion depending on size and surgeon preference. Adjuvant chemotherapy via a cisplatin-based regimen with mitotane is indicated for those tumors that are unresectable or metastatic, although long-term outcomes for these patients remain poor.[25]

Cancer surveillance for neonates known to have LFS begins at birth with a complete abdominopelvic ultrasound, and follow-up abdominopelvic ultrasound imaging is recommended every 3 to 4 months along with detailed physical examinations. Special attention should be paid to blood pressure, weight, height, and examination findings concerning for Cushing syndrome or androgen excess. Furthermore, peripheral blood biochemical markers including total testosterone, dehydroepiandrosterone sulfate, and androstenedione are obtained along with surveillance ultrasounds for more in-depth ACC evaluation.

In addition to the risk for ACC, neonates with LFS are at increased risk for the development of sarcomas and brain tumors. As such, annual brain MRI (the first of which should be obtained with contrast) and annual whole-body MRI are also recommended, with surveillance ultrasounds starting when the syndrome diagnosis is made.[22,26]

RHABDOID TUMOR

Rhabdoid tumors are rare, highly aggressive malignant tumors that can arise in any soft tissue, but most often do so in the kidney (rhabdoid tumor of the kidney [RTK]) or the brain, where they are classified as atypical teratoid rhabdoid tumors (ATRT).[27] Most often identified in very young children, with a median age at diagnosis of approximately 15 to 18 months, rhabdoid tumors can present in infancy as multiple primary malignancies with a dismal prognosis. In one Canadian study, median survival time for infants age 6 months and younger was 3 months.[28] Generally, these very young patients are found to have a central nervous system ATRT and an RTK, or an ATRT and a lung or liver tumor. As such, brain and spine imaging should be undertaken for all patients with an RTK or other soft tissue rhabdoid tumor diagnosis. Treatment of rhabdoid tumors is intensive, and typically uses a combination of chemotherapy, surgery, and radiation.[29] High-dose chemotherapy with autologous stem cell transplant may be considered for very young patients with ATRT, because delaying, or potentially avoiding, cranial radiation therapy has important implications for minimizing negative long-term neuropsychological outcomes.[30]

It is estimated that approximately 25% to 30% of all patients with a rhabdoid tumor have an underlying predisposition syndrome, the likelihood of which increases with younger age at diagnosis and in the metachronous setting. Most of these individuals have a loss of function germline pathogenic alteration in the *SMARCB1* gene (also called *INI1*) located on chromosome 22q11.2, consistent with a diagnosis of rhabdoid tumor predisposition syndrome, type 1. A much smaller percentage of rhabdoid malignancies are detected in the context of a germline *SMARCA4* gene (chromosome

19p13.2) loss of function mutation, or rhabdoid tumor predisposition syndrome, type 2.[27,31]

Although no formal guidelines are in place for infants with known rhabdoid tumor predisposition syndrome, suggested surveillance has been proposed for germline carriers of loss of function *SMARCB1* variants and begins at birth. In light of the aggressive nature of rhabdoid malignancies, and the propensity for development of ATRT over other tumor locations, brain MRI screening is recommended every 3 months until the age of 5 years. Abdominal ultrasounds should also be obtained every 3 months through age 5 years for RTK surveillance. Whole-body MRI may be considered, but there is a lack of data to guide the imaging timing, frequency, and risk/benefit ratio to help guide parents in decision making regarding this aggressive strategy.[32] For the small number of *SMARCA4* germline mutation carriers, data are not available to recommend brain or abdominal imaging surveillance in infancy, and the risk for rhabdoid tumors is thought to be low. Instead, the focus for these patients is on ovarian surveillance in early adult years because of a risk of small cell carcinoma of the ovary, hypercalcemic type.[32]

PLEUROPULMONARY BLASTOMA

Pleuropulmonary blastoma (PPB) is the most common primary malignancy of the lung in childhood.[33] First described as a distinct entity in 1988, it was not until 2009 that heterozygous germline mutations in the *DICER1* gene (chromosome 14q32.13) were identified as causative in most PPB cases.[34] Three types of PPB have been defined, reflecting the progressive course of the disease over time, from a cystic lung lesion in infancy to a highly aggressive, sarcomatous malignancy by the age of 3 to 4 years. Type I PPB, a purely cystic entity with malignant cells limited to the cyst septa, may develop into a more aggressive type II PPB, combined solid and cystic PPB, and further still into the most aggressive type III PPB, a completely solid, often anaplastic, high-grade malignancy. Both type II and type III PPB diagnoses require careful metastatic disease evaluation and the quick initiation of chemotherapy as part of intensive, multimodal treatment.[34] A separate cystic lesion, type 1r PPB, is labeled as a "nonprogressed/regressed" benign version of the type 1 PPB, diagnosed as such only after careful pathologic tissue evaluation without identification of the small layer of primitive, malignant cells within the cyst septa.[35]

Classically, an infant is diagnosed with a multicystic lesion in the chest either incidentally or based on respiratory symptoms. Pulmonary cysts later found to be PPB have been identified on prenatal imaging at 23 weeks gestational age.[34,36] Types 1 and 1r PPB are extremely difficult to differentiate from other congenital lung cysts, and the distinction is essentially impossible based on radiologic imaging alone. As a result, the general recommendation is for early surgical resection of lung cysts diagnosed in infancy as opposed to observation or treatment with nonoperative strategies.[37]

For those fetuses who are at risk for DICER1 syndrome via a known maternal or paternal diagnosis and for those who have been confirmed to harbor a pathogenic mutation via prenatal testing, a third trimester ultrasound is advised to evaluate for large lung cysts that may need early intervention following birth.[35,38] Postnatally, a chest radiograph is recommended at birth to again screen for large pulmonary cysts, and a chest computed tomography should be obtained between 3 and 6 months of age.[38] In addition to chest imaging, an abdominal ultrasound early in infancy should be performed to evaluate for potential renal tumors known to be associated with DICER1 syndrome, specifically cystic nephroma and Wilms tumor.[35,38] Chest

HEMATOLOGIC MALIGNANCIES

Leukemia is the most common malignancy in childhood and is usually diagnosed after infancy. However, in many cases, the molecular events leading to hematologic malignancy occur in utero and neonates and infants can present with acute leukemia. In addition, there are syndromes associated with benign and malignant myeloproliferative neoplasms that can present in neonates and infants.

The most common neonatal hematologic neoplasm is transient abnormal myelopoiesis (TAM) associated with trisomy 21 (T21).[50] TAM is suspected when blasts, immature hematopoietic progenitors, are circulating in the peripheral blood at high levels, and is confirmed by the presence of specific *GATA1* gene mutations. In a prospective study, 8.5% of neonates with T21 had TAM defined by greater than 10% circulating blasts and *GATA1* mutations detectable by Sanger sequencing. *GATA1* mutations is detected by more sensitive, high-throughput sequencing methods, even in neonates with lower levels of circulating blasts.[51] As implied by the name, TAM generally resolves over time without intervention, usually within a few weeks. However, some neonates are quite ill with impaired liver, lung, and/or kidney function, necessitating intervention with cytoreductive chemotherapy. After resolution, about 20% of infants with overt TAM develop acute myeloid leukemia by the age of 5 years. All neonates with T21 should have a complete blood count with differential to assess for the presence of TAM and molecular testing for *GATA1* mutations should be considered when the blast count is greater than or equal to 10%.[52]

Neonates with Noonan syndrome are at risk for a similar, transient myeloproliferative disorder (Noonan syndrome–myeloproliferative disorder [NS-MPD]), which may be a harbinger of frank malignancy in the form of juvenile myelomonocytic leukemia.[53] Noonan syndrome is characterized by short stature, typical facies, and cardiac anomalies and is caused by mutation in one of several genes involved in *RAS* signaling pathways, most commonly *PTPN11* (chromosome 12q24.13).[54,55] One specific variant in *PTPN11* (Thr73Ile) is particularly associated with NS-MPD, although other variants in *PTPN11* and one *KRAS* variant have been described in infants with NS-MPD.[56,57] NS-MPD is characterized by splenomegaly and myeloid leukocytosis without cytogenetic abnormalities, along with the features of Noonan syndrome. In contrast to the TAM in T21, circulating blasts are not observed in NS-MPD, but thrombocytopenia is present.[58] Although most cases resolve spontaneously, some require cytoreduction, and approximately 10% develop clonal cytogenetic abnormalities consistent with juvenile myelomonocytic leukemia. A complete blood count with differential should be obtained at the time of diagnosis and 6 to 12 months later in all infants with Noonan syndrome, and more frequent physical examinations and with blood count evaluations may be considered for those variants at highest risk of NS-MPD.[59]

Nonsyndromic acute leukemia in neonates and infants accounts for less than 1% of childhood leukemia and is of myeloid, lymphoid, or mixed phenotypes, with most being acute myeloid leukemia. Neonates and infants typically have hyperleukocytosis, anemia, thrombocytopenia, hepatosplenomegaly, and often skin lesions. Rearrangement of the *KMT2A* gene (chromosome 11q23.3) is the most common somatic genetic abnormality within the leukemic cells and is associated with a poor prognosis in those with infant acute lymphoblastic leukemia.[60] Because of its unique aggressiveness, particularly in those patients diagnosed between birth and 3 months of age, infant leukemia is biologically distinct from acute leukemia in older children. Although there are several leukemia predisposition syndromes caused by germline genetic variants, most present across all age ranges of children and adults.[61,62] Some of these leukemia predisposition syndromes may manifest in other ways in neonates and infants, including hematologic abnormalities. Thus, persistent cytopenias in the first year of life, with or without congenital abnormalities, should prompt consideration of bone marrow failure and leukemia predisposition syndromes.

GENETIC TESTING IN NEONATES

Germline genetic testing in neonates is performed on blood samples or buccal swabs. In cases where the patient has an active hematologic malignancy, skin punch biopsy may be necessary for fibroblast culture, because buccal tissue is usually contaminated by DNA from circulating blasts and any variants identified may be somatic. The genetic testing process should involve pretest and posttest counseling by a genetic counselor with expertise in pediatric cancer predisposition. In most cases, test results are available within 3 to 6 weeks of testing. If families are not ready to pursue germline genetic testing at present, but may consider doing so in the future, DNA banking is an option and typically involves sending blood or tissue to a genetic testing laboratory for DNA extraction and storage. In most cases, this involves an annual fee to maintain storage of the DNA.

PRECONCEPTION AND PRENATAL TESTING

Historically, prenatal genetic testing has been limited to pregnancies identified to be at a significantly increased risk for aneuploidy, or chromosomal abnormalities. However, this paradigm has shifted because germline genetic testing is now available for families with a known genetic syndrome caused by single-gene variants or pregnancies with a suspected single-gene disorder based on prenatal ultrasound findings. A fetal sample for genetic evaluation is obtained through chorionic villus sampling between 11 and 14 weeks gestation or via amniocentesis later in pregnancy, from 15 to 20 weeks gestation.

Preconception testing is achieved by way of in vitro fertilization with preimplantation genetic testing. This is a process overseen by reproductive endocrinology specialists through which an egg is removed from an ovary and then fertilized externally. The resulting embryo can undergo genetic analysis before transfer to the uterus, with preferential transfer of those embryos that do not harbor the specific familial mutation. Importantly, this technology can only be used in cases where the pathogenic mutation responsible for the known cancer predisposition syndrome has been previously identified.

SUMMARY

Development of malignancy in the neonatal or infant period is an extremely rare event. However, when a patient does present with cancer at such a young age, it is crucial to consider the potential for an underlying cancer predisposition syndrome, even more so in the setting of specific types of malignancy, bilateral or multifocal disease, additional congenital anomalies, or a history of cancer in close relatives. Early involvement of a genetic counselor with expertise in a pediatric oncology setting is critical, because diagnosis of a cancer predisposition syndrome may have profound implications for not only the patient, but also for immediate and extended family members in the forms of genetic testing, surveillance protocol initiation, risk-reduction procedures, and future family planning.

DISCLOSURES

The authors have no conflicts of interest to disclose.

REFERENCES

1. Desandes E, Guissou S, Ducassou S, et al. Neonatal solid tumors: incidence and survival in France. Pediatr Blood Cancer 2016;63:1375–80.
2. Chandrasekaran A. Neonatal solid tumors. Pediatr Neonatol 2018;59:65–70.
3. Zhang J, Walsh MF, Wu G, et al. Germline mutations in predisposition genes in pediatric cancer. N Engl J Med 2015;373:2336–46.
4. Brodeur GM, Nichols KE, Plon SE, et al. Pediatric cancer predisposition and surveillance: an overview, and a tribute to Alfred G. Knudson Jr. Clin Cancer Res 2017;23:e1–5.
5. Alfaar AS, Hassan WM, Bakry MS, et al. Neonates with cancer and causes of death; lessons from 615 cases in the SEER databases. Cancer Med 2017;6: 1817–26.
6. Orbach D, Sarnacki S, Brisse HJ, et al. Neonatal cancer. Lancet Oncol 2013;14: e609–20.
7. Interiano RB, Davidoff AM. Current management of neonatal neuroblastoma. Curr Pediatr Rev 2015;11:179–87.
8. Hero B, Simon T, Spitz R, et al. Localized infant neuroblastomas often show spontaneous regression: results of the prospective trials NB95-S and NB97. J Clin Oncol 2008;26:1504–10.
9. Twist CJ, Schmidt ML, Naranjo A, et al. Maintaining outstanding outcomes using response- and biology-based therapy for intermediate-risk neuroblastoma: a report from the children's oncology group study ANBL0531. J Clin Oncol 2019; 37:3243–55.
10. Kamihara J, Bourdeaut F, Foulkes WD, et al. Retinoblastoma and neuroblastoma predisposition and surveillance. Clin Cancer Res 2017;23:e98–106.
11. Ritenour LE, Randall MP, Bosse KR, et al. Genetic susceptibility to neuroblastoma: current knowledge and future directions. Cell Tissue Res 2018;372: 287–307.
12. Park JR, Eggert A, Caron H. Neuroblastoma: biology, prognosis, and treatment. Hematol Oncol Clin North Am 2010;24:65–86.
13. Scollon S, Anglin AK, Thomas M, et al. A comprehensive review of pediatric tumors and associated cancer predisposition syndromes. J Genet Couns 2017; 26:387–434.
14. Leiderman YI, Kiss S, Mukai S. Molecular genetics of RB1: the retinoblastoma gene. Semin Ophthalmol 2007;22:247–54.
15. Shields CL, Shields JA. Basic understanding of current classification and management of retinoblastoma. Curr Opin Ophthalmol 2006;17:228–34.
16. Knudson AG Jr. Mutation and cancer: statistical study of retinoblastoma. Proc Natl Acad Sci U S A 1971;68:820–3.
17. Friend SH, Bernards R, Rogelj S, et al. A human DNA segment with properties of the gene that predisposes to retinoblastoma and osteosarcoma. Nature 1986; 323:643–6.
18. Gombos DS. Retinoblastoma in the perinatal and neonatal child. Semin Fetal Neonatal Med 2012;17:239–42.
19. Gallie B. Canadian guidelines for retinoblastoma care. Can J Ophthalmol 2009; 44:639–42.
20. Soliman SE, Dimaras H, Khetan V, et al. Prenatal versus postnatal screening for familial retinoblastoma. Ophthalmology 2016;123:2610–7.
21. Li FP, Fraumeni JF Jr. Soft-tissue sarcomas, breast cancer, and other neoplasms. A familial syndrome? Ann Intern Med 1969;71:747–52.

22. Kratz CP, Achatz MI, Brugieres L, et al. Cancer screening recommendations for individuals with Li-Fraumeni syndrome. Clin Cancer Res 2017;23:e38–45.
23. Tatsi C, Stratakis CA. Neonatal Cushing syndrome: a rare but potentially devastating disease. Clin Perinatol 2018;45:103–18.
24. Chen QL, Su Z, Li YH, et al. Clinical characteristics of adrenocortical tumors in children. J Pediatr Endocrinol Metab 2011;24:535–41.
25. Rodriguez-Galindo C, Figueiredo BC, Zambetti GP, et al. Biology, clinical characteristics, and management of adrenocortical tumors in children. Pediatr Blood Cancer 2005;45:265–73.
26. Rednam SP. Updates on progress in cancer screening for children with hereditary cancer predisposition syndromes. Curr Opin Pediatr 2019;31:41–7.
27. Geller JI, Roth JJ, Biegel JA. Biology and treatment of rhabdoid tumor. Crit Rev Oncog 2015;20:199–216.
28. Fossey M, Li H, Afzal S, et al. Atypical teratoid rhabdoid tumor in the first year of life: the Canadian ATRT registry experience and review of the literature. J Neurooncol 2017;132:155–62.
29. Mitchell SG, Pencheva B, Porter CC. Germline genetics and childhood cancer: emerging cancer predisposition syndromes and psychosocial impacts. Curr Oncol Rep 2019;21:85.
30. Cohen BH, Geyer JR, Miller DC, et al. Pilot study of intensive chemotherapy with peripheral hematopoietic cell support for children less than 3 years of age with malignant brain tumors, the CCG-99703 Phase I/II Study. A report from the children's oncology group. Pediatr Neurol 2015;53:31–46.
31. Eaton KW, Tooke LS, Wainwright LM, et al. Spectrum of SMARCB1/INI1 mutations in familial and sporadic rhabdoid tumors. Pediatr Blood Cancer 2011;56:7–15.
32. Foulkes WD, Kamihara J, Evans DGR, et al. Cancer surveillance in Gorlin syndrome and rhabdoid tumor predisposition syndrome. Clin Cancer Res 2017;23: e62–7.
33. Dehner LP, Schultz KA, Hill DA. Pleuropulmonary blastoma: more than a lung neoplasm of childhood. Mo Med 2019;116:206–10.
34. Messinger YH, Stewart DR, Priest JR, et al. Pleuropulmonary blastoma: a report on 350 central pathology-confirmed pleuropulmonary blastoma cases by the international pleuropulmonary blastoma registry. Cancer 2015;121:276–85.
35. Schultz KAP, Williams GM, Kamihara J, et al. DICER1 and associated conditions: identification of at-risk individuals and recommended surveillance strategies. Clin Cancer Res 2018;24:2251–61.
36. Mechoulan A, Leclair MD, Yvinec M, et al. [Pleuropulmonary blastoma: a case of early neonatal diagnosis through antenatal scan screening]. Gynecol Obstet Fertil 2007;35:437–41.
37. Miniati DN, Chintagumpala M, Langston C, et al. Prenatal presentation and outcome of children with pleuropulmonary blastoma. J Pediatr Surg 2006;41: 66–71.
38. Schultz KAP, Rednam SP, Kamihara J, et al. PTEN, DICER1, FH, and their associated tumor susceptibility syndromes: clinical features, genetics, and surveillance recommendations in childhood. Clin Cancer Res 2017;23:e76–82.
39. Wasserman JD, Tomlinson GE, Druker H, et al. Multiple endocrine neoplasia and hyperparathyroid-jaw tumor syndromes: clinical features, genetics, and surveillance recommendations in childhood. Clin Cancer Res 2017;23:e123–32.
40. Wells SA Jr, Asa SL, Dralle H, et al. Revised American Thyroid Association guidelines for the management of medullary thyroid carcinoma. Thyroid 2015;25: 567–610.

41. Isaacs H Jr. Fetal and neonatal hepatic tumors. J Pediatr Surg 2007;42: 1797–803.
42. Ng K, Mogul DB. Pediatric liver tumors. Clin Liver Dis 2018;22:753–72.
43. Calvisi DF, Solinas A. Hepatoblastoma: current knowledge and promises from preclinical studies. Transl Gastroenterol Hepatol 2020;5:42.
44. Meyers RL, Maibach R, Hiyama E, et al. Risk-stratified staging in paediatric hepatoblastoma: a unified analysis from the Children's Hepatic Tumors International Collaboration. Lancet Oncol 2017;18:122–31.
45. Achatz MI, Porter CC, Brugieres L, et al. Cancer screening recommendations and clinical management of inherited gastrointestinal cancer syndromes in childhood. Clin Cancer Res 2017;23:e107–14.
46. Leclair MD, El-Ghoneimi A, Audry G, et al. The outcome of prenatally diagnosed renal tumors. J Urol 2005;173:186–9.
47. Wang KH, Kupa J, Duffy KA, et al. Diagnosis and management of Beckwith-Wiedemann syndrome. Front Pediatr 2019;7:562.
48. Cullinan N, Villani A, Mourad S, et al. An eHealth decision-support tool to prioritize referral practices for genetic evaluation of patients with Wilms tumor. Int J Cancer 2020;146:1010–7.
49. Kalish JM, Doros L, Helman LJ, et al. Surveillance recommendations for children with overgrowth syndromes and predisposition to Wilms tumors and hepatoblastoma. Clin Cancer Res 2017;23:e115–22.
50. Roberts I, Izraeli S. Haematopoietic development and leukaemia in Down syndrome. Br J Haematol 2014;167:587–99.
51. Roberts I, Alford K, Hall G, et al. GATA1-mutant clones are frequent and often unsuspected in babies with Down syndrome: identification of a population at risk of leukemia. Blood 2013;122:3908–17.
52. Bull MJ, Committee on G. Health supervision for children with Down syndrome. Pediatrics 2011;128:393–406.
53. Niemeyer CM. RAS diseases in children. Haematologica 2014;99:1653–62.
54. Tartaglia M, Niemeyer CM, Fragale A, et al. Somatic mutations in PTPN11 in juvenile myelomonocytic leukemia, myelodysplastic syndromes and acute myeloid leukemia. Nat Genet 2003;34:148–50.
55. Tartaglia M, Kalidas K, Shaw A, et al. PTPN11 mutations in Noonan syndrome: molecular spectrum, genotype-phenotype correlation, and phenotypic heterogeneity. Am J Hum Genet 2002;70:1555–63.
56. Kratz CP, Niemeyer CM, Castleberry RP, et al. The mutational spectrum of PTPN11 in juvenile myelomonocytic leukemia and Noonan syndrome/myeloproliferative disease. Blood 2005;106:2183–5.
57. Schubbert S, Zenker M, Rowe SL, et al. Germline KRAS mutations cause Noonan syndrome. Nat Genet 2006;38:331–6.
58. Choong K, Freedman MH, Chitayat D, et al. Juvenile myelomonocytic leukemia and Noonan syndrome. J Pediatr Hematol Oncol 1999;21:523–7.
59. Villani A, Greer MC, Kalish JM, et al. Recommendations for cancer surveillance in individuals with RASopathies and other rare genetic conditions with increased cancer risk. Clin Cancer Res 2017;23:e83–90.
60. Dreyer ZE, Hilden JM, Jones TL, et al. Intensified chemotherapy without SCT in infant ALL: results from COG P9407 (Cohort 3). Pediatr Blood Cancer 2015;62:419–26.
61. Porter CC. Germ line mutations associated with leukemias. Hematology Am Soc Hematol Educ Program 2016;2016:302–8.
62. Porter CC, Druley TE, Erez A, et al. Recommendations for surveillance for children with leukemia-predisposing conditions. Clin Cancer Res 2017;23:e14–22.

Neonatal Leukemia

Patrick A. Brown, MD[a,b],*

KEYWORDS

- Leukemia • ALL • AML • KMT2A • JMML • RAS • TAM • Down syndrome

KEY POINTS

- Neonatal leukemia includes infant acute leukemia (acute lymphoblastic leukemia and acute myeloid leukemia [AML]), juvenile myelomonocytic leukemia, and transient abnormal myelopoiesis (TAM) of Down syndrome.
- Infant acute leukemia frequently harbors *KMT2A* rearrangements and is associated with a poor prognosis relative to childhood acute leukemia.
- Juvenile myelomonocytic leukemia is caused by mutations that activate Ras pathway signaling and can either be sporadic or arise in the setting of predisposing constitutional syndromes, such as neurofibromatosis type 1 or Noonan syndrome.
- Neonates with Down syndrome are at high risk of TAM, which typically is self-resolving but carries a substantial risk of early mortality and subsequent progression to AML.

DEFINITIONS AND SCOPE

For the purposes of this article, *neonatal leukemia* encompasses 3 distinct disorders diagnosed prior to 1 year of age: (1) acute leukemia (referred to hereafter as *infant leukemia*), subclassified as acute lymphoblastic leukemia (ALL), acute myeloid leukemia (AML), and acute leukemia of ambiguous lineage (ALAL); (2) juvenile myelomonocytic leukemia (JMML), which is a mixed myelodysplastic/myeloproliferative disorder (MDS); and (3) transient abnormal myelopoiesis (TAM), which is a preleukemic disorder occurring in neonates with Down syndrome (DS) (**Table 1**). Each of these is described separately.

INFANT LEUKEMIA
Epidemiology

Fortunately, infant acute leukemia is rare, with an estimated incidence of approximately 40 cases per million in the United States, which equates to approximately 160 cases of infant leukemia per year. Within the infant age group, neuroblastoma, brain tumors, and acute leukemia all occur with similar frequency. Of the cases of

[a] Department of Oncology, Johns Hopkins Kimmel Cancer Center, Baltimore, MD, USA;
[b] Department of Pediatrics, Johns Hopkins Kimmel Cancer Center, Baltimore, MD, USA
* Johns Hopkins Oncology, 1650 Orleans Street, CRB1 Room 2M51, Baltimore, MD 21231.
E-mail address: pbrown2@jhmi.edu

Clin Perinatol 48 (2021) 15–33
https://doi.org/10.1016/j.clp.2020.11.002
0095-5108/21/© 2020 Elsevier Inc. All rights reserved.

Table 1
Classification of neonatal leukemia

Disorder	Epidemiology	Comments
Infant acute leukemia (includes ALL, AML, and rare mixed phenotype or undifferentiated)	• Incidence approximately 40 per million infants (160 cases/y in the US) • Slightly more ALL than AML • Female predominance (1.2:1) • Sporadic	• Infant ALL nearly always B-lineage, rarely T-lineage • *KMT2A* rearrangements in 75% of ALL and 50% of AML • Generally worse prognosis relative to acute leukemia in older children
JMML	• Incidence 10 per million infants (40 cases per year in the US) • 50% of JMML cases occur in infants, and nearly all JMML occurs in patients <5 years old • Male predominance (2.5:1) • 75% of cases are sporadic, 25% of cases occur in setting of predisposition syndromes (NF1, NS)	• Driven by Ras signaling pathway mutations • Characterized by proliferation of myeloid precursors and widespread organ infiltration (especially spleen, lungs, intestines) • Generally fatal without HSCT
TAM of DS	• Incidence approximately150 per million infants (600 cases/y in the US) • Occurs exclusively in patients with DS; incidence is 10%–15% in newborns with DS	• Driven by *GATA1* mutations • Characterized by proliferation of megakaryoblasts and organ infiltration (especially liver) • Spontaneously resolves, but may be clinically severe, with 10%–20% mortality due to multiorgan failure • Of survivors of TAM, approximately 10% subsequently develop AML 1–4 y later

infant leukemia, there is slight predominance of ALL over AML. Rarely, cases are not clearly classifiable as ALL or AML. These cases collectively are referred to as ALAL and are subclassified either as mixed phenotype acute leukemia (MPAL) or acute un-differentiated leukemia (AUL). Of infant ALL cases, nearly all are B-lineage, with fewer than 5% T-lineage. The incidence of ALL in infants is lower than in children aged 1 year to 14 years old and approximately the same as the incidence of ALL in adolescents. In contrast, the incidence of AML in infants is approximately twice the incidence of AML in older children and adolescents. Both infant ALL and AML demonstrate a female pre-dominance (approximately 1.2:1), in contrast to the male predominance (approxi-mately 1.2:1) seen in acute leukemia diagnosed beyond the first birthday.[1]

Clinical Features and Diagnostic Approach

Compared with older children, infants with acute leukemia tend to present with more aggressive features, including high white blood cell (WBC) counts, hepatosplenome-galy, central nervous system (CNS) involvement, and leukemia cutis (skin infiltra-tion).[2,3] Otherwise, the clinical features that characterize acute leukemia in infants are no different from those associated with acute leukemia occurring in older children. The same diagnostic challenges that confront pediatricians when dealing with the infant patient in general apply to diagnosing infant leukemia. Bone and joint pain, for example, a common complaint of older children with leukemia, is difficult to elicit in babies. The most common findings that ultimately lead to the diagnosis of leukemia in infants (poor feeding, decreased energy, pallor, rash, and fever) are highly nonspecific and are associated with a broad differential diagnosis.

The diagnostic criteria and required testing to make a diagnosis of acute leukemia in infants—namely, the demonstration of at least 20% leukemic blasts in the bone marrow—is identical to that in older children. Because infants often present clinically with very high WBC counts with a high percentage of circulating leukemic blasts and may be very ill, however, a diagnostic bone marrow aspiration may not be necessary. All of the standard diagnostic testing (flow cytometry for immunophenotyping, karyotype, fluorescence in situ hybridization, and so forth) may be performed on peripheral blood.

Molecular Pathogenesis

A high proportion of infant leukemias are characterized cytogenetically by balanced chromosomal translocations involving the histone lysine methyltransferase 2A gene (*KMT2A*, formerly known as mixed lineage leukemia [*MLL*] gene) at chromosome 11q23. *KMT2A* rearrangements (*KMT2A*-r) occur in approximately 5% of childhood ALL cases overall[4] but in 70% to 80% of ALL in infants.[2,5] In childhood AML, *KMT2A*-r is more common overall (15%–20%) but is more common in the infant age group (approximately 50%).[6]

KMT2A-r results in the fusion of the N-terminus of the *KMT2A* gene with the C-terminus of a partner gene. Remarkably, approximately 100 different *KMT2A* partner genes now have been identified.[7] In infant ALL, 4 partner genes account for 93% of cases: *AFF1* (formerly *AF4*; 49%), *MLLT1* (formerly *ENL*; 22%), *MLLT3* (formerly *AF9*; 17%), and *MLLT10* (formerly *AF10*; 5%). In infant AML, 3 partner genes account for 66% of cases: *MLLT3* (22%), *MLLT10* (27%), and *ELL* (17%).

Various lines of evidence (retrospective analyses of neonatal samples[8] and twin concordance studies,[9] for example) have shown that *KMT2A* rearrangements are acquired in hematopoietic precursors in utero, and, compared with other oncogenic fusions, such as *ETV6-RUNX1*, initiate a strikingly rapid progression to leukemia. One intriguing aspect of leukemia epidemiology is that *KMT2A*-r leukemias occur with high frequency in 2 very different clinical situations: (1) infants with de novo acute leukemia and (2) patients with treatment-related secondary myelodysplastic syndrome/AML after exposure to potent DNA topoisomerase II (DNAt2) inhibitors (eg, etoposide). This has led to a hypothesis, with supporting evidence from case-control[10,11] and laboratory[12] studies, that maternal exposure to environmental DNAt2 inhibitors (eg, dietary flavonoids) during pregnancy may contribute to the risk of *KMT2A*-r infant leukemia. Germline genetic susceptibility also may play a role, because candidate gene studies[13,14] and genome-wide association studies[15,16] have identified several single-nucleotide polymorphisms that correlate with risk of developing infant leukemia.

In ALL, *KMT2A*-r is associated with CD10 negativity and coexpression of one or more myeloid antigens, suggesting that these leukemias arise from very immature lymphoid progenitors.[17] In AML, *KMT2A*-r is associated with monocytic differentiation.[3] Infant leukemia cases can be of ambiguous lineage, due to either a mixed phenotype (MPAL) or to lack of differentiation markers (AUL).

Prognostic Factors and Risk Stratification

The prognostic significance of infant age differs between ALL and AML. In ALL, infants fare far worse than older children. The 4 year event-free survival (EFS) in Interfant-99, the largest trial of infant ALL to date, was 47%.[5] Recent trials for childhood ALL report long-term EFS rates exceeding 85%.[18,19] In AML, outcomes for infants are similar to those for older children.[3]

The prognostic significance of *KMT2A*-r also differs between infant ALL and AML. In infant ALL, *KMT2A*-r is clearly associated with poorer outcome. In the Children's Cancer Group protocol CCG-1953, the 5-year EFS for *KMT2A*-r infants was 34% versus 60% with germline (nonrearranged) *KMT2A* (*KMT2A*-g).[2] In Interfant-99, 4-year EFS rates in *KMT2A*-r and *KMT2A*-g infants were 37% and 74%, respectively.[5] In infant AML, *KMT2A*-r is not a significant risk factor. In a combined analysis of AML-BFM-98 and AML-BFM-2004, 5-year EFS rates were 43% and 52% for *KMT2A*-r and *KMT2A*-g infants, respectively ($P = .59$).[3] There is, however, evidence that within *KMT2A*-r pediatric AML cases, certain *KMT2A* fusion partners may be associated with favorable (eg, *MLLT11*) or unfavorable (eg, *MLLT10*) prognosis, leading to the incorporation of *KMT2A* fusion partner into pediatric AML risk stratification algorithms.[20,21]

Among infants with *KMT2A*-r ALL, additional independent prognostic factors include age and WBC count at diagnosis, with younger infants and those with the higher WBC count having poorer outcomes.[2,5,22] In the context of a 7-day prophase of single-agent prednisone given prior to intensive induction chemotherapy in the Interfant-99 protocol, a poor response (greater than or equal to 1000 blasts per microliter in the peripheral blood on day 8) also was an independent negative prognostic factor.[5]

As discussed previously, infant *KMT2A*-g ALL patients are considered to be low risk and have favorable clinical features (lower WBC counts and older age at presentation). The outcome of *KMT2A*-g infants, however, clearly is inferior to ALL patients diagnosed after 1 year of age. This is likely due, in part, to differences in distribution of favorable genetic features, because infants with *KMT2A*-g ALL are much less likely to harbor the favorable genetic features high hyperdiploidy and *ETV6–RUNX1* fusions compared with older children.[23,24]

Among infant AML cases without *KMT2A*-r, there is a rare subset that presents with megakaryocytic (platelet) differentiation, known as acute megakaryoblastic leukemia (AMKL). A variety of oncogenic fusions, of which the first to be described was the *RBM15-MKL1* fusion resulting from the t(1;22)(p13;q13) translocation, drive this rare subset of infant leukemia. The prognosis generally is unfavorable due to a high risk of chemotherapy resistance and relapse, although outcomes do vary according to the specific oncogenic fusion.[25] This infant AMKL subset, which is sporadic, is different from the AMKL that occurs commonly in patients with DS. DS-related myeloid leukemia (ML-DS), as discussed later, also typically presents with megakaryoblastic differentiation. ML-DS, however, usually is diagnosed beyond the first year of life and before 4 years of age, typically is preceded by TAM in the newborn period, and has a favorable prognosis.[26]

Current Treatment

The infant patient's unique vulnerability to complications and toxicities presents a challenge in treating infant acute leukemia. There are limited data to guide how the distinct and rapidly changing physiology of infants (in terms of body composition, binding of drugs by plasma proteins, cytochrome p450 activity, renal function, immunocompetence, and so forth) should be considered in designing chemotherapy treatment protocols. The data that do exist differ by chemotherapy drug. For example, no age dependency was found for the pharmacokinetics of daunorubicin[27] whereas the systemic clearance rate of methotrexate tended to increase with age during infancy.[28]

Infant leukemia protocols have encountered problems with excessive toxicity, both in ALL[29] and AML.[30] Survivors of infant leukemia also demonstrate an increased risk of late effects, particularly in cases of treatment that included cranial radiation or hematopoietic stem cell transplantation (HSCT).[31]

Given the similar prognosis and response to therapy for infants with AML compared with older children, infants with AML generally are treated on the same clinical trial protocols as older children, which typically include intensive multiagent chemotherapy to induce remission followed by consolidation with either additional chemotherapy courses (for patients with favorable prognostic features) or allogeneic HSCT (for patients with unfavorable prognostic features). Gemtuzumab ozogamicin, an antibody-drug conjugate targeting the myeloid antigen CD33, increasingly is considered a standard component of AML induction therapy based on favorable results, in both older pediatric patients overall[32] and infants specifically.[33]

Treatment of infant ALL, on the other hand, is quite different from that for childhood ALL generally. There are 3 major cooperative groups conducting specific clinical trials for infant ALL: Interfant, based in Europe; the Children's Oncology Group (COG), based in North America; and the Japanese Pediatric Leukemia/Lymphoma Study Group (JPLSG). All have adopted an identical induction strategy based on Interfant-99 (**Table 2**).[5] In recently completed trials, all used a prospective risk-stratified approach that incorporates *KMT2A*-r status and age (**Table 3**). **Table 4** summarizes the postinduction treatment approaches for infant ALL by the major cooperative groups. Interfant-06 tested whether consolidation with myeloid-style chemotherapy with cytarabine, daunorubicin, mitoxantrone, and etoposide is superior to lymphoid-style consolidation with cyclophosphamide, cytarabine, and 6-mercaptopurine in *KMT2A*-r infants. The testing of myeloid-style chemotherapy stems from the hypothesis that these leukemias derive from an early hematopoietic precursor with myeloid differentiation potential and, therefore, may respond better to chemotherapy regimens developed for AML. COG AALL0631 tested whether the addition of a FLT3 tyrosine kinase inhibitor (lestaurtinib) to postinduction chemotherapy would enhance the effectiveness of chemotherapy, based on data showing aberrant activation of the FLT3 pathway in *KMT2A*-r ALL. The JPLSG MLL-10 protocol tested early consolidation with high-dose cytarabine and intensive supportive care measures. The use of

Table 2 Interfant induction		
Drug	**Route**	**Days**
Predniso(lo)ne	PO/NG	1–7
Daunorubicin	IV	8 & 9
Cytarabine	IV	8–21
Dexamethasone	PO/NG/IV	8–28
Vincristine	IV	8, 15, 22 & 29
Pegaspargase	IV	12
Methotrexate	IT	1 & 29
Cytarabine	IT	15
Hydrocortisone	IT	15 & 29

Dosing is age-dependent. Check protocol for specific dosing.
Abbreviations: IT, intrathecal; IV, intravenous; NG, nasogastric tube; PO, oral.

Table 3
Risk stratification of infant acute lymphoblastic leukemia/lymphoma

	Europe-Based Cooperative Group for Infant Acute Lymphoblastic Leukemia Trials	Children's Oncology Group	Japanese Pediatric Leukemia Study Group	Approximate Event-Free Survival
High risk	KMT2A-r and age <6 mo and WBC ≥ 300,000/µL	KMT2A-r and age <3 mo	KMT2A-r and (age <6 mo or CNS leukemia)	20%
Intermediate risk	KMT2A-r and not high risk	KMT2A-r and not high risk	KMT2A-r and not high risk	50%
Low risk	KMT2A-g	KMT2A-g	KMT2A-g	75%

HSCT in infant ALL differed among the groups, reflecting uncertainty regarding the risk/benefit ratio of HSCT in this population.[34] There does appear to be a subset of KMT2A-r patients at high risk of relapse (very young age, very high WBC counts, and persistence of disease after chemotherapy) who may benefit from HSCT in first remission.[35,36] **Table 5** summarizes consensus recommendations regarding the treatment of infant leukemia.[37]

Future Directions

Infant leukemia has a poor prognosis compared with leukemia occurring in older children, due both to increased risk of relapse and increased risk of severe therapy-related toxicity. There is a pressing need to identify novel treatment strategies. The importance of collaborative and innovative clinical trials for this disease cannot be overemphasized. To that end, the 3 major cooperative groups are collaborating to test novel treatment approaches and improve the standard of care. The unique

Table 4
Postinduction approaches for infant acute lymphoblastic leukemia/lymphoma in 3 major cooperative groups on most recent trials

	Interfant	Children's Oncology Group	Japanese Pediatric Leukemia Study Group
Trial	Interfant-06	AALL0631	MLL-10
Randomized postinduction intervention	Protocol IB vs ADE/MAE	± Lestaurtinib (FLT3 TKI)	None (single arm)
HSCT	All high risk, plus MRD + after MARMA	None	All high risk

Abbreviations: ADE/MAE: cytarabine, 100 mg/m² every 12 h, d 1 to 10; daunorubicin, 50 mg/m² d 1, 3, and 5; etoposide 100 mg/m², d 1 to 5/mitoxantrone 12 mg/m² d 1, 3, and 5; cytarabine, 100 mg/m² every 12 h, d 1 to 10; etoposide, 100 mg/m² days 1 to 5; MARMA: methotrexate, 5000 mg/m² d 1 and 8; 6-mercaptopurine, 25 mg/m² d 1 to 14; cytarabine, 3000 mg/m² every 12 h, d 15, 16, 22, and 23; PEG asparaginase, 2500 IU/m² day 23; MRD, minimal residual disease; Protocol IB consolidation: cyclophosphamide, 1000 mg/m², d 1 and 29; cytarabine, 75 mg/m², d 3 to 6, 10 to 13, 17 to 20, and 24 to 27; 6-mercaptopurine, 60 mg/m², d 1 to 28 consolidation; TKI, tyrosine kinase inhibitor.

Table 5
Summary of consensus recommended treatment strategies for infant leukemia subtypes

Risk Group	Defined on the Basis of...	Recommended Treatment Approach
Infant ALL		
High risk	KMT2A-r, younger age, late MRD clearance	Interfant induction, then intensive chemotherapy consolidation, then strongly consider HSCT (prefer non-TBI based, prefer age at HSCT at least 6 mo); continued consolidation and maintenance if HSCT unavailable
Intermediate risk	KMT2A-r, older age, early MRD clearance	Interfant induction, then intensive chemotherapy consolidation and maintenance
Low risk	KMT2A-g	Interfant induction, then identical approach as pediatric ALL (risk-stratified chemotherapy based on genetics and MRD response)
Infant AML	Identical approach as pediatric AML (intensive chemotherapy/gemtuzumab induction, then risk-based consolidation with chemotherapy/gemtuzumab for low risk and HSCT for high risk)	

Abbreviations: MRD, minimal residual disease; TBI, total body irradiation.

molecular biology of *KMT2A*-r leukemia has suggested novel treatment approaches, several of which are in various stages of clinical investigation. **Table 6** summarizes these approaches.

JUVENILE MYELOMONOCYTIC LEUKEMIA
Epidemiology

The epidemiology of JMML is strikingly different from ALL or AML. The estimated annual incidence of JMML is 1.3 cases per million children under the age of 15 years, which equates to approximately 80 cases per year in the United States. JMML occurs almost exclusively in children less than 5 years old, and approximately half of the cases occur in infants. Thus, in the first year of life, the annual incidence is approximately 10 per million. There is a significant male predominance in JMML (approximately 2.5:1).[1] Most cases of JMML are sporadic. As discussed later, a subset of cases arises in the setting of germline mutations in the Ras signaling pathway that predispose to JMML.

Clinical Features and Diagnostic Approach

The clinical signs and symptoms of JMML are the result of the aggressive proliferation and organ infiltration of myeloid precursor cells originating the in the bone marrow. The most frequent clinical findings in JMML are splenomegaly (which often is massive) and abnormal blood counts. The WBC count usually is high, and there nearly always is a striking left shift of myeloid cells, with prominent populations of myelocytes, metamyelocytes, monocytes, and nucleated red cells. Unlike acute leukemia, blasts typically are not present in large numbers in the blood. Low platelets are common, especially when splenomegaly is prominent. Hepatomegaly generally is less prominent than splenomegaly. Infiltration of the lungs is common, resulting in cough, tachypnea, and infiltrates on imaging that are indistinguishable from respiratory infections. Intestinal infiltration can result in diarrhea, which can be bloody. Leukemic skin lesions are

Table 6
Targeted therapeutics for infant leukemia

Biologic Target	Agent(s)	Summary of Rationale	Clinical Trials	References
FLT3	FLT3 tyrosine kinase inhibitors (lestaurtinib, midostaurin)	Constitutive activation of FLT3 signaling via overexpression of FLT3 and autocrine signaling	NCT00557193	54–61
Hypermethylation	Demethylating agents (azacitidine)	CpG hypermethylation	NCT02828358	62–65
Microenvironment	CXCR4 inhibitors (plerixafor)	Stromal-mediated chemoprotection	NCT01319864	66–70
Surface antigens (immunotherapy)	BiTE antibodies (blinatumomab), CAR T cells (tisagenlecleucel)	CD19 expression	EudraCT:2016–004674–17; NCT04276870	71,72
DOT1L (H3K79 methyltransferase)	DOT1L inhibitors (pinometostat)	Dependence for leukemogenesis in KMT2A-r models	NCT02141828	73–79
KMT2A-Menin interaction	Menin inhibitors (SNDX-5613)	Dependence for leukemogenesis is KMT2A-r models	Syndax trials (in development)	80–83
BCL2	BCL2 inhibitors (venetoclax)	BCL2 overexpression	AALL2021 (in development)	84–87

common and may mimic several common rashes of infancy. Constitutional symptoms, such as fever and lethargy, frequently are present.[38]

The diagnosis is suggested by the clinical findings, but bone marrow aspirate and biopsy are needed to exclude acute leukemia. The typical marrow of JMML is hypercellular with low blast percentage and reduced numbers of megakaryocytes. Karyotyping is normal in approximately two-thirds of cases, shows monosomy 7 in approximately one-quarter of cases, and shows other clonal abnormalities in approximately 10%.[39] The finding of elevated levels of fetal hemoglobin (HbF) in blood is supportive of a diagnosis of JMML. Ultimately, the demonstration of one of the characteristic mutations involving the Ras signaling pathway (discussed later) is the gold standard for making the diagnosis of JMML.

Molecular Pathogenesis

JMML is driven by hyperactive Ras pathway signaling (**Fig. 1**) on the basis of mutations in one of several genes, including *PTPN11* (which encodes the SHP-2 protein), *KRAS*, *NRAS*, *NF1*, and *CBL*. Approximately 75% of JMML cases are sporadic, arising from somatic mutations in the bone marrow of patients with no germline mutations in the Ras pathway. The remaining 25% of cases arise in patients with germline mutations leading to JMML predisposition syndromes, including neurofibromatosis type 1 (NF1) (caused by germline *NF1* mutations), Noonan syndrome (NS) (caused by germline mutations in one of several genes, most commonly *PTPN11*), and NS-like disorder (caused by germline mutations in *CBL*).[40]

Prognostic Factors and Risk Stratification

Most cases of JMML are rapidly fatal without treatment. Even with optimal treatment, long-term survival in JMML is achieved in only approximately 50% of patients. Relapse after treatment occurs in 35% of patients and is the most common cause of treatment failure.[41] There is, however, significant clinical heterogeneity among JMML cases, and several risk factors have been identified, most of which are linked to the mutational landscape (**Table 7**). Some cases of JMML are not uniformly associated with fatal progression in the absence of treatment and may even spontaneously regress, allowing a watchful waiting strategy for a subset of patients. In addition to these genetic factors, several clinical factors, such as age greater than or equal to 2 years at diagnosis, platelet count less than or equal to 33×10^9/L, and HbF level greater than or equal to 10% have been associated with worse prognosis.[42]

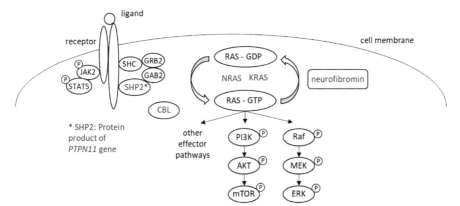

Fig. 1. Ras pathway. JMML mutations highlighted in red.

Table 7
Genetics and risk stratification in JMML

Genetic Subset	Clinical Features, Risk Factors and Treatment Implications
Noonan syndrome (germline *PTPN11* and other mutations)	• Spontaneous resolution possible • Minimal treatment, no HSCT unless progression
Neurofibromatosis type 1 (germline *NF1* mutations)	• Older age at diagnosis • Higher platelet count • Higher percentage of BM blasts • Fatal without allogeneic HSCT
Noonan syndrome-like disorder (germline *CBL* mutations)	• Value of HSCT uncertain • Frequent occurrence of mixed chimerism after HSCT
Somatic *PTPN11* mutations	• Rapidly fatal without allogeneic HSCT • High probability of relapse
Somatic *KRAS* mutations	• Mostly infants • Frequent association with monosomy 7 • Aggressive at presentation but low risk of relapse after allogeneic HSCT

Somatic NRAS mutations	• Heterogeneous subtype
	  ◦ In older children with high levels of HbF: rapid progression, high relapse rate after HSCT
	  ◦ In infants or in cases with G12S mutation: indolent course with spontaneous regression possible

Current Treatment

The only proved curative therapy for JMML is HSCT, and, for most JMML patients, the goal is to proceed to HSCT as soon as feasible.[41] There are exceptions to this, as noted in **Table 5**. For example, JMML associated with NS and NL-like disorder often spontaneously regress with time.[40] There also are rare cases with somatic NRAS mutations that can survive without HSCT. For all other cases, HSCT should be pursued once a diagnosis is established.

Efforts to demonstrate an improvement in JMML survival outcomes by incorporating pre-HSCT treatment largely have been unsuccessful. Cytoreductive chemotherapy with mercaptopurine, cytarabine, and/or 13-*cis*-retinoic acid may be useful as a temporizing measure in certain cases but should not be considered standard.[41] Splenectomy also has been studied but without clear benefit.[43] Farnesyl transferase inhibitors, such as tipifarnib, were studied enthusiastically as Ras-targeted therapy in JMML, but no survival benefit was demonstrated.[44]

Future Directions

Comprehensive molecular profiling, preclinical studies of targeted therapies, and anecdotal clinical evidence have suggested novel treatment strategies for JMML. The obvious importance of the Ras signaling pathway as a driver of JMML biology has led to a clinical trial of trametinib, an inhibitor of MEK, a downstream effector of Ras signaling (ClinicalTrials.gov NCT03190915). Studies demonstrating a pattern of CpG hypermethylation among JMML cases with high-risk features, such as older age and PTPN11 somatic mutations, have led to a clinical trial of the demethylating agent azacitidine (ClinicalTrials.gov NCT02447666). Given the suboptimal survival and significant toxicity associated with HSCT, there is an urgent need to develop improved therapies for JMML, and prospective trials of these novel approaches hopefully will represent a step in that direction.

TRANSIENT ABNORMAL MYELOPOIESIS
Epidemiology

Of the 6000 or so babies born each year with DS (constitutional trisomy 21) in the United States, approximately 10% to 15% develop TAM.[45]

Clinical Features and Diagnostic Approach

The clinical presentation of TAM varies tremendously, from an asymptomatic condition, detected only as an incidental finding due to abnormal blood counts, to a critical illness, with massive hepatosplenomegaly with jaundice and transaminase elevation, pleural/pericardial effusions, coagulopathy, and multiorgan failure due to widespread leukemic infiltration.[46,47] Blood count abnormalities (high WBC counts and low platelets, anemia) and circulating megakaryoblasts are among the most common signs, so it is essential to review a peripheral blood smear for all neonates with DS.[48] Jaundice also is common but also is common in DS newborns without TAM. The most severe cases are associated with persistent, progressive jaundice and a risk of hepatic fibrosis and failure that may be fatal.[48] Most cases of TAM present in the first week of life, but TAM also may develop prenatally as hydrops fetalis. A diagnosis of TAM is suspected based on clinical features and is confirmed by demonstrating the characteristic GATA1 mutation (discussed later).

Molecular Pathogenesis

TAM is unique to DS and is caused by cooperation between constitutional trisomy 21 and acquired N-terminal truncating mutations in the myeloid transcription factor gene GATA1 (Fig. 2).[49] GATA1 mutations are acquired during fetal myeloid hematopoiesis in approximately 30% of DS neonates.[50] Approximately half of DS neonates with GATA1 mutations are diagnosed with TAM due to clonal expansion of the mutant clone, and approximately half are clinically silent, showing no signs or symptoms of TAM, presumably due to lack of clinically significant clonal expansion. In patients with TAM, the GATA1 mutant clone typically spontaneously regresses without specific treatment. Approximately 5% to 10% of DS neonates with GATA1 mutations (regardless of whether they were diagnosed clinically with TAM), however, subsequently acquire additional oncogenic mutations, most commonly in cohesin or epigenetic regulator genes, and develop AML, usually between the ages of 1 year and 4 years.[51,52] This form of AML is known as ML-DS.

Prognostic Factors and Risk Stratification

The prognosis is excellent for most neonates with TAM, because most cases spontaneously resolve without treatment. There are several clinical features, however, that indicate a more aggressive presentation, and these cases account for observation that the overall mortality of TAM is 15% to 20%. High-risk features include hydrops fetalis, leukocytosis (WBC count >100 × 10^9/L), massive hepatomegaly, liver transaminase elevation, disseminated intravascular coagulation with bleeding, and renal and/or cardiac failure.[48]

Current Treatment

Patients with TAM and high-risk clinical features may benefit from chemotherapy in an effort to reduce risk of early mortality, which results most commonly from progressive liver failure due to leukemic infiltration and/or fibrosis.[53] TAM megakaryoblasts appear to be very sensitive to cytarabine, and low-dose cytarabine is the treatment of choice in

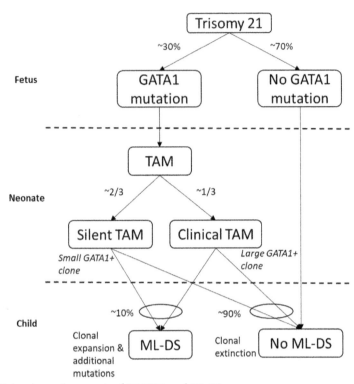

Fig. 2. Molecular pathogenesis of DS TAM and ML-DS.

high-risk cases. Although there is good evidence that low dose cytarabine can reduce the risk of mortality due to TAM, there is no evidence that treatment with cytarabine has a significant impact on the likelihood of subsequent development of ML-DS.[48]

Future Directions

Despite detailed understanding of the molecular pathogenesis of the development of TAM and its progression in some cases to ML-DS, there remain several unsolved clinical problems that require further study. Among the most important of these is the practical matter of how to evaluate DS neonates for TAM and *GATA1* mutations. It now is recognized that the incidence of *GATA1* mutations in DS neonates is approximately 30%, only half of which show clinical signs of TAM. Because all DS neonates with *GATA1* mutations, whether or not they have clinical TAM, have a substantial (approximately 10%) risk of developing ML-DS later in childhood, should all DS neonates be screened with *GATA1* sequencing on peripheral blood, so that *GATA1* mutant patients can be monitored for the development of ML-DS? If so, how should such a screening strategy be implemented?

Another important question is whether there are predictive biomarkers to identify the approximately 10% of GATA1-mutant DS neonates who are destined to progress to ML-DS. It is tempting to think that, if there are predictable molecular events driving the progression, this may point to targeted therapeutic strategies to prevent the development of ML-DS in this subset.

Finally, the high rate of mortality for TAM patients with high-risk clinical features suggests that the current strategy of identifying and treating these patients is not sufficiently effective. A better understanding of the biological processes leading to liver failure, which results from infiltration and fibrosis and is the most common cause of early mortality, many point to more effective and targeted treatment strategies than the empiric use of cytarabine.

SUMMARY

Neonatal leukemia is rare but is among the most common malignancies in infancy and is associated with high rates of morbidity and mortality. Each of the 3 major forms of neonatal leukemia (infant acute leukemia, JMML and DS-associated TAM) is driven at a molecular level by unique constitutional and acquired genetic events. Evolving understanding of these diseases at a molecular level is facilitating better diagnostics, more refined risk assessment and prognostication, and suggesting novel therapeutic strategies that have the potential to be more effective and less toxic than traditional treatments that rely on cytotoxic chemotherapy and HSCT.

DISCLOSURES

No relevant conflicts of interest.

CLINICAL CARE POINTS

- Newborns with Down syndrome should be screened for transient abnormal myelopoiesis. Minimal screening includes complete blood count to assess for circulating myeloblasts and thrombocytopenia and physical exam to assess for hepatomegaly; optimal screening also includes *GATA1* mutation testing.
- Neonates with leukemia are at high risk of infections and fevers should be managed with aggressive empiric antimicrobial therapy.
- Signs and symptoms of neonatal leukemia are non-specific, so complete blood counts should be included in the work up of infants presenting with failure to thrive, lethargy, poor feeding, abdominal distension, pallor, rash and fever.
- Neonates with leukemia should be referred to tertiary care centers with multidisciplinary subspecialty expertise, including but not limited to pediatric hematology/oncology.

Best Practices

What is the current practice for neonatal leukemia?
  Best Practice/Guideline/Care Path Objective(s)
  For infant acute leukemia, treatment includes risk-based multiagent chemotherapy, with risk factors including age, genetics (presence or absence of *KMT2A* gene rearrangement), and early response to therapy. The role of stem cell transplant is controversial.
  For juvenile myelomonocytic leukemia, management is also risk-based, with risk determined largely by genetic subset. For most subset, stem cell transplant is treatment of choice.
  For transient abnormal myelopoiesis of Down syndrome, most cases can be managed with supportive care only, with chemotherapy reserved for aggressive cases causing liver and other organ dysfunction. Close follow up over the ensuing years is important due to substantial risk of subsequent myeloid leukemia of Down syndrome.

What changes in current practice are likely to improve outcomes?
  For infant acute leukemia and juvenile myelomonocytic leukemia, the development of novel molecularly targeted therapies are most likely to improve outcomes
  For transient abnormal myelopoiesis of Down syndrome, more widespread screening for GATA1 mutations and more aggressive evaluation to identify high risk patients in need of treatment are most likely to improve outcomes.

Is there a Clinical Algorithm? If so, please include
See **Tables 4** and **6.**

Major Recommendations
Neonatal leukemia requires highly specialized multidisciplinary care
Comprehensive genetic testing is required for optimal management of neonatal leukemia
All newborns with Down syndrome should be screened for transient abnormal myelopoiesis
with a complete blood count and physical exam (minimally) and *GATA1* mutation testing
(optimally)

References/Source(s): Reference numbers. [37,41,47.]

REFERENCES

1. Howlader N, Noone AM, Krapcho M, et al, editors. SEER cancer statistics review, 1975-2017. Bethesda (MD): National Cancer Institute; 2020. Available at: https://seer.cancer.gov/csr/1975_2017/. based on November 2019 SEER data submission, posted to the SEER web site.

2. Hilden JM, Dinndorf PA, Meerbaum SO, et al. Analysis of prognostic factors of acute lymphoblastic leukemia in infants: report on CCG 1953 from the Children's Oncology Group. Blood 2006;108(2):441–51.

3. Creutzig U, Zimmermann M, Bourquin JP, et al. Favorable outcome in infants with AML after intensive first- and second-line treatment: an AML-BFM study group report. Leukemia 2012;26(4):654–61.

4. Behm FG, Raimondi SC, Frestedt JL, et al. Rearrangement of the MLL gene confers a poor prognosis in childhood acute lymphoblastic leukemia, regardless of presenting age. Blood 1996;87(7):2870–7.

5. Pieters R, De Lorenzo P, Ancliffe P, et al. Outcome of infants younger than 1 year with acute lymphoblastic leukemia treated with the interfant-06 protocol: results from an international phase III randomized study. J Clin Oncol 2019;37(25):2246–56.

6. Harrison CJ, Hills RK, Moorman AV, et al. Cytogenetics of childhood acute myeloid leukemia: United Kingdom Medical Research Council Treatment trials AML 10 and 12. J Clin Oncol 2010;28(16):2674–81.

7. Meyer C, Burmeister T, Groger D, et al. The MLL recombinome of acute leukemias in 2017. Leukemia 2018;32(2):273–84.

8. Gale KB, Ford AM, Repp R, et al. Backtracking leukemia to birth: identification of clonotypic gene fusion sequences in neonatal blood spots. Proc Natl Acad Sci U S A 1997;94(25):13950–4.

9. Ford AM, Ridge SA, Cabrera ME, et al. In utero rearrangements in the trithorax-related oncogene in infant leukaemias. Nature 1993;363(6427):358–60.

10. Alexander FE, Patheal SL, Biondi A, et al. Transplacental chemical exposure and risk of infant leukemia with MLL gene fusion. Cancer Res 2001;61(6):2542–6.

11. Spector LG, Xie Y, Robison LL, et al. Maternal diet and infant leukemia: the DNA topoisomerase II inhibitor hypothesis: a report from the children's oncology group. Cancer Epidemiol Biomarkers Prev 2005;14(3):651–5.

12. Strick R, Strissel PL, Borgers S, et al. Dietary bioflavonoids induce cleavage in the MLL gene and may contribute to infant leukemia. Proc Natl Acad Sci U S A 2000;97(9):4790–5.

13. Smith MT, Wang Y, Skibola CF, et al. Low NAD(P)H:quinone oxidoreductase activity is associated with increased risk of leukemia with MLL translocations in infants and children. Blood 2002;100(13):4590–3.

14. Wiemels JL, Smith RN, Taylor GM, et al. Methylenetetrahydrofolate reductase (MTHFR) polymorphisms and risk of molecularly defined subtypes of childhood acute leukemia. Proc Natl Acad Sci U S A 2001;98(7):4004–9.

15. Ross JA, Linabery AM, Blommer CN, et al. Genetic variants modify susceptibility to leukemia in infants: a Children's Oncology Group report. Pediatr Blood Cancer 2013;60(1):31–4.

16. Valentine MC, Linabery AM, Chasnoff S, et al. Excess congenital non-synonymous variation in leukemia-associated genes in MLL- infant leukemia: a Children's Oncology Group report. Leukemia 2014;28(6):1235–41.

17. Basso G, Rondelli R, Covezzoli A, et al. The role of immunophenotype in acute lymphoblastic leukemia of infant age. Leuk Lymphoma 1994;15(1–2):51–60.

18. Hunger SP, Lu X, Devidas M, et al. Improved survival for children and adolescents with acute lymphoblastic leukemia between 1990 and 2005: a report from the children's oncology group. J Clin Oncol 2012;30(14):1663–9.

19. Pui CH, Campana D, Pei D, et al. Treating childhood acute lymphoblastic leukemia without cranial irradiation. N Engl J Med 2009;360(26):2730–41.

20. Cooper TM, Ries RE, Alonzo TA, et al. Revised risk stratification criteria for children with newly diagnosed acute myeloid leukemia: a report from the Children's Oncology Group. Blood 2017;130:407.

21. Balgobind BV, Raimondi SC, Harbott J, et al. Novel prognostic subgroups in childhood 11q23/MLL-rearranged acute myeloid leukemia: results of an international retrospective study. Blood 2009;114(12):2489–96.

22. Tomizawa D, Koh K, Sato T, et al. Outcome of risk-based therapy for infant acute lymphoblastic leukemia with or without an MLL gene rearrangement, with emphasis on late effects: a final report of two consecutive studies, MLL96 and MLL98, of the Japan Infant Leukemia Study Group. Leukemia 2007;21(11):2258–63.

23. Lorenzo P, Moorman A, Pieters R, et al. Cytogenetics and outcome of infants with acute lymphoblastic leukemia and absence of MLL rearrangements. Leukemia 2014;28(2):428–30.

24. Linden M, Boer J, Schneider P, et al. Clinical and molecular genetic characterization of wild-type MLL infant acute lymphoblastic leukemia identifies few recurrent abnormalities. Haematologica 2016;101(3):e95–9.

25. de Rooij JD, Branstetter C, Ma J, et al. Pediatric non-Down syndrome acute megakaryoblastic leukemia is characterized by distinct genomic subsets with varying outcomes. Nat Genet 2017;49(3):451–6.

26. Hitzler JK, Zipursky A. Origins of leukaemia in children with Down syndrome. Nat Rev Cancer 2005;5(1):11–20.

27. Hempel G, Relling MV, de Rossi G, et al. Pharmacokinetics of daunorubicin and daunorubicinol in infants with leukemia treated in the interfant 99 protocol. Pediatr Blood Cancer 2010;54(3):355–60.

28. Lonnerholm G, Valsecchi MG, De Lorenzo P, et al. Pharmacokinetics of high-dose methotrexate in infants treated for acute lymphoblastic leukemia. Pediatr Blood Cancer 2009;52(5):596–601.

29. Salzer WL, Jones TL, Devidas M, et al. Decreased induction morbidity and mortality following modification to induction therapy in infants with acute lymphoblastic leukemia enrolled on AALL0631: a report from the Children's Oncology Group. Pediatr Blood Cancer 2015;62(3):414–8.

30. Gibson BE, Webb DK, Howman AJ, et al. Results of a randomized trial in children with Acute Myeloid Leukaemia: medical research council AML12 trial. Br J Haematol 2011;155(3):366–76.
31. Leung W, Hudson M, Zhu Y, et al. Late effects in survivors of infant leukemia. Leukemia 2000;14(7):1185–90.
32. Gamis AS, Alonzo TA, Meshinchi S, et al. Gemtuzumab ozogamicin in children and adolescents with de novo acute myeloid leukemia improves event-free survival by reducing relapse risk: results from the randomized phase III Children's Oncology Group trial AAML0531. J Clin Oncol 2014;32(27):3021–32.
33. Guest EM, Aplenc R, Sung L, et al. Gemtuzumab ozogamicin in infants with AML: results from the Children's Oncology Group trials AAML03P1 and AAML0531. Blood 2017;130(7):943–5.
34. Sison EAR, Brown P. Does hematopoietic stem cell transplantation benefit infants with acute leukemia? Hematology Am Soc Hematol Educ Program 2013;2013(1): 601–4.
35. Mann G, Attarbaschi A, Schrappe M, et al. Improved outcome with hematopoietic stem cell transplantation in a poor prognostic subgroup of infants with mixed-lineage-leukemia (MLL)-rearranged acute lymphoblastic leukemia: results from the Interfant-99 Study. Blood 2010;116(15):2644–50.
36. Van der Velden VHJ, Corral L, Valsecchi MG, et al. Prognostic significance of minimal residual disease in infants with acute lymphoblastic leukemia treated within the Interfant-99 protocol. Leukemia 2009;23(6):1073–9.
37. Brown P, Pieters R, Biondi A. How I treat infant leukemia. Blood 2019;133(3): 205–14.
38. Hasle H. Myelodysplastic and myeloproliferative disorders of childhood. Hematology Am Soc Hematol Educ Program 2016;2016(1):598–604.
39. Niemeyer CM, Flotho C. Juvenile myelomonocytic leukemia: who's the driver at the wheel? Blood 2019;133(10):1060–70.
40. Niemeyer CM. JMML genomics and decisions. Hematology Am Soc Hematol Educ Program 2018;2018(1):307–12.
41. Locatelli F, Niemeyer CM. How I treat juvenile myelomonocytic leukemia. Blood 2015;125(7):1083–90.
42. Niemeyer CM, Arico M, Basso G, et al. Chronic myelomonocytic leukemia in childhood: a retrospective analysis of 110 cases. European Working Group on Myelodysplastic Syndromes in Childhood (EWOG-MDS). Blood 1997;89(10): 3534–43.
43. Locatelli F, Nollke P, Zecca M, et al. Hematopoietic stem cell transplantation (HSCT) in children with juvenile myelomonocytic leukemia (JMML): results of the EWOG-MDS/EBMT trial. Blood 2005;105(1):410–9.
44. Stieglitz E, Ward AF, Gerbing RB, et al. Phase II/III trial of a pre-transplant farnesyl transferase inhibitor in juvenile myelomonocytic leukemia: a report from the Children's Oncology Group. Pediatr Blood Cancer 2015;62(4):629–36.
45. Bhatnagar N, Nizery L, Tunstall O, et al. Transient abnormal myelopoiesis and AML in Down syndrome: an update. Curr Hematol Malig Rep 2016;11(5):333–41.
46. Roy A, Roberts I, Vyas P. Biology and management of transient abnormal myelopoiesis (TAM) in children with Down syndrome. Semin Fetal Neonatal Med 2012; 17(4):196–201.
47. Tunstall O, Bhatr N, James B, et al. Guidelines for the investigation and management of transient leukaemia of Down syndrome. Br J Haematol 2018;182(2): 200–11.

48. Gamis AS, Alonzo TA, Gerbing RB, et al. Natural history of transient myeloproliferative disorder clinically diagnosed in Down syndrome neonates: a report from the Children's Oncology Group Study A2971. Blood 2011;118(26):6752–9 [quiz: 6996].

49. Mundschau G, Gurbuxani S, Gamis AS, et al. Mutagenesis of GATA1 is an initiating event in Down syndrome leukemogenesis. Blood 2003;101(11):4298–300.

50. Roberts I, Alford K, Hall G, et al. GATA1-mutant clones are frequent and often unsuspected in babies with Down syndrome: identification of a population at risk of leukemia. Blood 2013;122(24):3908–17.

51. Yoshida K, Toki T, Okuno Y, et al. The landscape of somatic mutations in Down syndrome-related myeloid disorders. Nat Genet 2013;45(11):1293–9.

52. Nikolaev SI, Santoni F, Vannier A, et al. Exome sequencing identifies putative drivers of progression of transient myeloproliferative disorder to AMKL in infants with Down syndrome. Blood 2013;122(4):554–61.

53. Klusmann JH, Creutzig U, Zimmermann M, et al. Treatment and prognostic impact of transient leukemia in neonates with Down syndrome. Blood 2008; 111(6):2991–8.

54. Armstrong SA, Kung AL, Mabon ME, et al. Inhibition of FLT3 in MLL. Validation of a therapeutic target identified by gene expression based classification. Cancer Cell 2003;3(2):173–83.

55. Taketani T, Taki T, Sugita K, et al. FLT3 mutations in the activation loop of tyrosine kinase domain are frequently found in infant ALL with MLL rearrangements and pediatric ALL with hyperdiploidy. Blood 2004;103(3):1085–8.

56. Brown P, Levis M, Shurtleff S, et al. FLT3 inhibition selectively kills childhood acute lymphoblastic leukemia cells with high levels of FLT3 expression. Blood 2005; 105(2):812–20.

57. Brown P, Levis M, McIntyre E, et al. Combinations of the FLT3 inhibitor CEP-701 and chemotherapy synergistically kill infant and childhood MLL-rearranged ALL cells in a sequence-dependent manner. Leukemia 2006;20(8):1368–76.

58. Stam RW, den Boer ML, Schneider P, et al. Targeting FLT3 in primary MLL-gene-rearranged infant acute lymphoblastic leukemia. Blood 2005;106(7):2484–90.

59. Chillon MC, Gomez-Casares M, Lopez-Jorge C, et al. Prognostic significance of FLT3 mutational status and expression levels in MLL-AF4+ and MLL-germline acute lymphoblastic leukemia. Leukemia 2012;26(11):2360–6.

60. Stam RW, Schneider P, de Lorenzo P, et al. Prognostic significance of high-level FLT3 expression in MLL-rearranged infant acute lymphoblastic leukemia. Blood 2007;110(7):2774–5.

61. Brown P, Kairalla J, Wang C, et al. SIOP 2016 scientific programme+index. Pediatr Blood Cancer 2016;63(Supplement S3):S7.

62. Schafer E, Irizarry R, Negi S, et al. Promoter hypermethylation in MLL-r infant acute lymphoblastic leukemia: biology and therapeutic targeting. Blood 2010; 115(23):4798–809.

63. Stumpel DJ, Schneider P, van Roon EH, et al. Specific promoter methylation identifies different subgroups of MLL-rearranged infant acute lymphoblastic leukemia, influences clinical outcome, and provides therapeutic options. Blood 2009; 114(27):5490–8.

64. Stumpel, Dominique JPM, Schneider P, et al. Absence of global hypomethylation in promoter hypermethylated Mixed Lineage Leukaemia-rearranged infant acute lymphoblastic leukaemia. Eur J Cancer 2013;49(1):175–84.

65. Stumpel DJ, Schotte D, Lange-Turenhout E, et al. Hypermethylation of specific microRNA genes in MLL-rearranged infant acute lymphoblastic leukemia: major matters at a micro scale. Leukemia 2011;25(3):429–39.

66. Sison EAR, Rau RE, McIntyre E, et al. MLL-rearranged acute lymphoblastic leukaemia stem cell interactions with bone marrow stroma promote survival and therapeutic resistance that can be overcome with CXCR 4 antagonism. Br J Haematol 2013;160(6):785–97.

67. Sison EAR, McIntyre E, Magoon D, et al. Dynamic chemotherapy-induced upregulation of CXCR4 expression: a mechanism of therapeutic resistance in pediatric AML. Mol Cancer Res 2013;11(9):1004–16.

68. Sison EAR, Magoon D, Li L, et al. Plerixafor as a chemosensitizing agent in pediatric acute lymphoblastic leukemia: efficacy and potential mechanisms of resistance to CXCR4 inhibition. Oncotarget 2014;5(19):8947.

69. Sison EAR, Magoon D, Li L, et al. POL5551, a novel and potent CXCR4 antagonist, enhances sensitivity to chemotherapy in pediatric ALL. Oncotarget 2015; 6(31):30902.

70. Cooper TM, Sison EAR, Baker SD, et al. A phase 1 study of the CXCR4 antagonist plerixafor in combination with high-dose cytarabine and etoposide in children with relapsed or refractory acute leukemias or myelodysplastic syndrome: a Pediatric Oncology Experimental Therapeutics Investigators' Consortium study (POE 10-03). Pediatr Blood Cancer 2017;64(8). https://doi.org/10.1002/pbc.26414.

71. von Stackelberg A, Locatelli F, Zugmaier G, et al. Phase I/phase II study of blinatumomab in pediatric patients with relapsed/refractory acute lymphoblastic leukemia. J Clin Oncol 2016;34(36):4381–9.

72. Maude SL, Laetsch TW, Buechner J, et al. Tisagenlecleucel in children and young adults with B-cell lymphoblastic leukemia. N Engl J Med 2018;378(5):439–48.

73. Bernt KM, Zhu N, Sinha AU, et al. MLL-rearranged leukemia is dependent on aberrant H3K79 methylation by DOT1L. Cancer Cell 2011;20(1):66–78.

74. Nguyen AT, Taranova O, He J, et al. DOT1L, the H3K79 methyltransferase, is required for MLL-AF9-mediated leukemogenesis. Blood 2011;117(25):6912–22.

75. Deshpande AJ, Chen L, Fazio M, et al. Leukemic transformation by the MLL-AF6 fusion oncogene requires the H3K79 methyltransferase Dot1l. Blood 2013; 121(13):2533–41.

76. Daigle SR, Olhava EJ, Therkelsen CA, et al. Potent inhibition of DOT1L as treatment of MLL-fusion leukemia. Blood 2013;122(6):1017–25.

77. Daigle SR, Olhava EJ, Therkelsen CA, et al. Selective killing of mixed lineage leukemia cells by a potent small-molecule DOT1L inhibitor. Cancer Cell 2011;20(1): 53–65.

78. Stein EM, Garcia-Manero G, Rizzieri DA, et al. The DOT1L inhibitor EPZ-5676: safety and activity in relapsed/refractory patients with MLL-rearranged leukemia. Blood 2014;124(21):387.

79. Shukla N, O'Brien MM, Silverman LB, et al. Preliminary report of the phase 1 study of the DOT1L inhibitor, pinometostat, EPZ-5676, in children with relapsed or refractory MLL-r acute leukemia: safety, exposure and target inhibition. Blood 2015;126(23):3792.

80. Yokoyama A, Somervaille TC, Smith KS, et al. The menin tumor suppressor protein is an essential oncogenic cofactor for MLL-associated leukemogenesis. Cell 2005;123(2):207–18.

81. Caslini C, Yang Z, El-Osta M, et al. Interaction of MLL amino terminal sequences with menin is required for transformation. Cancer Res 2007;67(15):7275–83.

82. Klossowski S, Miao H, Kempinska K, et al. Menin inhibitor MI-3454 induces remission in MLL1-rearranged and NPM1-mutated models of leukemia. J Clin Invest 2020;130(2):981–97.

83. Krivtsov AV, Evans K, Gadrey JY, et al. A menin-MLL inhibitor induces specific chromatin changes and eradicates disease in models of MLL-rearranged leukemia. Cancer Cell 2019;36(6):660–73.e11.

84. Robinson BW, Behling KC, Gupta M, et al. Abundant anti-apoptotic BCL-2 is a molecular target in leukaemias with t(4;11) translocation. Br J Haematol 2008; 141(6):827–39.

85. Jayanthan A, Incoronato A, Singh A, et al. Cytotoxicity, drug combinability, and biological correlates of ABT-737 against acute lymphoblastic leukemia cells with MLL rearrangement. Pediatr Blood Cancer 2011;56(3):353–60.

86. Benito JM, Godfrey L, Kojima K, et al. MLL-rearranged acute lymphoblastic leukemias activate BCL-2 through H3K79 methylation and are sensitive to the BCL-2-specific antagonist ABT-199. Cell Rep 2015;13(12):2715–27.

87. Khaw SL, Suryani S, Evans K, et al. Venetoclax responses of pediatric ALL xenografts reveal sensitivity of MLL-rearranged leukemia. Blood 2016;128(10): 1382–95.

Neonatal Central Nervous System Tumors

Shubin Shahab, MD, PhD[a,b,*], Jason Fangusaro, MD[c,d]

KEYWORDS

- Neonatal brain tumor • Neonatal CNS tumor • Congenital brain tumor
- Congenital CNS tumor • Fetal brain tumor • Fetal CNS tumor

KEY POINTS

- Neonatal brain tumors represent less than 2% of all childhood central nervous system (CNS) tumors; however, they are associated with significant morbidity and mortality.
- The most common neonatal CNS tumor is teratoma; however, other histologies, such as astrocytoma and glioma, ependymoma, atypical teratoid/rhabdoid tumors, medulloblastoma, choroid plexus tumors, and craniopharyngiomas, also can be seen.
- Management options for neonatal CNS tumors often are limited due to the ability of newborns to tolerate surgery, radiation, and/or chemotherapy.
- A multidisciplinary approach is critical to address the psychosocial and medical challenges of these cases.

INTRODUCTION

Central nervous system (CNS) tumors are the most common solid tumors among children, but they are relatively rare in newborns. Although cooperative group studies generally have considered tumors occurring in children under the age of 3 years infant tumors, neonatal brain tumors are a unique entity that deserve more scrutiny. Multiple prior studies have more specifically established neonatal brain tumors as tumors diagnosed prenatally or in the first 2 months of life.[1,2] For the purpose of this review, the terms, *neonatal*, *perinatal*, and *congenital*, are used to refer to this same entity. Most reports suggest only approximately 0.5% to 1.9% of brain tumor cases occur during the perinatal period,[3,4] with an incidence ranging from 0.3 to 2.9 cases per 100,000 live births.[5] Biologically, congenital brain tumors are distinct from those occurring in older children. Supratentorial tumors are much more common than

^a Aflac Cancer and Blood Disorders Center, Children's Healthcare of Atlanta, Atlanta, GA, USA;
^b Emory University School of Medicine, 1760 Haygood Drive Northeast HSRB E397, Atlanta, GA 30322, USA; ^c Aflac Cancer and Blood Disorders Center, Children's Healthcare of Atlanta, 1405 Clifton Road Northeast, Atlanta, GA 30322, USA; ^d Department of Pediatrics, Emory University School of Medicine, Atlanta, GA, USA
* Corresponding author.
E-mail address: sshahab@emory.edu

Clin Perinatol 48 (2021) 35–51
https://doi.org/10.1016/j.clp.2020.11.003
0095-5108/21/© 2020 Elsevier Inc. All rights reserved.

infratentorial tumors in neonates, and the prognosis and survival outcomes in this age group are much worse compared with those in older children.[6] Management is difficult with limited options for surgery and radiotherapy, given the concern for mortality and acute and late morbidities. The true rate of perinatal brain tumors may be underestimated because many may go undiagnosed due to intrauterine fetal demise. Although gliomas are the most common type of brain tumor in children of all ages, including infants (less than 3 years old [**Fig. 1**][7]), teratomas are the most common brain tumors in neonates, with astrocytoma, choroid plexus papilloma (CPP), embryonal tumors, and craniopharyngioma seen less frequently.

PRENATAL DIAGNOSIS AND IMAGING

With advanced fetal ultrasonography (US), many neonatal brain tumors are diagnosed prenatally, although histologic confirmation still typically has to be done after birth. Routine US examinations may miss fetal brain tumors as the brain undergoes rapid growth and development near the end of the third trimester. Teratomas and hamartomas may be detected before 22 weeks, germinal tumors between 22 weeks and 32 weeks, and gliomas after 32 weeks.[4] Prenatally, tumors can cause hydrocephalus, although the fetal skull can expand to a remarkable extent leading to macrocrania, or local skull swelling. For large tumors, this may lead to fetal hydrops requiring cranial decompression to permit vaginal delivery. Cesarean section is necessary in approximately two-thirds of these cases.[3]

Hydrocephalus, secondary to tumor growth or intracranial hemorrhage and obstruction of the ventricular system, often leads to symptoms of irritability and vomiting after birth. The fetus also may experience high-output heart failure, which can lead to stillbirth. Newborns also can present with seizures and somnolence. Occasionally, congenital brain tumors can be accompanied by other malformations, such as cleft lip/palate and cardiac and urinary tract defects. A recent population-based cohort study of 5.2 million children in Norway and Sweden revealed an increased risk of brain/CNS malignancy, specifically in children with oral clefts in the cohort from Sweden. In both countries, the risk for CNS cancer in the first year of life was increased in children with multiple birth defects. Birth defects also were found to have an increased association with medulloblastoma (MB), primitive neuroectodermal tumor, and germ cell tumors in a separate retrospective study of 3733 patients with brain tumors in the California Cancer Registry.[8]

US is the imaging modality used most commonly in the prenatal period; however, once a diagnosis of a brain tumor is suspected, fetal magnetic romance imaging (MRI) may help determine the exact location of the tumor, involvement of adjacent structures, and the developmental state of the remainder of the brain, which can help with prognosis and preparation for potential surgical intervention.[3] US may demonstrate a heterogeneous pattern with destruction of normal structures and mass effect and document the presence of hydrocephalus or calcifications in the case of teratomas. Importantly, prenatal diagnosis can help determine timing and route of delivery, prepare health care teams for postnatal management, and allow time for prenatal parental counseling regarding prognosis and therapeutic options.

TYPES OF NEONATAL BRAIN TUMORS
Germ Cell Tumors

Histologically, intracranial germ cell tumors are composed of germinomas and nongerminomatous germ cell tumors (NGGCTs). The NGGCT category comprises of multiple histologies, including teratomas, teratomas with malignant transformation, yolk

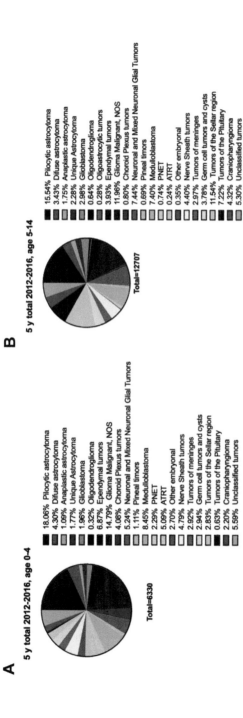

Fig. 1. Distribution of brain tumor diagnoses among children between the ages of (*A*) 0 to 4 years and (*B*) 5 years to 14 years based on the incidence of CNS tumor diagnosed in the US population from 2012 to 2016 and presented in the Central Brain Tumor Registry of the United States (CBTRUS) statistical report.[7] Note the higher incidence of embryonal tumors (AT/RT, ETMR, pineal tumors, MB, and other embryonal) and choroid plexus tumors among the younger age group.

A

5 y total 2012-2016, age 0-4

Total=6330

18.06% Pilocytic astrocytoma
4.30% Difuse astrocytoma
1.09% Anaplastic astrocytoma
1.77% Unique Astrocytoma
1.96% Glioblastoma
0.32% Oligodendroglioma
6.87% Ependymal tumors
14.79% Glioma Malignant, NOS
4.06% Choroid Plexus tumors
1.11% Neuronal and Mixed Neuronal Glial Tumors
8.45% Pineal timors
2.29% Medulloblastoma
5.09% PNET
2.70% ATRT
2.92% Other embryonal
2.94% Nerve Sheath tumors
2.83% Tumors of meninges
0.63% Germ cell tumors and cysts
2.20% Tumors of the Sellar region
5.59% Tumors of the Pituitary
        Craniopharyngioma
        Unclassified tumors

B

5 y total 2012-2016, age 5-14

Total=12707

15.54% Pilocytic astrocytoma
3.43% Difuse astrocytoma
1.75% Anaplastic astrocytoma
2.28% Unique Astrocytoma
2.98% Glioblastoma
0.64% Oligodendroglioma
0.28% Oligoastrocytic tumors
3.93% Ependymal tumors
11.96% Glioma Malignant, NOS
0.80% Choroid Plexus tumors
7.44% Neuronal and Mixed Neuronal Glial Tumors
0.69% Pineal timors
7.40% Medulloblastoma
0.74% PNET
0.24% ATRT
0.35% Other embryonal
4.40% Nerve Sheath tumors
2.97% Tumors of meninges
3.78% Germ cell tumors and cysts
11.54% Tumors of the Sellar region
7.22% Tumors of the Pituitary
4.32% Craniopharyngioma
5.30% Unclassified tumors

sac tumors, choriocarcinoma, embryonal carcinoma, and mixed germ cell tumors.[9] Teratomas are the most common brain tumors in the neonatal period, constituting 33% to 50% of all cases.[10,11] They are derived from all 3 germ layers (ectoderm, mesoderm, and endoderm) and can present as mature or immature forms. Neonatal teratomas can be located anywhere along the midline, with the sacrococcygeal region being most common.[10] In the brain, they often are located in the pineal region or the neurohypophysis or adjacent to the third ventricle.[4,12] These also can involve the hemispheres in neonates. Sometimes teratomas may be associated with elevation of alpha-fetoprotein (AFP) and/or human chorionic gonadotropin (beta-HCG) in the serum and cerebrospinal fluid (CSF).[13] Symptoms vary based on location and extent of the tumor; however, even mature teratomas can be devastating in the neonatal period because they can interfere with the most critical period of brain development. Due to their midline location, resection may be difficult.

Imaging typically reveals a heterogenous mixture of solid and cystic components, mineralization, and fatty tissue. The solid components and the rim of the cystic regions usually are contrast-enhancing. The mainstay of treatment of teratomas remains maximal surgical resection. Mature teratomas are not sensitive to chemotherapy, but chemotherapy may be beneficial for immature teratomas.[14] Unfortunately, the prognosis remains dismal for infants. Radiation typically is avoided in this age due to long-term effect on neurodevelopmental outcome and because doses of radiation needed to treat mature teratoma are not feasible, particularly in the CNS. Overall survival rates have been reported to be less than 10% at 1 year,[3,15] often because the tumor is very extensive at the time of presentation.

Astrocytomas

Astrocytomas are the most common brain tumor overall in both adults and children; however, they are less common in infants. Most pediatric astrocytomas are low-grade glioma (LGG) (World Health Organization [WHO] grades I and II), with only approximately 10% high-grade glioma (HGG) (WHO grades III and IV). Conversely, a recent review revealed that a majority of neonatal cases were high grade. In a review of 101 cases, Isaacs[16] found that the majority of tumors in this age range were HGGs (55% HGG vs 45% LGG), with the majority glioblastoma multiforme (GBM) (44.6%), a WHO grade IV tumor. Other studies have reported a much lower percentage of GBM among neonatal brain tumors.[17] HGGs in children can be associated with Li-Fraumeni syndrome (inherited *TP53* mutation [**Table 1**]), and LGGs can occur in association with neurofibromatosis type 1 or neurofibromatosis type 2.

The most common presenting symptoms are macrocephaly, hydrocephalus, and intracranial hemorrhage.[16] In some cases, astrocytomas also have been found on routine prenatal US, and a majority of these cases were diagnosed in the 3rd trimester. In the Isaacs[16] study of 101 perinatal astrocytomas, 9% of the cases were stillborn and overall survival was reported to be 46.5%.

Children with LGGs often are treated successfully by surgery alone, when feasible, and, in some cases, chemotherapy is added for patients with residual disease. For HGGs, surgery and radiation therapy commonly are used, but the role of chemotherapy is less clear. In the neonatal population, however, surgery remains the mainstay of treatment, regardless of grade. Chemotherapy can be given for LGGs, if necessary, and some patients may get delayed or salvage radiation if they survive beyond infancy. In the case series by Isaacs, the survival rate for neonates with GBM was 50%,[16] which is higher than reported for older children.[18] The survival rate for fetal cases, however, was only 6.5%.[16] Neonatal HGGs may have a better prognosis than their pediatric or adult counterparts,[5,17,19–22] including sporadic cases

Table 1
Common genetic syndromes associated with pediatric brain tumors

Genetic Syndrome and Incidence	Mutation	Type of Brain Tumor	Other Findings
Ataxia telangiectasia 1:20,000–1:100,000	*ATM*	Meningioma	Progressive cerebellar atrophy, telangiectasias, radiosensitivity, immunodeficiency, cancer predisposition
Cowden syndrome 1:250,000	*PTEN*	Dysplastic cerebellar gangliocytoma Glial tumors (gliosarcoma)	Mucocutaneous papillomatous lesions, multiple hamartomas, cancer predisposition
Turcot syndrome	*APC* (FAP) *MLH1, MSH2, MSH6, PMS2* (HNPCC)	MB Glioma	Adenomatous colorectal polyps, colorectal cancer
Gardner syndrome 1:8000	*APC*	MB	Intestinal polyposis, colorectal cancer as well as cancers of small bowel, stomach, pancreas, thyroid, CNS, liver, bile duct, adrenal glands. Dental abnormalities, osteomas, skin fibromas, dermoid tumors
Gorlin syndrome 1:57,000–1:164,000	*PTCH*	MB Meningioma	Eye anomalies, macrocephaly, cleft lip/palate, bridging of the sella, odontogenic keratocysts, dural/falcine calcifications, basal cell carcinoma
Li-Fraumeni 1:5000	*TP53*	Glioma MB CPC	Multiple cancers (adrenocortical carcinomas, sarcomas, breast cancer)
Multiple endocrine neoplasia type 1 1:30,000	*MEN1*	Pituitary adenoma	Pancreas, pituitary, parathyroid tumors, gastrinomas, carcinoid tumors of the duodenum
Familial retinoblastoma	*RB*	Pineoblastoma	Bilateral retinoblastoma, osteosarcoma
von Hippel-Lindau 1:36,000	*VHL*	Hemangioblastoma	Multiple tumors, (renal angiomas, clear cell renal cell carcinomas; pheochromocytomas, serous cystadenomas, endolymphatic sac tumors)

(*continued on next page*)

Table 1 (continued)			
Genetic Syndrome and Incidence	Mutation	Type of Brain Tumor	Other Findings
Neurofibromatosis type 1 1:2500–1:3000	NF1	Gliomas	Multiple CNS and peripheral nervous system tumors (schwannomas, neurofibromas); vascular dysplasias (moyamoya, stenosis), café au lait spots
Neurofibromatosis type 2 1:33,000–1:37,000	NF2	Bilateral vestibular schwannomas Meningiomas Ependymomas	Café au lait spots
Tuberous sclerosis 1:6000–1:10,000	TSC1/TSC2	Subependymal giant cell astrocytomas	CNS subependymal nodules, cortical tubers, white matter changes. Cardiac rhabdomyomas, ash leave macules. Benign hamartomas in multiple organs
Rhabdoid tumor predisposition syndrome <1:1000000	SMARCB1, SMARCA4	AT/RTs	Extracranial rhabdoid tumors often before age 3 y
Aicardi syndrome 1:100000–1:167000	unknown	Choroid plexus tumors	Infantile spasms, agenesis of corpus callosum, chorioretinal abnormalities

of spontaneous resolution.[23,24] This suggests a difference in underlying biology. Some reports suggest a lower mutational burden in congenital high-grade tumors compared with those in older children.[23,25,26] Many pediatric HGGs are characterized by histone *H3F3A* mutations (H3K27 M or H3.3G34 R/V) or *PDGFRA* amplifications as well as amplifications in *EGFR*, *MYC*, *MYCN*, and *MDM4*.[27] Chromosomal aberrations include 1q gain and, less frequently, 7q gain and 10q loss. In a recent study of HGG in very young children,[26] focal amplifications of *PDGFRA* and *EGFR* were absent and histone H3F3A K27 M mutation was present in only 2 cases (6%), whereas *CDKN2A* amplifications were seen in 2 children. In this study, 1q gain and 10q loss were seen as well. In a separate study of 11 very young infants, Paugh and colleagues[28] reported absence of 1q gain and only 1 case of 10q loss. Some infant HGGs also demonstrate loss of *SNORD,* the gene encoding small nucleolar RNA.[26,27] Additionally, infant HGGs can display recurrent fusion of the kinase domain of NTRK1-3, which typically is not seen in older pediatric HGGs, and may be targetable given the availability of novel NTRK-targeting agents.[22,29,30]

Unfortunately, even with improved surgical techniques and less radiation, neonates with HGG are at increased risk of long-term effects. Seizures, developmental delay, neurocognitive dysfunction, motor disability, and endocrinopathies are common. The Children's Cancer Group CCG-945 study was a phase III trial from 1985 to 1992 that evaluated chemotherapy in children with HGG under 6 years of age with radiation avoidance for those less than 3 years of age and with radiation for those between ages 3 and 6. Children older than 3 years were randomized to either receive pCV (prednisone, lomustine, and vincristine) or an 8-drugs-in-1-day (8-in-1) regimen (lomustine, vincristine, hydroxyurea, procarbazine, cisplatin, cytosine arabinoside, methylprednisolone, and dacarbazine), and those younger than 3 years old were nonrandomly assigned to the 8-in-1 chemotherapy arm. Despite avoidance of radiation, study survivors diagnosed before 3 years of age had lower IQ, lower visual memory, slower processing speed, and poorer visual motor integration compared with those diagnosed between 3 years and 6 years of age, although the patient populations were too small for statistical analyses.[25] These findings need to be confirmed in larger cohorts but suggest the insult to critical regions of the brain regardless of cause during the neonatal period may lead to worse late effects compared with older children.

Subependymal giant cell astrocytomas (SEGAs) are a unique group of astrocytomas that usually occur in children with tuberous sclerosis complex (TSC) in their first or second decade of life, but, rarely, they may present in neonates. TSC is an autosomal dominant condition that arises as a result of mutations in either the *TSC1* (encoding hamartin) or the *TSC2* (encoding tuberin) gene and typically is characterized by hamartomas in the brain, skin, heart, liver, lung, and kidneys. Under normal circumstances, hamartin and tuberin negatively regulate the mTORC1 complex (mTOR = mammalian target of rapamycin) by preventing substrate use in unfavorable conditions. In patients with *TSC1* and/or *TSC2* mutations, however, this complex is hyperactivated, leading to a downstream kinase signaling cascade that subsequently leads to cell-cycle progression, transcription, translation, and, ultimately, hamartoma formation.[31] Neonates with TSC often present with cardiac rhabdomyomas, causing outflow obstruction as well as arrhythmias, rather than neurologic symptoms from SEGAs. A study from Kotulska and colleagues[32] identified 2.2% of patients with TSC who developed congenital SEGAs. Other common manifestations of TSC include seizures, developmental delay, skin lesions, and extra-CNS hamartomas. On US, SEGAs often appear as echogenic subependymal nodules along the ventricles. They also can have intratumoral calcifications. Treatment of SEGAs have come a long way since the discovery of mTOR inhibitors, with patients showing excellent long-term response. In a multicenter retrospective study by Saffari and colleagues,[33] the mTOR inhibitor everolimus was found to be safe and efficacious for patients under 2 years of age with TSC.

Choroid Plexus Tumors

Tumors developing from the epithelial lining of the choroid plexus of the ventricles are called choroid plexus tumors. They can be CPPs or choroid plexus carcinomas (CPCs). Choroid plexus tumors can be associated with Aicardi syndrome, an X-linked syndrome, characterized by agenesis of corpus callosum, chorioretinitis, and spasms, or with Li-Fraumeni syndrome, characterized by predisposition to multiple tumors secondary to *TP53* mutation. Although papillomas usually are surgically resectable and have a good prognosis, carcinomas have an extremely poor outcome. There is a third group of tumors identified by the WHO called atypical CPPs, which have an intermediate prognosis. Choroid plexus tumors in general are rare (0.4%–0.6% of all pediatric brain tumors) and often occur in infancy (approximately 50% in the first year of life). Most choroid plexus tumors are CPPs, accounting for 10% to 20% of neonatal brain tumors,[1,34] although some reports suggest this number could be higher.[35] Due to their location often associated with or adjacent to the ventricular surface, they often lead to ventriculomegaly and hydrocephalus from overproduction of CSF and blocked drainage. Although papillomas have a very good outcome with surgical resection alone in pediatric patients, in general, there is a significant surgical risk of hemorrhage and poor outcome in neonates due to immature brain and fragile vascularity. Recently, embolization prior to resection has led to improved surgical outcomes. In some cases, atypical papillomas are treated with neoadjuvant chemotherapy to decrease tumor vascularity and increase the chance of maximal surgical resection.[36] Occasionally, these tumors become very large and lead to massive ventriculomegaly and cortical atrophy.

Choroid plexus tumors typically are detected near the end of the third trimester on fetal US. They appear as fine nodular lesions in the lateral ventricles and modern imaging modalities usually can discriminate them from intracranial hemorrhage. CT scans typically show a large isodense to hyperdense mass with well demarcated margins and avid contrast enhancement.[10] MRI may show a well delineated T1 isointense and T2 hyperintense mass with frondlike appearance and contrast enhancement (**Fig. 2**).

CPCs have a much worse outcome compared with CPPs. These highly invasive tumors can metastasize along the neuroaxis with leptomeningeal spread and, rarely, extracranially into the lungs or abdomen.[15] CPCs also are characterized by frequent *TP53* mutations, which can be somatic (approximately 60% of the cases) or germline and associate with Li-Fraumeni syndrome in approximately 24% of cases[36] (see **Table 1**).

Embryonal Tumors

Embryonal tumors are derived from undifferentiated or poorly differentiated neuroepithelial cells and include MBs, which are common among older children, as well as tumors seen more commonly in the neonatal age group, including atypical teratoid/rhabdoid tumors (AT/RTs) and embryonal tumors with multilayered rosettes (ETMRs) (**Fig. 3**).

Medulloblastoma

MBs are the most common malignant brain tumor of childhood but are less common in neonates. Histologically, they are classified into classic, desmoplastic/nodular, or large cell/anaplastic variants. These are composed of small round blue cells often with Homer-Wright pseudorosettes, necrosis, and increased mitotic activity. In general, classic histology is associated with intermediate prognosis, desmoplastic with

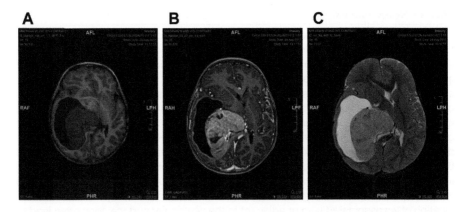

Fig. 2. Infant brain MRIs: (*A*) axial noncontrast T1, (*B*) axial postcontrast T1, and (*C*) axial noncontrast T2 demonstrating the T1/T2 isointense contrast-enhancing CPC arising from the right posterior lateral ventricle.

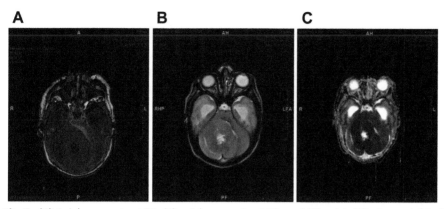

Fig. 3. (A) Axial noncontrast T1, (B) axial noncontrast T2, and (C) axial diffusion-weighted MRIs of infant brain with embryonal tumor, not otherwise specified.

good prognosis and large cell/anaplastic with bad prognosis.[37] More recently, MB has been divided into 4 different molecular subgroups that have implications for prognosis. These include WNT Wingless-type (WNT), the most favorable subtype; Sonic hedgehog (SHH), an intermediate prognosis group (the most common subtype in infants); group 3, which carries the worst prognosis; and group 4, which also has an intermediate prognosis.[38] These highly aggressive tumors are usually treated with a combination of surgery, radiation, and chemotherapy. In neonates and young infants, high-dose chemotherapy with autologous stem cell rescue often is used in lieu of or to delay radiation. Obtaining sufficient numbers of autologous stem cells may be challenging in neonates, however, due to their small size and low blood volume.[39]

MB now is widely accepted to be a tumor exclusive to the posterior fossa. On MRI, MBs usually are isointense on T1-weighted and T2-weighted images and slightly hypointense on diffusion-weighted imaging. They can spread along the neuroaxis requiring spine imaging and lumbar cytology at diagnosis. Prognosis for infant MB has improved with combinatorial approaches to therapy. Prior to the era of high-dose chemotherapy with autologous stem cell rescue, infants with MB had a survival rate of approximately 44% at 12 months.[19] The recently concluded Head Start III trial revealed a 5-year overall survival of 46% ± 5% for all patients, whereas for infants with desmoplastic histology, the 5-year overall and event-free survival rates were greater than 80%.[40]

Although most cases are sporadic, SHH-driven MBs can be associated with Gorlin syndrome characterized by mutation in *PTCH1* gene and development of skin cancers along with MB (see **Table 1**). Some SHH- MBs also are associated with Li-Fraumeni syndrome. WNT-MBs can be associated with Gardner syndrome, an autosomal dominant disorder characterized by intestinal polyposis and colorectal adenocarcinoma due to mutation in the *APC* gene.

Atypical teratoid/rhabdoid tumors

AT/RTs are rare tumors that disproportionately affect young children. Classically they are characterized by loss of INI1, a member of the SWI/SNF chromatin remodeling complex. Those with germline mutations in the *SMARCB1* (encoding INI1) or *SMARCA4* (encoding BRG1) genes, that is, those with rhabdoid tumor predisposition syndrome, tend to develop AT/RTs earlier in life,[41] even as early as the neonatal period (see **Table 1**). AT/RTs genetically are relatively silent tumors, although recently they have been subclassified into at least 3 different molecular subgroups.[42,43] Primarily located in the supratentorial compartment, AT/RTs are characterized by a rapidly growing large heterogenous solid and cystic mass with necrosis, mineralization, and hemorrhage. They also can occur in the infratentorium, including the cerebellum, brainstem, cerebellopontine angle, or the spinal cord. CNS dissemination is present at diagnosis in approximately one-third of the cases. AT/RTs are treated similar to MBs with a combination of surgery, high-dose chemotherapy, and radiation if children are older. Prognosis has improved with multimodal therapy, although median survival in the infant age group still is only approximately 9 months.[19,44–46]

Embryonal tumors with multilayered rosettes

ETMRs are another extremely rare group of brain tumors occurring primarily in young infants. Molecularly, these tumors are characterized by amplification of the chromosome 19q region C19 MC coding for a miRNA cluster as well as overexpression of the protein LIN28 A. Histology demonstrates high cellularity with abundant neuropil and cells arranged around vessels forming rosettes (**Fig. 4**). Most of these occur in the first 2 years of life, and approximately two-thirds are supratentorial. Like other embryonal tumors, these often can present with CNS metastasis at diagnosis, and they are associated with extremely poor prognosis, with average survival of approximately 12 months.[47]

Because of the need for multimodal therapy, infants with embryonal tumors are at increased risk of neurologic, cognitive, and endocrine toxicities even when they survive. In a study of 27 infants with CNS tumors from St. Jude Children's Research Hospital, a substantial fraction of survivors had audiovisual deficits, speech and cognitive delays, or growth delays; required hormone replacemen; or developed seizure disorders requiring antiepileptics.[21]

Craniopharyngioma

Craniopharyngiomas arise from remnants of Rathke pouch and typically have excellent overall survival in older children; however, they often are associated with significant morbidities. They are divided into papillary and adamantinomatous histologies. The adamantinomatous subtype is the predominant variant and can occur at any age. Conversely, the papillary subtype is seen almost exclusively in adults.[48] On US, they appear as a large intracranial mass in the suprasellar region, often indistinguishable from a teratoma. MRI may help further delineate the tumor and its impact on normal brain parenchyma.

Although rare, craniopharyngiomas in neonates carry a worse prognosis due to limited treatment options in this age group. Because of their location in the neurohypophysis, children may develop long-term endocrinopathies requiring hormone replacement or management of diabetes insipidus. Occasionally, they may have developmental delay and/or seizures. Surgically, tumors less than 6 cm in diameter are considered to be more likely to undergo gross total resection, whereas those greater than 8 cm usually are associated with a poor outcome.[49] Although radiation often is utilized in older children, because of the significant risk of neurocognitive devastation,[50] it is avoided in neonates.

Neuronal and Mixed Neuroglial Tumors

Desmoplastic infantile astrocytoma (DIA) and desmoplastic infantile ganglioglioma (DIG) are 2 WHO grade I tumors that are very rare, accounting for less than 1% of all pediatric brain tumors. They both, however, are relatively common in neonates. DIGs are seen almost entirely in infants less than 6 months of age and in most cases are considered congenital. They carry a favorable prognosis with surgical resection

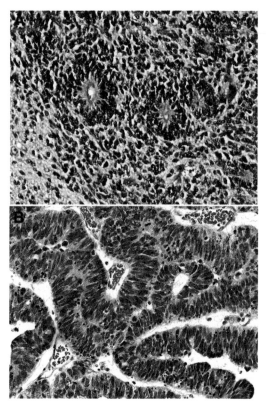

Fig. 4. (*A*) Characteristic pathology of ETMR tumor displaying high cellularity with abundant neuropil and cells arranged around vessels forming rosettes. (*B*) An ETMR tumor displaying medulloepithelioma histology resembling embryonic neural tube with papillary arrangement without obvious multilayered rosettes.

alone. These usually are large cystic supratentorial tumors that can involve the superficial cerebral cortex and leptomeninges. The cysts can grow to massive size with relatively little edema.[10] Multiple lobes commonly are involved with a predilection for frontal and parietal lobes. Rapid head growth with bulging fontanelle are common presenting features. Histologically, both have a stroma rich in collagen and spindle-shaped fibroblastic elements, but DIGs have a prevalence of neuronal elements whereas DIAs have astrocytic components exclusively.[51] On MRI, solid components are T1 and T2 hypointense, whereas the cystic components are classically T1 hypointense but T2 hyperintense.

Treatment primarily is surgical removal. Even with partial resection, long disease-free intervals are achieved without tumor progression. Chemotherapy can be considered in cases of recurrence or growth of residual tumor. Recent studies suggest DIGs may be MAP kinase pathway driven tumors, suggesting a potential role for MEK inhibitors in this disease.[52]

ETHICAL CHALLENGES IN NEONATAL BRAIN TUMOR MANAGEMENT

A brain tumor diagnosis in a neonate presents significant medical and ethical challenges for the medical team, parents, and family. If a diagnosis occurs prenatally, although still significant, preparations can be made to ensure safe delivery, and consideration given to possible treatment options versus withdrawal of care. If, however, diagnosis is made after birth, the decision process becomes more challenging. One such example is illustrated in **Fig. 5**, where a newborn presented with severe macrocrania at birth and was found to have a large intracranial tumor with minimal residual brain, leaving the family and the medical team with difficult choices. Families frequently are overwhelmed, making it difficult to fully participate in medical decision making. Hospitals without subspecialty care may not be prepared to identify appropriate treatment options, expected side effects, and outcomes or to comment on prognosis.[53] Even when diagnosed at large academic medical centers, accurate prediction of outcomes for intracranial tumors not always is possible. Parents expect clinicians to be knowledgeable experts who can provide objective, evidence-based opinions, but, given the rarity of neonatal tumors, limited data may be available to guide clinicians. Parents also may be asked to make difficult decisions while fatigued, stressed, and grieving. At times, even when the prognosis is expected to be grim, families still may opt to pursue aggressive treatments. Non–tumor-directed therapies, such as hospice and palliative care, are essential when available, as discussed later. Racine and colleagues[54] argue that clinicians may have inherent biases about long-term neurologic outcome that affect their evidence-based prognostication. They suggest a set of 5 practice principles: reflection, humility, open-mindedness, partnership, and engagement. These principles may assist clinicians and help guide their approach in such difficult situations.

An additional issue is the lack of availability of palliative care for neonatal patients. In a recent study, Rosenberg and colleagues[55] found that a palliative care consult was obtained in only 16 of 90 neonates diagnosed with HGG, suggesting an underutilization of palliative care services in the neonatal intensive care unit. The investigators suggest that the reasons may be multifactorial, including a lack of palliative care resources, competing physician and patient priorities, diffusion of responsibility among multiple caregivers, lack of standardized pathways, discomfort among physicians and patients surrounding discussion of these issues, unpredictable timing of disease progression, and lack of patients' awareness of their prognosis.[55]

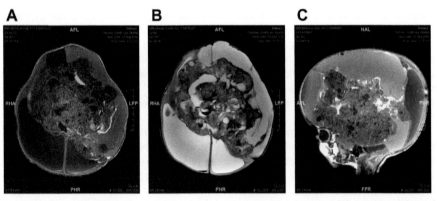

Fig. 5. Illustrative images of a newborn with large intracranial tumor. (A) Axial T1, (B) axial T2, and (C) sagittal MRIs demonstrate very little brain tissue remaining. After a discussion with neurosurgery, neonatology, neuro-oncology, and the family, a decision was made to not intervene. Family chose to enroll in home hospice, where the neonate died peacefully within a few weeks.

GENETIC PREDISPOSITION

There are several rare genetic conditions that predispose to the development of brain tumors[56] (see **Table 1**); however, a majority of these do not present with brain tumors in the neonatal age group. It is essential that neonatologists be aware of these conditions and the potential for brain tumor development to help prepare families for future implications of these genetic diseases.

SUMMARY

Significant research has evaluated the underlying molecular genetic make-up of pediatric brain tumors, with the most recent WHO classification putting more emphasis on molecular characteristics and removing some previously used nomenclature based on histologic architecture alone.[9] Despite advances in understanding and management of pediatric brain tumors, there remains a relative paucity of studies looking specifically at the neonatal population.

This review highlights the most common brain tumors seen in the neonatal population. Neonates are a unique population having a different epidemiologic distribution and tumor biology.[22] Prognosis in general, however, for all neonatal brain tumors remains poor, partly due to the inability of neonates to tolerate significant toxicity that often accompanies treatment regimens, including surgery, chemotherapy, and radiotherapy. With advances in supportive care, innovative therapies, and better diagnostics, this outlook gradually is changing. Key challenges, however, remain. Because of the rarity of these tumors, prospective clinical trials are almost impossible. As a result, clinicians often have to depend on case reports, tumor registries, and clinical experience to guide treatments. Given the lack of prospective clinical data, it is not always clear which patients should receive intervention and whether the toll on future neurocognitive impact is justified. These and other difficult issues make it imperative that, whenever possible, a multidisciplinary team be involved in these rare cases, including neuro-oncologists, neonatologist, neurosurgeons, neurologists, palliative care physicians, and social workers.

Best practices

What is the current practice for neonatal brain tumors?

- Currently, this is not standardized because these are relatively rare. Practice also largely varies based on specific histologic diagnosis (see text).

Best practice/guideline/care path objective(s)

- If diagnosed prenatally, referral may be made to a tertiary care center for anticipated complications during delivery as well as management of the infant.
- If diagnosed at birth, if feasible and safe, the infant should be transferred to a tertiary care center for multidisciplinary care.
- It is important to involve a multidisciplinary team, including neurosurgery, neuro-oncology, neonatology, palliative care, and radiation oncology as well as genetics, social work, and other ancillary services from the outset to consider all options before giving recommendations and to support the family.

What changes in current practice are likely to improve outcomes?

- Early involvement of palliative/supportive care has been shown to improve patient/family satisfaction regardless of outcome.
- Newer therapeutic options, such as targeted therapies, may be better tolerated by neonates as more is learned about the biology of these tumors.

Major recommendations

- Early referral to tertiary care center for multidisciplinary management is strongly encouraged.
- Early involvement of palliative/supportive care team regardless of anticipated outcome is strongly encouraged.
- Improvement in surgical techniques, supportive care, and targeted therapy has led to improvement in outcome for several subtypes of neonatal brain tumors; however, prognosis still remains dismal in general, necessitating the need for more research on this unique patient population and their underlying biological differences.

References/Source(s):[19,51,53]

ACKNOWLEDGEMENT

We would like to thank Dr. Matthew Schneiderjan for graciously providing us with the H&E images for **Figure 4**.

FINANCIAL DISCLOSURES

None.

REFERENCES

1. Mazewski CM, Hudgins RJ, Reisner A, et al. Neonatal brain tumors: a review. Semin Perinatol 1999;23:286–98.
2. SRaJJ Volpe. Brain tumors and vein of Galen malformations. In: Volpe JJ, editor. Volpe's neurology of the newborn. 6 edition. Philadelphia, PA: Elsevier, Inc; 2018. p. 1127–46.e1124.
3. Milani HJ, Araujo Junior E, Cavalheiro S, et al. Fetal brain tumors: prenatal diagnosis by ultrasound and magnetic resonance imaging. World J Radiol 2015;7: 17–21.
4. Sugimoto M, Kurishima C, Masutani S, et al. Congenital brain tumor within the first 2 months of life. Pediatr Neonatol 2015;56:369–75.
5. SaA S, Cancer T. Childhood brain tumors. Treasure Island (FL). StatPearls publishing; 2019. Available at: https://www.ncbi.nlm.nih.gov/books/NBK535415/.
6. Ostrom QT, de Blank PM, Kruchko C, et al. Alex's lemonade stand foundation infant and childhood primary brain and central nervous system tumors diagnosed in the United States in 2007–2011. Neuro Oncol 2014;16:x1–36.
7. Ostrom QT, Cioffi G, Gittleman H, et al. CBTRUS statistical report: primary brain and other central nervous system tumors diagnosed in the United States in 2012-2016. Neuro Oncol 2019;21:v1–100.
8. Partap S, MacLean J, Von Behren J, et al. Birth anomalies and obstetric history as risks for childhood tumors of the central nervous system. Pediatrics 2011;128: e652–7.
9. Louis DN, Perry A, Reifenberger G, et al. The 2016 World Health Organization classification of tumors of the central nervous system: a summary. Acta Neuropathol 2016;131:803–20.
10. Shekdar KV, Schwartz ES. Brain tumors in the neonate. Neuroimaging Clin N Am 2017;27:69–83.
11. Maghrabi Y, Kurdi ME, Baeesa SS. Infratentorial immature teratoma of congenital origin can be associated with a 20-year survival outcome: a case report and review of literature. World J Surg Oncol 2019;17:22.

12. Isaacs H Jr. Fetal intracranial teratoma. A review. Fetal Pediatr Pathol 2014;33: 289–92.
13. Qaddoumi I, Sane M, Li S, et al. Diagnostic utility and correlation of tumor markers in the serum and cerebrospinal fluid of children with intracranial germ cell tumors. Childs Nerv Syst 2012;28:1017–24.
14. Fukuoka K, Yanagisawa T, Suzuki T, et al. Successful treatment of hemorrhagic congenital intracranial immature teratoma with neoadjuvant chemotherapy and surgery. J Neurosurg Pediatr 2014;13:38–41.
15. Hwang SW, Su JM, Jea A. Diagnosis and management of brain and spinal cord tumors in the neonate. Semin Fetal Neonatal Med 2012;17:202–6.
16. Isaacs H Jr. Perinatal (fetal and neonatal) astrocytoma: a review. Childs Nerv Syst 2016;32:2085–96.
17. Shimamura N, Asano K, Ogane K, et al. A case of definitely congenital glioblastoma manifested by intratumoral hemorrhage. Childs Nerv Syst 2003;19:778–81.
18. Das KKaK, Raj. Pediatric glioblastoma. In: DV S, editor. Glioblastoma [internet]. Brisbane (Au): Codon Publications; 2017.
19. Bishop AJ, McDonald MW, Chang AL, et al. Infant brain tumors: incidence, survival, and the role of radiation based on surveillance, epidemiology, and end results (SEER) data. Int J Radiat Oncol Biol Phys 2012;82:341–7.
20. Fangusaro J. Pediatric high grade glioma: a review and update on tumor clinical characteristics and biology. Front Oncol 2012;2:105.
21. Qaddoumi I, Carey SS, Conklin H, et al. Characterization, treatment, and outcome of intracranial neoplasms in the first 120 days of life. J Child Neurol 2011;26: 988–94.
22. Clarke M, Mackay A, Ismer B, et al. Infant high grade gliomas comprise multiple subgroups characterized by novel targetable gene fusions and favorable outcomes. Cancer Discov 2020;10(7):942–63.
23. Davis T, Doyle H, Tobias V, et al. Case report of spontaneous resolution of a congenital glioblastoma. Pediatrics 2016;137:e20151241.
24. Thompson WD Jr, Kosnik EJ. Spontaneous regression of a diffuse brainstem lesion in the neonate. Report of two cases and review of the literature. J Neurosurg 2005;102:65–71.
25. Batra V, Sands SA, Holmes E, et al. Long-term survival of children less than six years of age enrolled on the CCG-945 phase III trial for newly-diagnosed high-grade glioma: a report from the Children's oncology group. Pediatr Blood Cancer 2014;61:151–7.
26. Gielen GH, Gessi M, Buttarelli FR, et al. Genetic analysis of diffuse high-grade astrocytomas in infancy defines a novel molecular entity. Brain Pathol 2015;25: 409–17.
27. El-Ayadi M, Ansari M, Sturm D, et al. High-grade glioma in very young children: a rare and particular patient population. Oncotarget 2017;8:64564–78.
28. Paugh BS, Qu C, Jones C, et al. Integrated molecular genetic profiling of pediatric high-grade gliomas reveals key differences with the adult disease. J Clin Oncol 2010;28:3061–8.
29. Wu G, Diaz AK, Paugh BS, et al. The genomic landscape of diffuse intrinsic pontine glioma and pediatric non-brainstem high-grade glioma. Nat Genet 2014;46:444–50.
30. Jones C, Karajannis MA, Jones DTW, et al. Pediatric high-grade glioma: biologically and clinically in need of new thinking. Neuro Oncol 2017;19:153–61.
31. Curatolo P, Moavero R. mTOR inhibitors in tuberous sclerosis complex. Curr Neuropharmacol 2012;10:404–15.

32. Kotulska K, Borkowska J, Mandera M, et al. Congenital subependymal giant cell astrocytomas in patients with tuberous sclerosis complex. Childs Nerv Syst 2014; 30:2037–42.
33. Saffari A, Brosse I, Wiemer-Kruel A, et al. Safety and efficacy of mTOR inhibitor treatment in patients with tuberous sclerosis complex under 2 years of age - a multicenter retrospective study. Orphanet J Rare Dis 2019;14:96.
34. Gupta P, Sodhi KS, Mohindra S, et al. Choroid plexus papilloma of the third ventricle: a rare infantile brain tumor. J Pediatr Neurosci 2013;8:247–9.
35. Anselem O, Mezzetta L, Grange G, et al. Fetal tumors of the choroid plexus: is differential diagnosis between papilloma and carcinoma possible? Ultrasound Obstet Gynecol 2011;38:229–32.
36. Crawford JR, Isaacs H Jr. Perinatal (fetal and neonatal) choroid plexus tumors: a review. Childs Nerv Syst 2019;35:937–44.
37. Borowska A, Jozwiak J. Medulloblastoma: molecular pathways and histopathological classification. Arch Med Sci 2016;12:659–66.
38. Taylor MD, Northcott PA, Korshunov A, et al. Molecular subgroups of medulloblastoma: the current consensus. Acta Neuropathol 2012;123:465–72.
39. Orbach D, Hojjat-Assari S, Doz F, et al. Peripheral blood stem cell collection in 24 low-weight infants: experience of a single centre. Bone Marrow Transplant 2003; 31:171–4.
40. Dhall G, O'Neil SH, Ji L, et al. Excellent outcome of young children with nodular desmoplastic medulloblastoma treated on "head start" III: a multi-institutional, prospective clinical trial. Neuro Oncol 2020. https://doi.org/10.1093/neuonc/noaa102.
41. Sredni ST, Tomita T. Rhabdoid tumor predisposition syndrome. Pediatr Dev Pathol 2015;18:49–58.
42. Torchia J, Golbourn B, Feng S, et al. Integrated (epi)-genomic analyses identify subgroup-specific therapeutic targets in CNS rhabdoid tumors. Cancer Cell 2016;30:891–908.
43. Johann PD, Erkek S, Zapatka M, et al. Atypical teratoid/rhabdoid tumors are comprised of three epigenetic subgroups with distinct enhancer landscapes. Cancer Cell 2016;29:379–93.
44. Chi SN, Zimmerman MA, Yao X, et al. Intensive multimodality treatment for children with newly diagnosed CNS atypical teratoid rhabdoid tumor. J Clin Oncol 2009;27:385–9.
45. Dufour C, Beaugrand A, Le Deley MC, et al. Clinicopathologic prognostic factors in childhood atypical teratoid and rhabdoid tumor of the central nervous system: a multicenter study. Cancer 2012;118:3812–21.
46. Lafay-Cousin L, Hawkins C, Carret AS, et al. Central nervous system atypical teratoid rhabdoid tumours: the Canadian paediatric brain tumour consortium experience. Eur J Cancer 2012;48:353–9.
47. Tariq MU, Ahmad Z, Minhas MK, et al. Embryonal tumor with multilayered rosettes, C19MC-altered: report of an extremely rare malignant pediatric central nervous system neoplasm. SAGE Open Med Case Rep 2017;5. 2050313X17745208.
48. Lithgow KP, Ute, Karavitaki Niki. Craniopharyngiomas. South Dartmouth (MA): MDText.com, Inc; 2019. Available at: https://www.ncbi.nlm.nih.gov/books/NBK538819/.
49. Arai T, Ohno K, Takada Y, et al. Neonatal craniopharyngioma and inference of tumor inception time: case report and review of the literature. Surg Neurol 2003;60: 254–9 [discussion 259].

50. Steinbok P. Craniopharyngioma in children: long-term outcomes. Neurol Med Chir (Tokyo) 2015;55:722–6.
51. Bianchi F, Tamburrini G, Massimi L, et al. Supratentorial tumors typical of the infantile age: desmoplastic infantile ganglioglioma (DIG) and astrocytoma (DIA). A review. Childs Nerv Syst 2016;32:1833–8.
52. Blessing MM, Blackburn PR, Krishnan C, et al. Desmoplastic infantile ganglioglioma: a MAPK pathway-driven and microglia/macrophage-rich neuroepithelial tumor. J Neuropathol Exp Neurol 2019;78:1011–21.
53. Olischar M, Stavroudis T, Karp JK, et al. Medical and ethical challenges in the case of a prenatally undiagnosed massive congenital brain tumor. J Perinatol 2015;35:773–5.
54. Racine E, Bell E, Farlow B, et al. The 'ouR-HOPE' approach for ethics and communication about neonatal neurological injury. Dev Med Child Neurol 2017; 59:125–35.
55. Rosenberg J, Massaro A, Siegler J, et al. Palliative care in patients with high-grade gliomas in the neurological intensive care unit. Neurohospitalist 2020. https://doi.org/10.1177/1941874419869714.
56. Vijapura C, Saad Aldin E, Capizzano AA, et al. Genetic syndromes associated with central nervous system tumors. Radiographics 2017;37:258–80.

Neonatal Retinoblastoma

Frank Y. Lin, MD, Murali M. Chintagumpala, MD*

KEYWORDS

- Retinoblastoma • Neonatal retinoblastoma • Leukocoria • RB1

KEY POINTS

- Loss of red reflex in one or both eyes on neonatal physical examination should prompt an immediate detailed ophthalmologic examination.
- Children born to at least one parent with a history of retinoblastoma should be evaluated at birth for retinoblastoma and at regular intervals as prescribed by the ophthalmologist.
- MRI of the orbits and brain at diagnosis is required to confirm intraocular tumor and to assess for extraocular extension if present.
- Genetic counseling is important when retinoblastoma is diagnosed, especially in the neonatal period.

INTRODUCTION

Retinoblastoma is the most common ocular malignancy of childhood, primarily affecting children of very young age. In countries with developed medical systems, most cases are diagnosed before the age of 2 years, and approximately 80% before 4 years of age. The incidence of retinoblastoma has remained steady over the past 40 years, with an estimated 300 cases annually in the United States,[1] or approximately 1 in 18,000 live births.[2,3] Cases within 4 weeks of life are uncommon[4]; however, an appropriate index of suspicion is critical for the neonatal specialist, because an understanding of at-risk patients and early detection of tumors allow for prompt multidisciplinary intervention and the possibility of minimizing treatment intensity and toxicity.

Retinoblastoma is universally lethal if left untreated and a risk to vision at advanced stages. However, modern management techniques and the understanding of retinoblastoma genetics have transformed the prognosis to among the most treatable and curable of pediatric cancers, provided the tumor is confined to the globe (intraocular).

A brief description of the following terms aids in the understanding of the fundamental concepts reviewed in this article.

- Intraocular versus extraocular retinoblastoma

Texas Children's Cancer Center, Baylor College of Medicine, 6701 Fannin Street, Suite 1510, Houston, TX 77030, USA
* Corresponding author.
E-mail address: ralic@bcm.edu

Clin Perinatol 48 (2021) 53–70
https://doi.org/10.1016/j.clp.2020.12.001
0095-5108/21/© 2020 Elsevier Inc. All rights reserved.

- o Intraocular: Tumor remains confined within the globe. Patients receiving therapy at this stage have a greater than 97% chance for cure.[1,5]
- o Extraocular: Extension of retinoblastoma beyond the globe. Therapy is intensified, whereas prognosis varies according to extent of disseminated disease. Delay in diagnosis or lack of access to medical care increases the risk of extraocular extension.
- Laterality
  - o Unilateral: One eye is affected by retinoblastoma.
  - o Bilateral: Both eyes are affected by retinoblastoma. Formation and growth of new tumors may occur at various time points.
  - o Trilateral: A primary intracranial embryonal tumor located in the suprasellar or pineal regions in conjunction with ocular tumors. Occurs in approximately 5% of patients with genetic predisposition for retinoblastoma.[6,7]
- Genetics
  - o Sporadic or nonheritable retinoblastoma: Tumors diagnosed in patients without a germline predisposition for retinoblastoma. Typically presents as unilateral retinoblastoma.
  - o Heritable (hereditary) or familial retinoblastoma: Patients with a family history of retinoblastoma or genetic predisposition (germline *RB1* pathogenic variant). Children with bilateral (or trilateral) disease are expected to have this genetic predisposition, and tumors may be detected in infancy.

CLINICAL FINDINGS

Leukocoria, or a white pupillary reflex, is the most frequent presenting sign of retinoblastoma in the United States, identified in more than half of patients.[8] Leukocoria results from the presence of a retinal mass located within the line of sight through the pupil and may obscure the red reflex. Often noticed first by a family member[8] or in a photograph (photoleukocoria),[9] leukocoria should prompt referral for an ophthalmologic examination. Importantly, assessment for red reflex is technically challenging by nondilated funduscopic examination of a young child,[10] and should be carefully attempted at every well child visit.

The second most common presenting sign of retinoblastoma is strabismus, occurring in approximately a quarter of patients and indicating loss of central vision.[8] Patients with more advanced disease may manifest less common changes in the appearance of the eye, including heterochromia (change in iris color) or rubeosis iridis (neovascularization of the iris), and in cases of extraocular retinoblastoma, proptosis (eye displacement) or buphthalmos (eye enlargement).[1,5,8]

Among neonates, the diagnosis of retinoblastoma is most likely made during proactive screening of at-risk newborns[4] or incidentally discovered during examination for other ocular etiologies.[11] In a reported series of 46 neonates with retinoblastoma, 67% were diagnosed because of positive family history, with 13% examined because of leukocoria.[4] Importantly, early identification of retinoblastoma tumors does not preclude advanced disease as an initial presentation.[4,12]

DIFFERENTIAL DIAGNOSIS

The differential diagnosis for retinoblastoma varies by age. In a large series of patients referred to an academic center, conditions that simulate retinoblastoma (pseudoretinoblastoma) in children less than 1 year of age included: persistent fetal vasculature (49%), Coats disease (20%), and vitreous hemorrhage (7%).[13]

More broadly, other differential considerations include: retinopathy of prematurity, toxocariasis, familial exudative vitreoretinopathy, rhegmatogenous retinal detachment, astrocytic hamartoma, medulloepithelioma, juvenile xanthogranuloma, coloboma, uveitis, congenital cataract, and Norrie disease.[1,14]

DIAGNOSTIC MODALITIES

The gold standard diagnostic approach for a child with retinoblastoma is direct visualization of tumor by an experienced ophthalmologist during an examination under anesthesia (EUA). An EUA includes dilated fundoscopy with indirect ophthalmoscopy and scleral depression.[14] The risks of anesthesia in a young child are balanced against the need to fully assess the retina, optic nerve, and anterior chamber. Use of ocular ultrasound (to detect findings consistent with calcific tumor)[14,15] or optical coherence tomography (to image small retinal lesions)[16] coordinated with the ophthalmic EUA may provide additional diagnostic evidence for retinoblastoma. Distinct from most pediatric tumors, tissue biopsy is avoided except in atypical cases to prevent nosocomial seeding of the tumor to an extraocular space. Emerging diagnostic techniques include sampling of aqueous humor[17,18] or plasma[19] to detect cell-free tumor DNA; however, the clinical role of these tests requires further investigation.

Imaging of the brain and orbits should be performed at the time of diagnosis to assess for orbital and optic nerve extension, and to rule out trilateral retinoblastoma (midline intracranial tumors in the suprasellar or pineal region).[6,7] In the pediatric patient, MRI has largely replaced computed tomography (CT) scanning to avoid radiation exposure.[20–22] In resource limited settings, however, CT detection of a calcified intraocular mass can help inform the diagnosis.[23] Importantly, CT or MRI findings alone are insufficient for a retinoblastoma diagnosis.[21]

Examination of cerebrospinal fluid by diagnostic lumbar puncture and marrow evaluation by bone marrow aspirate and core biopsy are typically performed in patients with extraocular or a high suspicion for metastatic disease.[24]

The utility of prenatal imaging of fetuses at risk for retinoblastoma is not yet certain, and literature is currently limited to small series and individual case reports. Retinal tumors have been detected by prenatal ultrasonography at 35 and 37 weeks gestation,[25,26] and by fetal MRI at 35 weeks gestation.[27] There are no clear recommendations regarding management of tumors detected prenatally. Management should be discussed by a multidisciplinary team and expedient postnatal examination by an ocular oncologist is critical. Canadian guidelines have suggested delivery as early as 36 weeks gestation to begin tumor-directed treatment[28]; however, this is not currently standard practice in the United States.

DISEASE CLASSIFICATION
Grouping of Intraocular Retinoblastoma

A classification schema for intraocular retinoblastoma was first published by Reese and Ellsworth[29] in 1963, and categorized disease severity according to predicted rates of ocular salvage and response to external beam radiation therapy. As new treatment options became available, particularly chemotherapy, new classification systems were developed. Most notably, the International Intraocular Retinoblastoma Classification led by Murphree, classified intraocular retinoblastoma into groups from A through E in order of disease severity based on size, location, and other features visualized on ophthalmologic examination.[1,30] Modifications have been made to the International Intraocular Retinoblastoma Classification over time by the Shields' group, known as the International Classification of Retinoblastoma (**Fig. 1**, **Table 1**).[1,31,32] This model

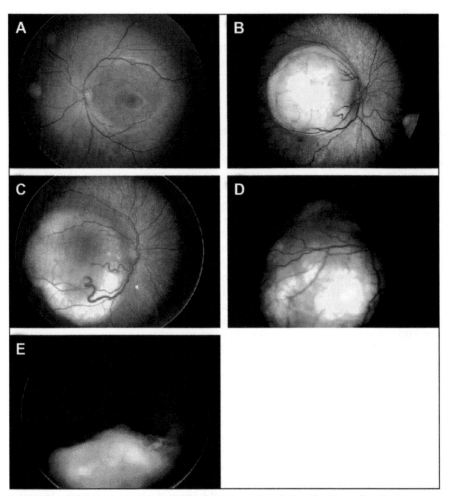

Fig. 1. Clinical features of each group in the International Classification of Retinoblastoma. (*A*) Group A retinoblastoma. Small extramacular tumor less than 3 mm in diameter. (*B*) Group B retinoblastoma. Medium-sized macular retinoblastoma with subtle surrounding subretinal fluid. (*C*) Group C retinoblastoma. Large retinoblastoma with localized subretinal seeds. (*D*) Group D retinoblastoma. Large retinoblastoma with extensive subretinal and vitreous seeds remote from the tumor. (*E*) Group E retinoblastoma. Extensive endophytic retinoblastoma with solid component of 14 mm thickness and involving more than 50% of the globe. (Shields CL, Shields JA. Basic understanding of current classification and management of retinoblastoma. Curr Opin Ophthalmol. 2006 Jun;17(3):228-34. doi:10.1097/01.icu. 0000193079.55240.18. PMID: 16794434. *Reproduced* with permission.)

of categorization has remained the general method for describing intraocular retinoblastoma and guiding therapy. Importantly, the variation between grouping systems should be acknowledged when patient cohorts are appraised in past clinical studies.

Staging Inclusive of Extraocular Retinoblastoma and Genetics

A recent classification system proposed by the American Joint Committee on Cancer used TNMH criteria (tumor, regional lymph node involvement, distant metastasis,

Table 1 International classification of retinoblastoma	
Group	**Features**
A	Retinoblastoma <3 mm in size
B	Retinoblastoma >3 mm in size or: Macular location (<3 mm to foveola) Juxtapapillary location (<1.5 mm to disk) Clear subretinal fluid <3 mm from margin
C	Retinoblastoma with (either or both): Subretinal seeds <3 mm from primary tumor Vitreous seeds <3 mm from primary tumor
D	Retinoblastoma with (either or both): Subretinal seeds >3 mm from primary tumor Vitreous seeds >3 mm from primary tumor
E	Extensive retinoblastoma with: Neovascular glaucoma Opaque media from hemorrhage in anterior chamber, vitreous, or subretinal space Invasion of postlaminar optic nerve, choroid (>3 mm), sclera, orbit, anterior chamber

Adapted from Shields CL, et al. The International Classification of Retinoblastoma predicts chemo-reduction success. Ophthalmology. Dec 2006;113(12):2277; with permission.

heritable trait), which included extraocular retinoblastoma (stage T4) and genetic status (H0 = wild-type germline *RB1* alleles; H1 = bilateral, trilateral, family history, or germline *RB1* pathogenic variant identified).[1,33–35] This staging system was validated using a sample of more than 2000 patients by the American Joint Committee on Cancer Ophthalmic Oncology Task Force, who concluded that it is a powerful clinical tool that can predict mortality, ocular salvage, and risk of metastasis.[33–35] Whether the American Joint Committee on Cancer classification gains wider adoption in clinical use and upcoming therapeutic trials will be of interest.

Histopathologic High-Risk Features

Extraocular dissemination of retinoblastoma is a significant negative prognostic factor. Enucleated eyes are examined for microscopic disease in regions of the eye vulnerable to metastatic extension. These histopathologic high-risk features include tumor invasion posterior to the lamina cribrosa of the optic nerve (postlaminar optic nerve invasion [PLONI]), which accesses the central nervous system (CNS), and extensive choroidal or scleral involvement, which can access vascular supply and orbital soft tissues (**Fig. 2**).[36–38] Although debate persists regarding defined criteria of high-risk features, these have generally been reported in approximately 15% to 40% of enucleated eyes with advanced retinoblastoma.[5] Patients treated with adjuvant chemotherapy have been demonstrated to have an excellent prognosis,[37] with a recently published prospective clinical trial of 94 patients conducted by the Children's Oncology Group reporting a 96% event-free survival at 2 years.[39]

Notably, the presence of histopathologic high-risk features has not reliably correlated with disease appearance on CT or MRI,[40,41] and consideration for adjuvant chemotherapy should be based on histopathologic findings.

TREATMENT OPTIONS

The long-standing principle of retinoblastoma care has been to maximize overall survival, and if possible, salvage the globe and vision without negatively impacting

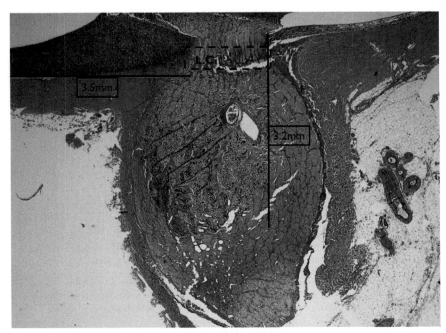

Fig. 2. Histopathologic high-risk features: greater than 3 mm of choroidal (massive) invasion around the optic nerve (peripapillary) and postlaminar (L.C.) optic nerve invasion of more than 1.5 mm (PLONI). The combination of more than 3-mm choroidal peripapillary invasion together with PLONI of more than 1.5 mm is the highest histopathologic risk for CNS recurrence after optic nerve cut end disease (hematoxylin and eosin, original magnification ×1.25). (*Courtesy of* Patricia Chévez-Barrios, MD.)

chance for cure. Uniquely, well-powered randomized controlled trials have not been conducted on optimal retinoblastoma care and are likely not feasible. However, modern methods for chemotherapy delivery have shifted the treatment paradigm away from radiation therapy over the past 25 years and maintained excellent survival outcomes,[42] including for neonates.[12]

Therapy is individualized to each patient according to: disease severity (grouping of intraocular retinoblastoma as described previously), laterality of tumors, and patient age. Therapeutic options range from focal consolidative modalities (laser hyperthermia/photocoagulation and cryotherapy), surgical enucleation, and chemotherapy, whereas radiation therapy is reserved for refractory cases.

Surgical Interventions

Focal consolidation of small retinal tumors

An important goal of screening at-risk neonates is to detect small tumors (group A or B) that may be amenable to focal control. During the course of an EUA, small retinal tumors (<4.5 mm width) may be treated with laser hyperthermia/photocoagulation,[43] and small peripheral tumors (<3.5 mm width) with cryotherapy.[1] Laser hyperthermia of tumors encroaching the fovea places vision at risk, and some institutions use chemotherapy to reduce tumor size before focal therapy.[44] These techniques have been demonstrated to improve disease in patients receiving chemotherapy for attempted ocular salvage,[45] and are coordinated with EUAs performed to assess treatment response.

The Toronto group reported a small series of infants with "invisible tumors" detected by optical coherence tomography and treated with laser hyperthermia. Two neonates less than 1 week of age were included in their study, but longer follow-up of a larger cohort would be of interest.[46]

Enucleation

Enucleation of an eye affected with advanced retinoblastoma remains an important and potentially curative intervention. Essentially, enucleation constitutes complete resection of a primary tumor. During the procedure, the eye is removed intact to avoid tumor spillage, and a long section of the optic nerve removed.[47] As previously discussed, enucleated eyes are examined for high-risk histopathologic features for assessment of metastatic risk, and if high-risk features are absent, adjuvant therapies are not indicated.

Upfront enucleation has long been recommended for patients with the most advanced intraocular retinoblastoma, group E (intraocular retinoblastoma replacing >50% of the glove with neovascular glaucoma, hemorrhage of the anterior chamber/vitreous/subretinal space, or invasion of postlaminar optic nerve/sclera/orbit/anterior chamber). Some institutions with significant technical expertise using novel chemotherapy-delivery approaches (discussed later) have reported early success in ocular salvage attempts of selective group E cases.[44] There has been suggestion that pretreatment of advanced group E eyes may result in delayed surgery and masking of histopathologic high-risk features.[48] Increasingly, eyes with group D retinoblastoma are offered attempted globe salvage with chemotherapy techniques, but enucleation is an accepted option particularly with eyes of poor visual potential.

Chemotherapy

The role of chemotherapy in retinoblastoma management has rapidly expanded over the past several decades as radiation therapy has been replaced as an upfront option. Chemotherapy to shrink intraocular tumors, or chemoreduction, is combined with focal consolidation as a strategy for ocular salvage. Three primary methods are used to deliver chemotherapy: (1) systemic administration, (2) intra-arterial/ophthalmic artery chemosurgery (OAC), and (3) intravitreal injection.

Systemic chemotherapy

Systemic administration has three distinct indications in retinoblastoma care: (1) chemoreduction of intraocular retinoblastoma, (2) adjuvant chemoprophylaxis of histopathologic high-risk features following enucleation (described previously), and (3) treatment of extraocular/metastatic retinoblastoma (discussed later).

The selection of agents for chemoreduction is guided by extent of disease, typically including a combination of carboplatin, etoposide, and vincristine. Standard dosing of these agents reliably salvaged eyes with less advanced tumors, including 93% of International Classification of Retinoblastoma group B and 90% of group C tumors. The ocular salvage rate of advanced disease was poor, however, with only 47% of group D eyes saved.[32] Systemic chemotherapy is not considered effective against the vitreous seeds of advanced tumors, and it was not until intravitreal chemotherapy (discussed later) was combined with systemic chemotherapy, that ocular salvage of group D eyes improved to approximately 75%.[49]

Special considerations in neonatal population

Neonates and infants less than 6 months old are at increased risk of toxicity from chemotherapy agents used in the backbone of frontline retinoblastoma regimens. In particular, the risk of ototoxicity related to carboplatin is heightened,[50] whereas peripheral neuropathy related to vincristine may be greater. Individualized dosing of carboplatin to a targeted area under the plasma concentration time curve can be considered.[51] Any child receiving chemotherapy should be closely monitored for changes in organ function, and if necessary, chemotherapy doses may require adjustment balanced against tumor response.

Intra-arterial chemotherapy/ophthalmic artery chemosurgery

Focused delivery of chemotherapy through the ophthalmic artery was first described by Kaneko in Japan more than 30 years ago[52] and introduced in the United States using a modified approach by Abramson et al[53] more than a decade ago. In intra-arterial chemotherapy (IAC)/OAC, a microcatheter is advanced via femoral artery catheterization to the ostium of the ophthalmic artery by fluoroscopic guidance, whereupon chemotherapy is gently infused by the operator (**Fig. 3**). The resultant concentration of chemotherapy delivered to the eye, most commonly melphalan in combination with carboplatin and/or topotecan, is amplified[54] while systemic exposure is minimized. Critically, IAC/OAC is reserved exclusively for patients with tumors confined to the globe. Patients with concern for extraocular or metastatic retinoblastoma require immediate systemic therapy.[55]

Although limited by institutional and operator experience, IAC/OAC is an increasingly used strategy for treatment of children with advanced intraocular retinoblastoma.[44,55,56] Two high-volume institutions reported ocular salvage rates of 72% at mean follow-up of 19 months,[57] and 96% at 1 year,[58] respectively. Outcomes at longer follow-up will be of interest. To mitigate inherent risks associated with IAC/OAC, the procedure should be performed by an experienced interventional radiologist or neurosurgeon in coordination with an anesthesiologist experienced with its unique needs.[56] Risks associated with IAC/OAC include transient eyelid edema, vitreous hemorrhage, ophthalmic artery occlusion, choroidal ischemia, and cerebral vascular accident.[59] Additionally, severe intraoperative cardiorespiratory instability has been observed in approximately 20% of cases, manifesting as hypotension, bradycardia, or decrease in respiratory compliance.[60] The causes for these cardiorespiratory events are uncertain, but possibly associated with perturbation of the autonomic reflex near the ophthalmic artery.

In the neonatal population, most institutions defer IAC/OAC until an infant is older than 3 to 6 months of age and weight greater than 7 kg to safely catheterize the femoral artery. One or multiple courses of systemic chemotherapy may be administered as "bridge therapy" until the patient grows into an age and weight appropriate for IAC/OAC (see **Fig. 3**).[61]

Intravitreal chemotherapy

Tumor deposits in the vitreous (seeds) have been challenging to control with systemic chemotherapy, likely because of lack of vascular access. A technique for direct intravitreal injection of chemotherapy described by Munier and coworkers[62] has been rapidly adopted across centers in combination with patients receiving systemic chemotherapy or IAC. Multiple groups have reported efficacy in tumor control[63–65] and more importantly, without evidence of extraocular tracking of tumor to date.[66] Chemotherapy agents used in intravitreal injection include melphalan and topotecan.[63,64,67]

Radiation Therapy

External beam radiation therapy was the first treatment modality used to achieve cure with ocular salvage. However, radiation therapy administered to very young children is

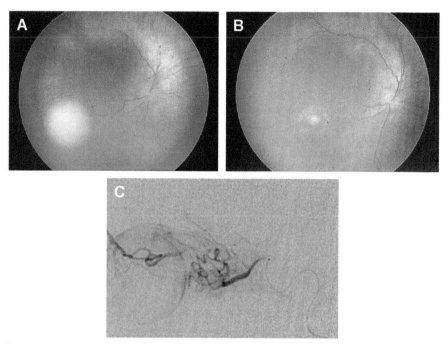

Fig. 3. (*A*) Fundus photograph of a neonate diagnosed with group B retinoblastoma before 3 weeks of age. Patient was treated with bridging chemotherapy until size and age were sufficient for IAC/OAC. (*B*) Fundus photograph following IAC/OAC therapy demonstrated stable regression. (*C*) Angiography of IAC/OAC with microcatheter at ostium of ophthalmic artery. ([*A, B*] *Courtesy of* Dan S. Gombos, MD; and [*C*] Stephen R. Chen, MD.)

associated with severe adverse effects, affecting orbital and skull development and significantly increasing the risk of secondary malignancies.[68,69] Among a large cohort of 963 patients with heritable retinoblastoma, the 50-year cumulative incidence of new malignancies was reported at 36%.[69] External beam radiation therapy is now avoided in favor of chemotherapy options, and reserved for patients with extraocular or metastatic retinoblastoma.

Episcleral plaque brachytherapy is a mechanism to locally deliver focused radiotherapy to a small tumor physically accessible to plaque placement.[70] This option has been reported to effectively control small retinoblastoma tumors refractory to other treatment modalities including chemotherapy and laser hyperthermia/cryotherapy.[71,72] In a series of 84 patients, 95% of treated eyes achieved tumor control at 5 years.[72]

Bilateral Retinoblastoma

Selection of treatment options for bilateral retinoblastoma is similarly individualized for the severity of each eye and therapy is initiated based on the eye with more advanced disease. Because of the risk of bilateral vision loss, extra attention should be made to design therapies that minimize treatment-associated ototoxicity. If both eyes are affected by advanced disease, attempted ocular salvage with systemic chemotherapy or tandem IAC/OAC is often considered.[14,44,73]

Extraocular Retinoblastoma

Extraocular extension of retinoblastoma significantly impacts survival outcome. Tumor extension can be confined to the orbit or can spread systemically to involve cervical lymph nodes, bone, and bone marrow. A more ominous development is CNS spread.

A multimodal approach inclusive of surgical resection, systemic chemotherapy, and consideration of external beam radiation therapy can result in cure in more than 70% of these children. The addition of high-dose chemotherapy plus autologous stem cell rescue is a published, potentially curative option for patients with distant metastasis without CNS involvement[74,75] and an important study question prospectively evaluated by the Children's Oncology Group study ARET0321 (NCT00554788). However, prognosis for children with CNS dissemination of retinoblastoma has remained dismal[76] and novel therapeutic approaches are needed.

Trilateral Retinoblastoma

Trilateral retinoblastoma refers to a primary intracranial, midline embryonal tumor in a patient with ocular retinoblastoma. These tumors are diagnosed in approximately 5% of patients with germline *RB1* pathologic variant, and most frequently affect young toddlers. An estimated 80% are located in the pineal region, followed by the suprasellar location.[7,77] Prognosis for patients with trilateral retinoblastoma is poor. One meta-analysis calculated a 48% survival at 5-years and median survival of 24 months, inclusive of patients treated with high-dose chemotherapy plus autologous stem cell rescue.[6]

Most institutions perform regular MRI of the brain to screen for trilateral retinoblastoma[78]; however, the efficacy of screening or survival benefit is uncertain.[79] Although the frequency of screening varies across institutions, evaluations every 6 months through age 5 or 6 years is common.

GENETICS OF RETINOBLASTOMA

The understanding of retinoblastoma biology and translation into clinical practice has provided an early model for individualized, genetics-informed patient care. Current clinical genetic tests detect greater than 90% of germline *RB1* alterations,[80] and guides acute screening and long-term counseling needs.[81]

That retinoblastoma was driven by two mutation events was first postulated by Knudson[82] in 1971, based on remarkable statistical analyses of phenotypic characteristics from 48 patients. The incidence and onset of tumors in younger infants, patients with multiple or bilateral tumors, or those with a positive family history were consistent with the presence of an underlying germline pathologic variant followed by a second acquired somatic defect,[83] in contrast to older patients with sporadic retinoblastoma who required two somatic events for tumorigenesis.[84–86] This gene, later discovered as the tumor suppressor *RB1* on chromosome 13,[87–89] plays a complex role in cell cycle regulation,[90] and biallelic loss of *RB1* function has been identified in greater than 95% of retinoblastoma tumors.[91] Patient *RB1* status has subsequently directed the genetic basis for management recommendations.

Approximately 40% percent of patients with retinoblastoma carry a germline *RB1* pathogenic variant (ie, heritable retinoblastoma), with up to 75% to 90% de novo occurrences with a negative family history.[1] Loss of a larger segment of chromosome 13q has been reported in 5% of patients with retinoblastoma, which can result in a characteristic syndrome according to genes affected, including craniofacial dysmorphism, psychomotor or speech delay, deafness, and heart anomalies.[92] Children with heritable retinoblastoma are at increased risk of subsequent malignancies, such as osteosarcoma, throughout their lifetime. However, a consensus screening algorithm for these secondary malignancies has not yet been established.[93,94]

Perinatal Genetics

A recent consensus statement published by the American Association of Ophthalmic Oncologists and Pathologists proposed a three-tier schedule for family members of a patient with retinoblastoma, stratified by pretest risk of a germline *RB1* pathogenic variant (**Figs. 4** and **5**).[95] Per this guideline, offspring born to parents with retinoblastoma should undergo dilated ophthalmic examination as soon as feasible after birth and repeated until germline *RB1* status is established.

Prenatal *RB1* genetic status of a fetus is determined from chorionic villus sampling or amniocentesis with high sensitivity and specificity.[28,96,97] In a survey study in the Netherlands, 11.8% of families with a germline *RB1* pathogenic variant pursued prenatal genetic testing.[98] However, potential clinical utility of these results is complex and families should be counseled on the absence of a consensus for intervention based on positive results. A small Canadian series reported 12 patients induced at 37 weeks gestation with successful treatment of smaller tumors.[97] Other countries,

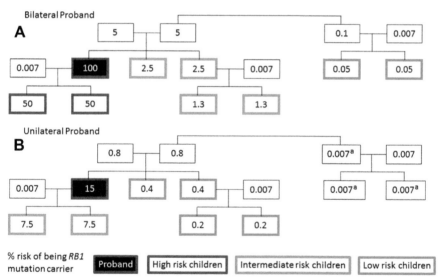

Fig. 4. Pretest risk for RB1 mutation in family members of affected child with retinoblastoma. (A) All probands with bilateral disease have a constitutional mutant RB1 allele. However, the RB1 mutation is frequently de novo in the child with retinoblastoma. Thus, most children with bilateral retinoblastoma are the first person in the family with disease. Before testing the patient, the risk for relatives to develop retinoblastoma can be estimated based on data from a large number of families. The percentage of risk for relatives to carry the mutant allele of the proband is shown. (B) Probands with unilateral disease and no family history of retinoblastoma have a 15% risk for carrying a mutant RB1 allele. The percentage of risk for relatives to carry that allele is shown. [a]Third- and fourth-degree relatives of unilateral probands have calculated risks of 0.003% and 0.001%, which are less than the normal population risk of 0.007% (1:15,000 live births); therefore, the risk is stated at 0.007%. (Adapted from Skalet, AH, et al. Screening Children at Risk for Retinoblastoma: Consensus Report from the American Association of Ophthalmic Oncologists and Pathologists. Ophthalmology. Mar 2018;125(3):454; with permission.)

Management Guidelines for Childhood Screening for Retinoblastoma Families									
Risk Category	% risk	Eye examination schedule based upon age of unaffected child							
		Birth to 8 wk[a]	>8 wk to 12 wk	>3 mo to 12 mo	>12 mo to 24 mo	>24 mo to 36 mo	>36 mo to 48 mo	>48 mo to 60 mo	5–7 y
High Risk	>7.5	Every 2–4 wk	Monthly		Every 2 mo	Every 3 mo	Every 4 mo	Every 6 mo	Every 6 mo
Intermediate Risk	1 – 7.5	Monthly		Every 2 mo		Every 3 mo		Every 4–6 mo	Every 6 mo
Low Risk	<1	Monthly		Every 3 mo	Every 4 mo		Every 6 mo		Annually
General population	0.007	Screening with pediatrician							

Non-sedated office examination preferred by most centers

Examination under anesthesia preferred by most centers

Fig. 5. Management guidelines for childhood screening for retinoblastoma. The presented schedules are general guidelines and reflect a schedule for examinations in which no lesions of concern are noted. It may be appropriate to examine some children more frequently. Decisions regarding examination method, EUA versus nonsedated examination in the office, are complex and best decided by the clinician in discussion with the patient's family. The preference of most clinical centers involved in the creation of this consensus statement is reflected, but individual centers may make policy decisions based on available resources and expert clinician preference. EUA is strongly considered for any child who is unable to participate in an office examination sufficiently to allow thorough examination of the retina. [a]A minority of clinical centers also prefer EUA for high- and intermediate-risk children (calculated risk >1%) from birth to 8 weeks of age. (*From* Skalet, AH, et al. Screening Children at Risk for Retinoblastoma: Consensus Report from the American Association of Ophthalmic Oncologists and Pathologists. Ophthalmology. Mar 2018;125(3):456; with permission.)

including the United States, have preferred immediate postnatal testing and screening without early induction of labor.[14]

Preimplantation genetic testing to identify embryos with a *RB1* pathologic variant has been performed as part of the in vitro fertilization process for prospective parents affected by heritable retinoblastoma. Multiple cases have been reported in the literature of children born without germline *RB1* gene defects by in vitro fertilization in this manner.[99]

LONG-TERM RECOMMENDATIONS

Survivors of childhood retinoblastoma should be monitored for long-term morbidities specific to therapies received. In many pediatric cancer centers, they are followed in specialty survivorship clinics with expertise in their screening and health care needs.[94,100–103]

SUMMARY POINTS

1. Retinoblastoma is a curable malignancy, but fatal if untreated. Among neonates, diagnosis is most frequently made by screening of at-risk patients by an experienced ophthalmologist.
2. Early detection of retinoblastoma tumors allows for the use of treatment modalities with minimal toxicity risk, including focal therapies performed by an ocular oncologist (laser hyperthermia or cryotherapy), and potentially avoids the need for surgical enucleation, chemotherapy, or radiation therapy.
3. If more intensive therapies are required, interventions are chosen to prioritize the best chance for cure, followed by preservation of the globe and remaining vision

if possible. Avoidance of radiation therapy is preferred because of adverse effects in a very young child.

4. A thorough family history plus *RB1* genetic testing is important to identify patients at risk for heritable retinoblastoma and inform screening recommendations for the patient and their family.

5. Prenatal diagnosis is achieved by fetal imaging or *RB1* genetic testing.

6. Rates of cure for patients with intraocular retinoblastoma are good where access to multidisciplinary medical care is readily available.

7. Long-term follow-up for potential comorbidities associated with therapy is important for survivors of childhood retinoblastoma.

DISCLOSURE

The authors have nothing to disclose.

REFERENCES

1. Leahey AM, Gombos DS, Chevez-Barrios P. Retinoblasotma. In: Blaney SM, Adamson PC, Helman LJ, editors. Pizzo and Poplack's pediatric oncology, 8th edition. Beaverton (OR): Ringgold Inc.; 2020. p. 868-88.

2. Broaddus E, Topham A, Singh AD. Incidence of retinoblastoma in the USA: 1975-2004. Br J Ophthalmol 2009;93(1):21–3.

3. Wong JR, Tucker MA, Kleinerman RA, et al. Retinoblastoma incidence patterns in the US Surveillance, Epidemiology, and End Results program. JAMA Ophthalmol 2014;132(4):478–83.

4. Abramson DH, Du TT, Beaverson KL. (Neonatal) retinoblastoma in the first month of life. Arch Ophthalmol 2002;120(6):738–42.

5. Dimaras H, Corson TW, Cobrinik D, et al. Retinoblastoma. Nat Rev Dis Primers 2015;1:15021.

6. de Jong MC, Kors WA, de Graaf P, et al. Trilateral retinoblastoma: a systematic review and meta-analysis. Lancet Oncol 2014;15(10):1157–67.

7. de Jong MC, Kors WA, Moll AC, et al. Screening for pineal trilateral retinoblastoma revisited: a meta-analysis. Ophthalmology 2020;127(5):601–7.

8. Abramson DH, Beaverson K, Sangani P, et al. Screening for retinoblastoma: presenting signs as prognosticators of patient and ocular survival. Pediatrics 2003; 112(6 Pt 1):1248–55.

9. Asensio-Sanchez VM, Diaz-Cabanas L, Martin-Prieto A. Photoleukocoria with smartphone photographs. Int Med Case Rep J 2018;11:117–9.

10. Butros LJ, Abramson DH, Dunkel IJ. Delayed diagnosis of retinoblastoma: analysis of degree, cause, and potential consequences. Pediatrics 2002; 109(3):E45.

11. Self J, Bush K, Baral VR, et al. Bilateral retinoblastoma presenting at retinopathy of prematurity screening. Arch Dis Child Fetal Neonatal Ed 2010;95(4):F292.

12. Camp DA, Dalvin LA, Schwendeman R, et al. Outcomes of neonatal retinoblastoma in pre-chemotherapy and chemotherapy eras. Indian J Ophthalmol 2019; 67(12):1997–2004.

13. Shields CL, Schoenberg E, Kocher K, et al. Lesions simulating retinoblastoma (pseudoretinoblastoma) in 604 cases: results based on age at presentation. Ophthalmology 2013;120(2):311–6.

14. Gombos DS. Retinoblastoma in the perinatal and neonatal child. Semin Fetal Neonatal Med 2012;17(4):239–42.

15. Kaste SC, Jenkins JJ 3rd, Pratt CB, et al. Retinoblastoma: sonographic findings with pathologic correlation in pediatric patients. AJR Am J Roentgenol 2000; 175(2):495–501.

16. Soliman SE, VandenHoven C, MacKeen LD, et al. Optical coherence tomography-guided decisions in retinoblastoma management. Ophthalmology 2017;124(6):859–72.

17. Berry JL, Xu L, Kooi I, et al. Genomic cfDNA analysis of aqueous humor in retinoblastoma predicts eye salvage: the surrogate tumor biopsy for retinoblastoma. Mol Cancer Res 2018;16(11):1701–12.

18. Gerrish A, Stone E, Clokie S, et al. Non-invasive diagnosis of retinoblastoma using cell-free DNA from aqueous humour. Br J Ophthalmol 2019;103(5):721–4.

19. Kothari P, Marass F, Yang JL, et al. Cell-free DNA profiling in retinoblastoma patients with advanced intraocular disease: an MSKCC experience. Cancer Med 2020;9(17):6093–101.

20. de Graaf P, Göricke S, Rodjan F, et al. Guidelines for imaging retinoblastoma: imaging principles and MRI standardization. Pediatr Radiol 2012;42(1):2–14.

21. de Jong MC, de Graaf P, Brisse HJ, et al. The potential of 3T high-resolution magnetic resonance imaging for diagnosis, staging, and follow-up of retinoblastoma. Surv Ophthalmol 2015;60(4):346–55.

22. Rodjan F, de Graaf P, van der Valk P, et al. Detection of calcifications in retinoblastoma using gradient-echo MR imaging sequences: comparative study between in vivo MR imaging and ex vivo high-resolution CT. AJNR Am J Neuroradiol 2015;36(2):355–60.

23. Char DH, Hedges TR 3rd, Norman D. Retinoblastoma. CT diagnosis. Ophthalmology 1984;91(11):1347–50.

24. Laurent VE, Torbidoni AV, Sampor C, et al. Minimal disseminated disease in non-metastatic retinoblastoma with high-risk pathologic features and association with disease-free survival. JAMA Ophthalmol 2016;134(12):1374–9.

25. Paquette LB, Miller D, Jackson HA, et al. In utero detection of retinoblastoma with fetal magnetic resonance and ultrasound: initial experience. AJP Rep 2012;2(1):55–62.

26. Stathopoulos C, Say EAT, Shields CL. Prenatal ultrasonographic detection and prenatal (prior to birth) management of hereditary retinoblastoma. Graefes Arch Clin Exp Ophthalmol 2018;256(4):861–2.

27. Staffieri SE, McGillivray G, Elder JE, et al. Managing fetuses at high risk of retinoblastoma: lesion detection on screening MRI. Prenatal Diagn 2015;35(2):174–8.

28. National Retinoblastoma Strategy Canadian Guidelines for Care: stratégie thérapeutique du rétinoblastome guide clinique Canadien. Can J Ophthalmol 2009; 44(Suppl 2):S1–88.

29. Reese AB, Ellsworth RM. The evaluation and current concept of retinoblastoma therapy. Trans Am Acad Ophthalmol Otolaryngol 1963;67:164–72.

30. Linn Murphree A. Intraocular retinoblastoma: the case for a new group classification. Ophthalmol Clin North Am 2005;18(1):41–53, viii.

31. Novetsky DE, Abramson DH, Kim JW, et al. Published international classification of retinoblastoma (ICRB) definitions contain inconsistencies: an analysis of impact. Ophthalmic Genet 2009;30(1):40–4.

32. Shields CL, Mashayekhi A, Au AK, et al. The International Classification of Retinoblastoma predicts chemoreduction success. Ophthalmology 2006;113(12):2276–80.

33. Mallipatna A, Gallie B, Chévez-Barrios P, et al. Retinoblastoma. In: Amin MB, Edge SB, Greene FL, editors. AJCC cancer staging manual. 8th edition. New York: Springer; 2017. p. 819–31.
34. Tomar AS, Finger PT, Gallie B, et al. A multicenter, international collaborative study for American Joint Committee on Cancer staging of retinoblastoma: Part II: treatment success and globe salvage. Ophthalmology 2020;127(12): 1733–46.
35. Tomar AS, Finger PT, Gallie B, et al. A multicenter, international collaborative study for American Joint Committee on Cancer staging of retinoblastoma: Part I: metastasis-associated mortality. Ophthalmology 2020;127(12):1719–32.
36. Sastre X, Chantada GL, Doz F, et al. Proceedings of the consensus meetings from the International Retinoblastoma Staging Working Group on the pathology guidelines for the examination of enucleated eyes and evaluation of prognostic risk factors in retinoblastoma. Arch Pathol Lab Med 2009;133(8):1199–202.
37. Kaliki S, Shields CL, Shah SU, et al. Postenucleation adjuvant chemotherapy with vincristine, etoposide, and carboplatin for the treatment of high-risk retinoblastoma. Arch Ophthalmol 2011;129(11):1422–7.
38. Shields CL, Shields JA, Baez KA, et al. Choroidal invasion of retinoblastoma: metastatic potential and clinical risk factors. Br J Ophthalmol 1993;77(9):544–8.
39. Chevez-Barrios P, Eagle RC Jr, Krailo M, et al. Study of unilateral retinoblastoma with and without histopathologic high-risk features and the role of adjuvant chemotherapy: a children's oncology group study. J Clin Oncol 2019;37(31): 2883–91.
40. Wilson MW, Rodriguez-Galindo C, Billups C, et al. Lack of correlation between the histologic and magnetic resonance imaging results of optic nerve involvement in eyes primarily enucleated for retinoblastoma. Ophthalmology 2009; 116(8):1558–63.
41. de Jong MC, de Graaf P, Noij DP, et al. Diagnostic performance of magnetic resonance imaging and computed tomography for advanced retinoblastoma: a systematic review and meta-analysis. Ophthalmology 2014;121(5):1109–18.
42. Broaddus E, Topham A, Singh AD. Survival with retinoblastoma in the USA: 1975-2004. Br J Ophthalmol 2009;93(1):24–7.
43. Shields CL, Santos MC, Diniz W, et al. Thermotherapy for retinoblastoma. Arch Ophthalmol 1999;117(7):885–93.
44. Abramson DH, Shields CL, Munier FL, et al. Treatment of retinoblastoma in 2015: agreement and disagreement. JAMA Ophthalmol 2015;133(11):1341–7.
45. Kim JW, Aziz HA, McGovern K, et al. Treatment outcomes of focal laser consolidation during chemoreduction for group B Retinoblastoma. Ophthalmol Retina 2017;1(5):361–8.
46. Soliman SE, VandenHoven C, MacKeen LD, et al. Secondary prevention of retinoblastoma revisited: laser photocoagulation of invisible new retinoblastoma. Ophthalmology 2020;127(1):122–7.
47. Shields JA, Shields CL, De Potter P. Enucleation technique for children with retinoblastoma. J Pediatr Ophthalmol Strabismus 1992;29(4):213–5.
48. Zhao J, Dimaras H, Massey C, et al. Pre-enucleation chemotherapy for eyes severely affected by retinoblastoma masks risk of tumor extension and increases death from metastasis. J Clin Oncol 1 2011;29(7):845–51.
49. Berry JL, Shah S, Bechtold M, et al. Long-term outcomes of Group D retinoblastoma eyes during the intravitreal melphalan era. Pediatr Blood Cancer 2017; 64(12). https://doi.org/10.1002/pbc.26696.

50. Qaddoumi I, Bass JK, Wu J, et al. Carboplatin-associated ototoxicity in children with retinoblastoma. J Clin Oncol 2012;30(10):1034–41.
51. Allen S, Wilson MW, Watkins A, et al. Comparison of two methods for carboplatin dosing in children with retinoblastoma. Pediatr Blood Cancer 2010;55(1):47–54.
52. Suzuki S, Yamane T, Mohri M, et al. Selective ophthalmic arterial injection therapy for intraocular retinoblastoma: the long-term prognosis. Ophthalmology 2011;118(10):2081–7.
53. Abramson DH, Dunkel IJ, Brodie SE, et al. A phase I/II study of direct intraarterial (ophthalmic artery) chemotherapy with melphalan for intraocular retinoblastoma initial results. Ophthalmology 2008;115(8):1398–404, 1404.e1391.
54. Schaiquevich P, Fabius AW, Francis JH, et al. Ocular pharmacology of chemotherapy for retinoblastoma. Retina (Phila) 2017;37(1):1–10.
55. Yousef YA, Soliman SE, Astudillo PPP, et al. Intra-arterial chemotherapy for retinoblastoma: a systematic review. JAMA Ophthalmol 2016;134(5):584–91.
56. Dalvin LA, Ancona-Lezama D, Lucio-Alvarez JA, et al. Ophthalmic vascular events after primary unilateral intra-arterial chemotherapy for retinoblastoma in early and recent eras. Ophthalmology 2018;125(11):1803–11.
57. Shields CL, Manjandavida FP, Lally SE, et al. Intra-arterial chemotherapy for retinoblastoma in 70 eyes: outcomes based on the international classification of retinoblastoma. Ophthalmology 2014;121(7):1453–60.
58. Francis JH, Levin AM, Zabor EC, et al. Ten-year experience with ophthalmic artery chemosurgery: ocular and recurrence-free survival. PLoS One 2018;13(5): e0197081.
59. De la Huerta I, Seider MI, Hetts SW, et al. Delayed cerebral infarction following intra-arterial chemotherapy for retinoblastoma. JAMA Ophthalmol 2016;134(6): 712–4.
60. Nghe MC, Godier A, Shaffii A, et al. Prospective analysis of serious cardiorespiratory events in children during ophthalmic artery chemotherapy for retinoblastoma under a deep standardized anesthesia. Paediatric Anaesth 2018;28(2): 120–6.
61. Gobin YP, Dunkel IJ, Marr BP, et al. Combined, sequential intravenous and intra-arterial chemotherapy (bridge chemotherapy) for young infants with retinoblastoma. PLoS One 2012;7(9):e44322.
62. Munier FL, Soliman S, Moulin AP, et al. Profiling safety of intravitreal injections for retinoblastoma using an anti-reflux procedure and sterilisation of the needle track. Br J Ophthalmol 2012;96(8):1084–7.
63. Francis JH, Abramson DH, Gaillard MC, et al. The classification of vitreous seeds in retinoblastoma and response to intravitreal melphalan. Ophthalmology 2015;122(6):1173–9.
64. Shields CL, Manjandavida FP, Arepalli S, et al. Intravitreal melphalan for persistent or recurrent retinoblastoma vitreous seeds: preliminary results. JAMA Ophthalmol 2014;132(3):319–25.
65. Amram AL, Rico G, Kim JW, et al. Vitreous seeds in retinoblastoma: clinicopathologic classification and correlation. Ophthalmology 2017;124(10):1540–7.
66. Francis JH, Abramson DH, Ji X, et al. Risk of extraocular extension in eyes with retinoblastoma receiving intravitreous chemotherapy. JAMA Ophthalmol 2017; 135(12):1426–9.
67. Rao R, Honavar SG, Sharma V, et al. Intravitreal topotecan in the management of refractory and recurrent vitreous seeds in retinoblastoma. Br J Ophthalmol 2018; 102(4):490–5.

68. Kleinerman RA, Schonfeld SJ, Sigel BS, et al. Bone and soft-tissue sarcoma risk in long-term survivors of hereditary retinoblastoma treated with radiation. J Clin Oncol 2019;37(35):3436–45.

69. Kleinerman RA, Tucker MA, Tarone RE, et al. Risk of new cancers after radiotherapy in long-term survivors of retinoblastoma: an extended follow-up. J Clin Oncol 2005;23(10):2272–9.

70. Shields CL, Shields JA, Cater J, et al. Plaque radiotherapy for retinoblastoma: long-term tumor control and treatment complications in 208 tumors. Ophthalmology 2001;108(11):2116–21.

71. Lucas JT, McGee R, Billups CA, et al. Prior non-irradiative focal therapies do not compromise the efficacy of delayed episcleral plaque brachytherapy in retinoblastoma. Br J Ophthalmol 2018. https://doi.org/10.1136/bjophthalmol-2018-311923.

72. Shields CL, Mashayekhi A, Sun H, et al. Iodine 125 plaque radiotherapy as salvage treatment for retinoblastoma recurrence after chemoreduction in 84 tumors. Ophthalmology 2006;113(11):2087–92.

73. Abramson DH, Marr BP, Francis JH, et al. Simultaneous bilateral ophthalmic artery chemosurgery for bilateral retinoblastoma (tandem therapy). PLoS One 2016;11(6):e0156806.

74. Dunkel IJ, Aledo A, Kernan NA, et al. Successful treatment of metastatic retinoblastoma. Cancer 2000;89(10):2117–21.

75. Palma J, Sasso DF, Dufort G, et al. Successful treatment of metastatic retinoblastoma with high-dose chemotherapy and autologous stem cell rescue in South America. Bone Marrow Transplant 2012;47(4):522–7.

76. Dunkel IJ, Chan HS, Jubran R, et al. High-dose chemotherapy with autologous hematopoietic stem cell rescue for stage 4B retinoblastoma. Pediatr Blood Cancer 2010;55(1):149–52.

77. de Jong MC, Kors WA, de Graaf P, et al. The incidence of trilateral retinoblastoma: a systematic review and meta-analysis. Am J Ophthalmol 2015;160(6): 1116–26.e5.

78. Kamihara J, Bourdeaut F, Foulkes WD, et al. Retinoblastoma and neuroblastoma predisposition and surveillance. Clin Cancer Res 2017;23(13):e98–106.

79. Qureshi S, Francis JH, Haque SS, et al. Magnetic resonance imaging screening for trilateral retinoblastoma: the Memorial Sloan Kettering Cancer Center experience 2006-2016. Ophthalmol Retina 2020;4(3):327–35.

80. Richter S, Vandezande K, Chen N, et al. Sensitive and efficient detection of RB1 gene mutations enhances care for families with retinoblastoma. Am J Hum Genet 2003;72(2):253–69.

81. Dhar SU, Chintagumpala M, Noll C, et al. Outcomes of integrating genetics in management of patients with retinoblastoma. Arch Ophthalmol 2011;129(11): 1428–34.

82. Knudson AG Jr. Mutation and cancer: statistical study of retinoblastoma. Proc Natl Acad Sci U S A 1971;68(4):820–3.

83. Hethcote HW, Knudson AG Jr. Model for the incidence of embryonal cancers: application to retinoblastoma. Proc Natl Acad Sci U S A 1978;75(5):2453–7.

84. Dryja TP, Cavenee W, White R, et al. Homozygosity of chromosome 13 in retinoblastoma. N Engl J Med 1984;310(9):550–3.

85. Godbout R, Dryja TP, Squire J, et al. Somatic inactivation of genes on chromosome 13 is a common event in retinoblastoma. Nature 1983;304(5925):451–3.

86. Dimaras H, Khetan V, Halliday W, et al. Loss of RB1 induces non-proliferative ret-inoma: increasing genomic instability correlates with progression to retinoblas-toma. Hum Mol Genet 2008;17(10):1363–72.
87. Hamosh A. RB transcriptional corepressor 1; RB1. In: OMIM 614041. 2020. Available at https://www.omim.org/entry/614041.
88. Friend SH, Bernards R, Rogelj S, et al. A human DNA segment with properties of the gene that predisposes to retinoblastoma and osteosarcoma. Nature 1986; 323(6089):643–6.
89. Lee WH, Bookstein R, Hong F, et al. Human retinoblastoma susceptibility gene: cloning, identification, and sequence. Science 1987;235(4794):1394–9.
90. Magnaghi-Jaulin L, Groisman R, Naguibneva I, et al. Retinoblastoma protein re-presses transcription by recruiting a histone deacetylase. Nature 1998; 391(6667):601–5.
91. Rushlow DE, Mol BM, Kennett JY, et al. Characterisation of retinoblastomas without RB1 mutations: genomic, gene expression, and clinical studies. Lancet Oncol 2013;14(4):327–34.
92. Mitter D, Ullmann R, Muradyan A, et al. Genotype-phenotype correlations in pa-tients with retinoblastoma and interstitial 13q deletions. Eur J Hum Genet 2011; 19(9):947–58.
93. Friedman DN, Hsu M, Moskowitz CS, et al. Whole-body magnetic resonance im-aging as surveillance for subsequent malignancies in preadolescent, adoles-cent, and young adult survivors of germline retinoblastoma: an update. Pediatr Blood Cancer 2020;67(7):e28389.
94. Tonorezos ES, Friedman DN, Barnea D, et al. Recommendations for long-term follow-up of adults with heritable retinoblastoma. Ophthalmology 2020; 127(11):1549–57.
95. Skalet AH, Gombos DS, Gallie BL, et al. Screening children at risk for retinoblas-toma: consensus report from the American Association of Ophthalmic Oncolo-gists and Pathologists. Ophthalmology 2018;125(3):453–8.
96. Lau CS, Choy KW, Fan DS, et al. Prenatal screening for retinoblastoma in Hong Kong. Hong Kong Med J 2008;14(5):391–4.
97. Soliman SE, Dimaras H, Khetan V, et al. Prenatal versus postnatal screening for familial retinoblastoma. Ophthalmology 2016;123(12):2610–7.
98. Dommering CJ, Henneman L, van der Hout AH, et al. Uptake of prenatal diag-nostic testing for retinoblastoma compared to other hereditary cancer syn-dromes in The Netherlands. Fam Cancer 2017;16(2):271–7.
99. Xu K, Rosenwaks Z, Beaverson K, et al. Preimplantation genetic diagnosis for retinoblastoma: the first reported liveborn. Am J Ophthalmol 2004;137(1):18–23.
100. Children's Oncology Group. Long-term follow-up guidelines for survivors of childhood, adolescent and young adult cancers, version 5.0. Monrovia, CA: Children's Oncology Group; October 2018. Available at http://www.survivorshipguidelines.org.
101. Landier W, Skinner R, Wallace WH, et al. Surveillance for late effects in child-hood cancer survivors. J Clin Oncol 2018;36(21):2216–22.
102. Friedman DN, Sklar CA, Oeffinger KC, et al. Long-term medical outcomes in sur-vivors of extra-ocular retinoblastoma: the Memorial Sloan-Kettering Cancer Cen-ter (MSKCC) experience. Pediatr Blood Cancer 2013;60(4):694–9.
103. Ford JS, Chou JF, Sklar CA, et al. Psychosocial outcomes in adult survivors of retinoblastoma. J Clin Oncol 2015;33(31):3608–14.

Neonatal Renal Tumors

Sei-Gyung K. Sze, MD

KEYWORDS

- Congenital mesoblastic nephroma • Wilms tumor
- Malignant rhabdoid tumor of the kidney • Clear cell sarcoma of the kidney • Neonatal

KEY POINTS

- Although Wilms tumor is the most common renal tumor of childhood, congenital meso-blastic nephroma is the most common neonatal renal tumor.
- Most renal tumors in neonates present as low stage and favorable histology, with very good outcomes.
- Treatment for most neonatal renal tumors is with primary radical nephrectomy alone; however, adjuvant chemotherapy or radiation may be indicated depending on the underlying histology or biology.
- Distant metastatic disease suggests a diagnosis of malignant rhabdoid tumor of the kidney or clear cell sarcoma of the kidney, and portends a poor prognosis.

INTRODUCTION

Renal tumors are rare in the neonatal period, accounting for approximately 5% to 7% of all neonatal tumors.[1,2] Although Wilms tumor (WT) is the most common renal malignancy of childhood overall, accounting for almost 90% of all pediatric renal tumors, different histopathologies are seen more frequently in the first few months of life.[1–3] Congenital mesoblastic nephroma is the most common renal neoplasm in neonates. Malignant rhabdoid tumor of the kidney, clear cell sarcoma of the kidney, and other rarer tumors are also seen in this younger age group with relatively greater frequency. There are some commonalities to the presentation and evaluation of renal tumors in this age group; this review begins with a general discussion and then highlights key aspects of specific diagnoses.

Prenatal ultrasound detects only approximately 15% of renal tumors.[2] Of the remainder, approximately half are identified by detection of an abdominal mass on physical examination. Other prenatal findings may include polyhydramnios due to increased urine production or less commonly fetal hydrops.[2–4] Other nonspecific signs that present after birth include vomiting, lethargy, pallor, abdominal distension, and failure to thrive. Laboratory evaluation may identify hematuria, anemia, hypercalcemia, or hyperreninism with associated hypertension.

Maine Children's Cancer Program, Department of Pediatrics, Maine Medical Center, Tufts School of Medicine, 100 Campus Drive, Suite 107, Scarborough, ME 04074, USA
E-mail address: ssze@mmc.org

Clin Perinatol 48 (2021) 71–81
https://doi.org/10.1016/j.clp.2020.11.004
0095-5108/21/© 2020 Elsevier Inc. All rights reserved.

perinatology.theclinics.com

When there is clinical suspicion for a renal mass, evaluation typically starts with abdominal ultrasound for initial investigation or for confirmation of findings on prenatal scans.[1,5] Ultrasound can be helpful to distinguish among cystic, solid, or mixed lesions. When a neoplasm is suspected, investigation should then proceed to cross-sectional imaging to better characterize the lesion, evaluate for metastatic disease, and guide treatment plans. Staging criteria for renal tumors are outlined in **Table 1**.

Decisions about initial biopsy or surgery for renal tumors are controversial and approaches differ between cooperative groups in the United States and Europe. However, protocols from both the National Wilms Tumor Study Group (NWTSG)/Children's Oncology Group (COG) and the International Society of Pediatric Oncology (SIOP) generally recommend upfront radical nephroureterectomy as initial treatment for unilateral renal tumors in children younger than 6 months.[1] This approach allows for accurate histologic diagnosis and staging, with collection of biologic material that has been unaltered by chemotherapy. In many cases, neonates may be cured by surgery alone and may be able to avoid cytotoxic chemotherapy. Exceptions to this approach include bilateral renal involvement, or situations in which upfront resection is deemed too risky for the infant. In these cases, an initial biopsy may be performed. If chemotherapy is indicated, doses are reduced based on weight to avoid the higher rates of toxicity observed in this young age group due to differences in drug metabolism and clearance.

Neonates with renal tumors generally have a very good prognosis, due to low stage at presentation and more favorable biologic features[1,2,5]; however, outcomes ultimately vary widely depending on the histologic diagnosis. Notably, malignant rhabdoid tumor of the kidney (MRTK), although extremely rare, tends to present aggressively, and carries a dismal prognosis. Van den Heuvel-Eibrink and colleagues[6] reported the largest, intercontinental retrospective analysis of renal tumors in infants younger than 7 months, treated on the most recent studies of the NWTSG, SIOP, the German Pediatric Hematology/Oncology group (GPOH), the French Pediatric Oncology Society, and the United Kingdom Children's Cancer Study Group. Among 10,430 children with a primary renal tumor, 750 were diagnosed before 7 months of age. Both overall survival (OS) and event-free survival (EFS) were significantly better for children diagnosed in the first month of life compared with those diagnosed

Table 1	
Staging criteria for renal tumors in the United States	
Stage	**Criteria**
I	Tumor confined to the kidney, completely resected
II	Regional extension of tumor (eg, penetration of renal capsule or extension into renal sinus), but completely resected • All sampled local lymph nodes are negative
III	Tumor extending outside the kidney but confined to the abdomen, incomplete resection • Preoperative biopsy • Preoperative or intraoperative tumor rupture • Intra-abdominal lymph node involvement • Peritoneal metastasis • Tumor thrombus at resection margin
IV	Distant metastatic disease (eg, lungs, liver, bone, brain, or lymph nodes outside of abdominopelvic region)
V	Bilateral renal involvement at diagnosis

between 1 and 7 months of age (EFS 92% vs 77%, P<.0001 and OS 92% vs 84, P = .01), likely reflecting the high proportion of benign congenital mesoblastic nephroma presenting in the younger cohort.

CONGENITAL MESOBLASTIC NEPHROMA
Epidemiology

Congenital mesoblastic nephroma (CMN) was first described by Bolande and colleagues[7] in 1967 as a clinical entity distinct from WT. CMN is the most common renal neoplasm in neonates and accounts for 54% to 66% of tumors in this age group (but only 2%–4% of pediatric renal tumors overall).[2,6] CMN occurs almost exclusively in infants, with a median age of diagnosis of 3.4 months, and more than 90% of cases are diagnosed in the first year of life.[8,9] Almost none occur after 2 years of age; therefore, a diagnosis of CMN should be questioned if applied to an older child. There is a slight male predominance (male:female 1.5:1.0).[1]

Presentation

CMN typically presents as a unilateral, solitary abdominal mass.[8] The mass may be detected on prenatal ultrasound, and in 70% of affected pregnancies are associated with polyhydramnios due to excess urine production.[10] Premature delivery and fetal hydrops also have been reported. Hypercalcemia has been described as a presenting feature of CMN, thought to be a paraneoplastic phenomenon due to the secretion of parathyroid hormone–like proteins or prostaglandins.[3] Elevated calcium does not appear to have prognostic significance, but can be followed as a tumor marker for some patients. Hypertension also may be seen; this finding is not specific to CMN, but in patients with CMN is thought to occur secondary to secretion of renin from entrapped juxtaglomerular cells.[11] Most CMNs presents as low stage; in the analysis from van den Heuvel-Eibrink and colleagues,[6] 74% were stage I/II at presentation, 13% were stage III, and no patients had metastatic disease.

Biology

CMN is classified as classic or cellular subtype based on histologic appearance,[12] and approximately 10% of cases have mixed classic and cellular features. Classic CMN accounts for approximately one-third of total cases. On gross appearance, these tumors have a firm, whorled appearance that is difficult to distinguish from normal kidney. The tumor consists of fibroblastic cells with elongated nuclei and low mitotic activity, which arrange themselves in fascicles that interdigitate between normal renal tissue. No clear capsule is formed; rather, the CMN tumor can penetrate the renal capsule and extend into perirenal fat and hilum.

In contrast, cellular CMN is typically soft and fleshy on gross appearance with cystic and hemorrhagic areas, and can often be clearly demarcated from normal kidney.[12] Cellular CMN is characterized by hypercellularity and high mitotic index with apoptotic cells and necrosis, and may be associated with a more aggressive presentation. The cellular variant is associated with the t(12;15) (p13;q25) translocation resulting in an ETV6-NTRK3 fusion protein.[13,14] The fusion results in constitutive activation of a tyrosine kinase growth signaling pathway. Interestingly, this translocation is identical to that seen in infantile fibrosarcoma (IFS), suggesting that IFS and cellular CMN may represent a single entity arising in different tissues. These molecular findings further suggest that it might be more appropriate to consider classic and cellular CMN distinct neoplasms, rather than different morphologic variants of the same neoplasm.

Treatment and Outcomes

The mainstay of treatment for CMN is primary surgical resection of the tumor by radical nephrectomy, followed by close observation with serial imaging.[8,15] Classic CMN typically presents as a low-grade tumor and can be effectively treated with surgery alone. Cellular and mixed variants can behave more aggressively and have greater potential to recur locally or metastasize.[16] Metastases, when they occur, have been reported to lungs, liver, heart, brain, and bone. Risk factors for recurrence are positive surgical margins or tumor rupture during resection, and recurrence is most likely within the first year after surgery.[16,17]

Adjuvant chemotherapy is generally reserved for children with higher-stage disease (stage III or greater), the cellular subtype of CMN, older age at presentation (older than 3 months), or evidence of disease recurrence after resection.[1,5] Treatment is typically adapted from the WT approach based on previous NWTSG or SIOP studies, and includes standard chemotherapeutic agents, such as vincristine, dactinomycin, doxorubicin, and cyclophosphamide.[9,15,16] The role of radiation therapy in the treatment of CMN has not been clearly established.

CMN of all stages typically carries an excellent prognosis, with EFS of 94% and OS of 96% reported in the largest international analysis of renal tumors in very young children.[6] The GPOH reported even higher survival rates (OS 100%) in children diagnosed with CMN before 3 months of age, compared with 83% in older children.[15]

WILMS TUMOR
Epidemiology and Presentation

WT is the second most common renal tumor presenting in the neonatal population, accounting for approximately 20% of all cases.[2] The clinical presentation of WT in this age group is similar to that of CMN, with approximately half presenting with an abdominal mass on examination, and roughly 16% with abdominal mass identified prenatally. Associated prenatal findings include polyhydramnios and fetal hydrops, although these are less common than with CMN.[2] CMN and WT are indistinguishable prenatally, however, and the finding of an abdominal mass on prenatal imaging requires postnatal follow-up. Findings on postnatal imaging that are more suggestive of a diagnosis of WT include tumor thrombus in the inferior vena cava or the renal vein, as well as pulmonary lesions, although these findings are less common overall in the neonatal period.[1] Hypertension also can be seen in neonates with WT and is thought to be due to excess renin production directly by the tumor cells.[3]

In fewer than 10% of cases, WT in the neonatal period is associated with congenital syndromes that may predispose children to tumorigenesis.[1] These include WAGR (Wilms Tumor, Aniridia, Genitourinary Abnormalities, Range of Developmental Delays) syndrome, Beckwith-Wiedemann syndrome, Denys-Drash syndrome, and Simpson-Golabi-Behmel syndrome. The risk of tumorigenesis varies depending on the syndrome, but WT is thought to arise from abnormalities at gene loci that dysregulate gene expression pathways necessary for renal morphogenesis and lead to aberrant stimulation of tissue-specific growth. Routine screening is recommended for children with these syndromes when the risk of tumor development is greater than 5%.[5] Screening is typically done by clinical examination and ultrasound evaluation every 3 months until the child is 5 years old.

Most WT in the neonatal period are low stage, with 80% presenting as stage I or II.[2,6] The vast majority are favorable histology (FH), which is consistent with the low stage presentation. Stage III tumors make up only 1% to 2% of all cases and stage IV metastatic disease is exceedingly rare. Bilateral disease (stage V) has also been reported in 8% to 12% of cases, depending on the series.

Treatment and Outcomes

Treatment considerations for neonatal WT are similar to those for WT presenting in other age groups. **Table 2** outlines the current COG-based treatment approach to WT. Upfront radical nephrectomy is the general rule.[1] Results of the COG study AREN0532 demonstrated that most patients deemed "very low risk" (younger than 2 years with tumors weighing <550 g and stage I FH) can be cured with surgery alone.[18] In cases of subsequent relapse, children are easily salvaged with a 2-drug chemotherapy regimen of vincristine and dactinomycin. With this approach, 4-year EFS was 90% and OS 100%. Within this group, molecular changes, including mutations of WT1 and loss of heterozygosity of 11p15, have been associated with an increased risk of relapse; therefore, it is recommended that children with these molecular changes receive adjuvant chemotherapy.[19]

All other children with WT not meeting the very low risk criteria are treated with chemotherapy after surgical resection, including all other stage I and II FH tumors.[18] Loss of heterozygosity (LOH) of chromosomes 1p and 16q have been identified as unfavorable molecular markers, and thus treatment is augmented with additional chemotherapy if these molecular changes are identified.[20] Patients with stage I or II FH tumors with LOH receive doxorubicin in addition to the vincristine/dactinomycin backbone, and treatment duration is also extended.

For children with synchronous bilateral involvement of WT, treatment begins with upfront chemotherapy using vincristine, dactinomycin, and doxorubicin for 6 to 12 weeks before definitive surgery.[1,21] Subsequent adjuvant therapy is modified based on the histologic response. This approach allows for reduction in tumor volume and thus preservation of renal parenchyma, with the long-term goal of preserving renal function. The COG study AREN0534 recently showed a 4-year EFS of 82% and OS of 95% with this approach, although these survival rates include patients of all ages.[21]

Radiation therapy is less likely to be required in the neonatal population, given the relatively higher frequency of low stage disease. However, when indicated, radiotherapy treatment requires careful consideration given the higher risk of toxicity and adverse late effects. Considerations include dose reduction or deferring radiotherapy until at least 6 months of age.[5,22] In general, radiation is directed to the affected flank for any positive lymph nodes, positive tumor margins, or intraoperative tumor spillage. Whole abdominal radiation is indicated for diffuse tumor spill or peritoneal seeding. Radiation is also recommended to any sites of distant metastases, such as the bone, brain, and liver. Whole lung irradiation for lung metastases can generally be avoided if lung nodules show complete response to upfront chemotherapy.[23]

WT in the neonatal population has a good prognosis overall, with EFS of 86% and OS 93%.[6]

MALIGNANT RHABDOID TUMOR
Epidemiology

MRTK accounts for approximately 11% of neonatal renal tumors.[2] MRTK presents primarily in the neonatal period and in infancy, and these younger age groups comprise almost 70% of all cases.[5] In contrast to other neonatal renal tumors, MRTK is very aggressive, presenting more frequently with stage III or IV disseminated disease.[6] Metastases can occur to the lung, bone, and brain, but also can be seen within the abdomen, and to lymph nodes, liver, and skin.

MRTK is one of the most aggressive pediatric cancers and outcomes are poor, owing to the early onset of both local and distant metastases and relative chemoresistance. Five-year EFS and OS are dismal, ranging from 8% to 16% in various series.[2,6] The presence of metastases at diagnosis and younger age at diagnosis are poor prognostic factors.

CLEAR CELL SARCOMA
Epidemiology

Clear cell sarcoma of the kidney (CCSK) is the least common neonatal renal tumor, accounting for only 3% of renal tumors in this age group.[1] The average age of presentation is 36 months, with a wide range from 2 months to 14 years.[30] There appears to be a male predominance, with a male-to-female ratio of 2:1.

Presentation

CCSK is also known as "bone metastasizing tumor of the kidney" owing to its original description in 1970; however, metastatic disease at the time of presentation is actually uncommon.[31] Distant metastatic disease is present in approximately 4% at diagnosis, and can be found most often to the bone, liver, lungs, or brain.[30] Local spread to regional lymph nodes (stage III) is more common and is found in 30%. Bilateral disease has not yet been reported.

Patients typically present with a palpable abdominal mass that is indistinguishable from other renal tumors on cross-sectional imaging.[2] Once a diagnosis is confirmed, bone scan is indicated to complete staging given the propensity for this tumor to spread to the bones.[1,5] Bone marrow involvement is relatively uncommon, however, and bone marrow aspiration is no longer routinely recommended as part of the staging evaluation.

Biology

The histogenesis and genetic etiology of CCSK are poorly understood. CCSK gets its name from the histologic appearance of cells within a pale myxoid stroma with open nuclei and finely dispersed chromatin, and sparse, clear cytoplasm.[30] Histologically, CCSK can show significant morphologic diversity, with 9 different histologic patterns described (classic, myxoid, sclerosing, cellular, epithelioid, palisading, spindle, storiform, and anaplastic). These histologic variants do not appear to have prognostic significance, but may contribute to difficulties in distinguishing CCSK from other renal tumors.[32]

Cytogenetics within CCSK are typically normal; however, a recurrent t(10;17) translocation has been reported in several cases.[33,34] The TP53 gene is located at the 17p breakpoint of these translocations; however, p53 is not thought to play a major role in the pathogenesis of CCSK.[35] Gene expression profiling of CCSK tumors has identified upregulation of neural markers within the SHH (sonic hedgehog) and PI3KA pathways.[36] EGFR in particular has been found to be amplified or mutated in small studies, and this may lend support to trialing EGFR inhibitors in patients with CCSK who are resistant or refractory to conventional chemotherapy.[37]

Treatment and Outcomes

Treatment of CCSK is similar to that of MRTK, and in the United States follows the intensified COG AREN0321 regimen for high-risk renal tumors. The addition of doxorubicin in particular appears to have improved outcomes in previous studies. In the last NWTS-5 study, children were treated with vincristine/doxorubicin/cyclophosphamide alternating with cyclophosphamide/etoposide for a total of 6 months, with radiation directed to affected sites. Five-year EFS and OS were reported to be 79% and 90%, respectively, although these values may be skewed by the older average age of children presenting with CCSK.[38] Data specifically in the neonatal population are limited; however, in the large collaborative study of infants up to 7 months of age treated in the United States and Europe, 5-year EFS was 49% and OS 51%.[6]

SUMMARY

Renal tumors are relatively uncommon in the neonatal period and are generally associated with a favorable prognosis, although outcomes vary widely based on histology. When not identified by prenatal ultrasound, these tumors will typically present with an incidental abdominal mass, abdominal distention, or hematuria. Although there are some exceptions, neonatal renal tumors are often associated with a lower stage, and local recurrence or metastatic disease are rare. Primary surgical resection is often the initial treatment of choice, with the need for adjuvant therapy dictated by histology and biology. Better understanding of the underlying molecular biology of these tumors may pave the way for novel therapeutic strategies, particularly for more challenging diagnoses such as MRTK or CCSK. Management of neonates with renal tumors, therefore, requires a careful multidisciplinary approach at a tertiary care center with experienced neonatology, pediatric oncology, pediatric surgery, radiology, and pathology.

CLINICS CARE POINTS

- Renal tumors are rare in the neonatal period and generally have a very good prognosis, with low-stage disease treated with primary nephrectomy alone.
- Tumors presenting with metastatic disease suggest a more aggressive histopathology and are associated with a poorer prognosis.
- Expanding knowledge of the molecular features of these tumors may offer opportunities for novel targeted therapies that may mitigate acute and long-term toxicities of conventional chemoradiation.
- Management of neonates with renal tumors requires a careful multidisciplinary approach with the input of pediatric oncology, surgery, neonatology, radiology, and pathology.

DISCLOSURE

The author has nothing to disclose.

REFERENCES

1. Powis M. Neonatal renal tumours. Early Hum Dev 2010;86:607–12.
2. Isaacs H Jr. Fetal and neonatal renal tumors. J Pediatr Surg 2008;43:1587–95.
3. Glick RD, Hicks MJ, Nuchtern JG, et al. Renal tumors in infants less than 6 months of age. J Pediatr Surg 2004;39:522–5.
4. Lamb MG, Aldrink JH, O'Brien SH, et al. Renal tumors in children younger than 12 months of age: a 65-year single institution review. J Pediatr Hematol Oncol 2017;39:103–7.
5. Shapiro E. Upper urinary tract anomalies and perinatal renal tumors. Clin Perinatol 2014;41:679–94.
6. van den Heuvel-Eibrink MM, Grundy P, Graf N, et al. Characteristics and survival of 750 children diagnosed with a renal tumor in the first seven months of life: a

collaborative study by the SIOP/GPOH/SFOP, NWTSG, and UKCCSG Wilms tumor study groups. Pediatr Blood Cancer 2008;50:1130–4.

7. Bolande RP, Brough AJ, Izant RJ. Congenital mesoblastic nephroma of infancy. A report of eight cases and the relationship to Wilms' tumor. Pediatrics 1967;40: 272–8.

8. Howell CG, Othersen HB, Kiviat NE, et al. Therapy and outcome in 51 children with mesoblastic nephroma: a report of the National Wilms' Tumor Study. J Pediatr Surg 1982;17:826–31.

9. England RJ, Haider N, Vujanic GM, et al. Mesoblastic nephroma: a report of the United Kingdom children's cancer and leukaemia group (CCLG). Pediatr Blood Cancer 2011;56:744–8.

10. Haddad B, Haziza J, Touboul C, et al. The congenital mesoblastic nephroma: a case report of prenatal diagnosis. Fetal Diagn Ther 1996;11:61–6.

11. Tsuchida Y, Shimizu K, Hata J, et al. Renin production in congenital mesoblastic nephroma in comparison with that in Wilms' tumor. Pediatr Pathol 1993;13: 155–64.

12. Gruver AM, Hansel DE, Luthringer DJ, et al. Congenital mesoblastic nephroma. J Urol 2010;183:1188–9.

13. Knezevich SR, Garnett MJ, Pysher TJ, et al. ETV6-NTRK3 gene fusions and trisomy 11 establish a histogenetic link between mesoblastic nephroma and congenital fibrosarcoma. Cancer Res 1998;58:5046–8.

14. Rubin B, Chen C, Morgan T, et al. Congenital mesoblastic nephroma t(12;15) is associated with ETV6-NTRK3 gene fusion: cytogenetic and molecular relationship to congenital (infantile) fibrosarcoma. Am J Pathol 1998;153:1451–8.

15. Furtwaengler R, Reinhard H, Leuschner I, et al. Mesoblastic nephroma–a report from the Gesellschaft Fur Padiatrische Onkologie und Hamatologie (GPOH). Cancer 2006;106:2275–83.

16. Loeb DM, Hill DA, Dome JS. Complete response of recurrent cellular congenital mesoblastic nephroma to chemotherapy. J Pediatr Hematol Oncol 2002;24: 478–81.

17. Beckwith JB, Weeks DA. Congenital mesoblastic nephroma. When should we worry? Arch Pathol Lab Med 1986;110:98–9.

18. Fernandez CV, Perlman EJ, Mullen EA, et al. Clinical outcome and biological predictors of relapse after nephrectomy only for very low-risk wilms tumor: a report from children's oncology group AREN0532. Ann Surg 2017;265:835–40.

19. Perlman EJ, Grundy PE, Anderson JR, et al. WT1 mutation and 11P15 loss of heterozygosity predict relapse in very low-risk wilms tumors treated with surgery alone: a children's oncology group study. J Clin Oncol 2011;29:698–703.

20. Grundy PE, Telzerow PE, Breslow N, et al. Loss of heterozygosity for chromosomes 16q and 1p in Wilms' tumors predicts an adverse outcome. Cancer Res 1994;54:2331–3.

21. Ehrlich P, Chi YY, Chintagumpala MM, et al. Results of the first prospective multi-institutional treatment study in children with bilateral wilms tumor (AREN0534): a report from the children's oncology group. Ann Surg 2017;266:470–8.

22. Thompson PA, Chintagumpala M. Renal and hepatic tumors in the neonatal period. Semin Fetal Neonatal Med 2012;17:216–21.

23. Dix DB, Seibel NL, Chi YY, et al. Treatment of stage IV favorable histology wilms tumor with lung metastases: a report from the children's oncology group AREN0533 study. J Clin Oncol 2018;36:1564–70.

24. Amar AM, Tomlinson G, Green DM, et al. Clinical presentation of rhabdoid tumors of the kidney. J Pediatr Hematol Oncol 2001;23:105–8.

25. Agrons G, Kingsman K, Wagner B, et al. Rhabdoid tumor of the kidney in children: a comparative study of 21 cases. Am J Roentgenol 1997;168:447–51.
26. Geller JI, Roth JJ, Biegel JA. Biology and treatment of rhabdoid tumor. Crit Rev Oncog 2015;20:199–216.
27. Biegel JA, Zhou J-Y, Rorke LB, et al. Germ-line and acquired mutations of INI1 in atypical teratoid and rhabdoid tumors. Cancer Res 1999; 59:74–9.
28. Sévenet N, Sheridan E, Amram D, et al. Constitutional mutations of the hSNF5/INI1 gene predispose to a variety of cancers. Am J Hum Genet 1999;65:1342–8.
29. Tomlinson GE, Breslow NE, Dome J, et al. Rhabdoid tumor of the kidney in the national wilms' tumor study: age at diagnosis as a prognostic factor. J Clin Oncol 2005;23:7641–5.
30. Argani P, Perlman EJ, Breslow NE, et al. Clear cell sarcoma of the kidney: a review of 351 cases from the National Wilms tumor study group pathology center. Am J Surg Pathol 2000;24:4–18.
31. Kidd JM. Exclusion of certain renal neoplasms from the category of Wilms' tumor. Am J Pathol 1970;59:16a (abstract).
32. Furtwängler R, Gooskens SL, van Tinteren H, et al. Clear cell sarcomas of the kidney registered on international society of pediatric oncology (SIOP) 93-01 and SIOP 2001 protocols: a report of the SIOP renal tumour study group. Eur J Cancer 2013;49:3497–506.
33. Punnett HH, Halligan GE, Zaeri N, et al. Translocation 10;17 in clear cell sarcoma of the kidney. A first report. Cancer Genet Cytogenet 1989;41:123–8.
34. Rakheja D, Weinberg AG, Tomlinson GE, et al. Translocation (10;17)(q22;p13): a recurring translocation in clear cell sarcoma of kidney. Cancer Genet Cytogenet 2004;154:175–9.
35. Hsueh C, Wang H, Gonzalez-Crussi F, et al. Infrequent p53 gene mutations and lack of p53 protein expression in clear cell sarcoma of the kidney: immunohistochemical study and mutation analysis of p53 in renal tumors of unfavorable prognosis. Mod Pathol 2002;15:606–10.
36. Cutcliffe C, Kersey D, Huang C-C, et al. Clear cell sarcoma of the kidney: upregulation of neural markers with activation of the sonic hedgehog and akt pathways. Clin Cancer Res 2005;11:7986–94.
37. Little SE, Bax DA, Rodriguez-Pinilla M, et al. Multifaceted dysregulation of the epidermal growth factor receptor pathway in clear cell sarcoma of the kidney. Clin Cancer Res 2007;13:4360–4.
38. Seibel NL, Chi Y-Y, Perlman EJ, et al. Impact of cyclophosphamide and etoposide on outcome of clear cell sarcoma of the kidney treated on the National Wilms Tumor Study-5 (NWTS-5). Pediatr Blood Cancer 2019;66:e27450.

Neonatal Liver Tumors

Howard M. Katzenstein, MD[a],*, Allison Aguado, MD[b],
Bradley Cheek, MD[c], Renee Gresh, DO[d]

KEYWORDS

- Neonatal • Liver • Cancer • Benign • Hepatoblastoma • Hemangioma
- Mesenchymal hamartoma • Focal nodular hyperplasia

KEY POINTS

- Metastatic malignancies are the most common neoplasm in the liver.
- Primary liver tumors require surgical resection for cure.
- Alpha fetoprotein is a biological marker for pediatric liver malignancy.
- Benign liver lesions are common and can often be discerned by radiographic findings.

Malignant liver lesions are uncommon and make up approximately 1% of all pediatric malignancies, comprising approximately 150 new diagnoses each year in the United States. The most common malignancy involving the liver is metastatic disease from neuroblastoma, leukemia, Langerhans cell histiocytosis, or hemophagocytic syndromes. Benign livers lesions often can be well characterized radiographically. Infectious processes are even more rare. The differential diagnosis of both malignant and benign lesions is age dependent. This article first provides a general approach to evaluating and managing liver tumors in infancy, and then discusses specific features of the most common types of liver tumor.

INTRODUCTION

Malignant liver lesions are uncommon and make up approximately 1% of all pediatric malignancies, comprising approximately 150 new diagnoses each year in the United States.[1] The most common malignancy involving the liver is metastatic disease from neuroblastoma, leukemia, Langerhans cell histiocytosis, or hemophagocytic

[a] Pediatric Hematology/Oncology and Bone Marrow Transplantation, Nemours Children's Specialty Care, Wolfson Children's Hospital, Mayo Clinic College of Medicine and Science, 807 Children's Way, Jacksonville, FL 32207, USA; [b] Interventional Radiology, Nemours/Alfred I. duPont Hospital for Children, 1600 Rockland Road, Wilmington, DE 19803, USA; [c] Wolfson Children's Hospital, Southeastern Pathology Associates, 800 Prudential Drive, Jacksonville, FL 32207, USA; [d] Pediatric Hematology/Oncology, Nemours/AI DuPont Hospital for Children, Sidney Kimmel Medical College at Thomas Jefferson University, 1600 Rockland Road, Wilmington, DE 19803, USA
* Corresponding author.
E-mail address: Howard.katzenstein@nemours.org

Clin Perinatol 48 (2021) 83–99
https://doi.org/10.1016/j.clp.2020.11.005
0095-5108/21/© 2020 Elsevier Inc. All rights reserved.

syndromes. Several benign livers lesions are common and often can be well characterized and diagnosed radiographically. Infectious processes can also occur in the liver but are even more rare and can usually be distinguished by fever, a specific exposure, and or a history of travel. The differential diagnosis of both malignant and benign lesions is age dependent.[2] Alpha fetoprotein (AFP) is a useful laboratory marker for malignancy. Surgical resection is the foundation of curative therapy for primary liver malignancies. Benign lesions can sometimes be observed, but some do harbor potential for transformation to a malignant lesion. Surgical resection is the typical treatment if a benign lesion is causing symptoms. This article first provides a general approach to evaluating and managing liver tumors in infancy, and then discusses specific features of the most common types of liver tumor.

Differential Diagnosis

The differential diagnosis of liver lesions is limited. Only a handful of primary malignant and benign liver lesions occur in the pediatric population regularly (**Table 1**).[3]

Work-up

The work-up of liver lesions depends on a good history and physical examination. A variety of syndromes and preexisting conditions[3,4] may point to the diagnosis, as might a positive family history (**Table 2**). Prematurity and the increasing survival among premature neonates have led to an increase in the diagnosis of hepatoblastoma (HB). There are no typically pathognomonic symptoms, especially in the neonatal and infant period. Jaundice is not a typical finding because primary tumors would need to be unusually and extraordinarily extensive to result in jaundice. Occasionally, the size of the tumor may result in obstructive/compressive symptoms compromising respiration. Furthermore, extensive liver involvement could result in reduced production of proteins that are synthesized in the liver (eg, coagulation factors), leading to altered hemostasis. Patients may present with a variety of nonspecific findings. However, the abdominal examination rarely helps clarify the specific pathologic diagnosis. The presence of obvious neonatal overgrowth or other syndrome stigmata may lead to the diagnosis (see **Table 2**). Hemihyperplasia (formerly called hemihypertrophy) is challenging to diagnose in the neonatal and infant population. Physical findings of portal hypertension can lead to the diagnosis of a liver tumor but are not necessarily specific.

The most important laboratory evaluation for a neonatal liver tumor includes measurement of the AFP (measured in nanograms per milliliter). Interpretation of AFP levels may be challenging, because the AFP level is normally increased in all newborns following birth. Tables exist that provide the normal AFP ranges based on age (discussed elsewhere in this issue, and see **Table 1**), but, in the first few months of

| Table 1 |||
| Liver lesion differential diagnosis based on age at diagnosis |||
Age Group	Malignant	Benign
Infant/toddler	Metastatic disease	Hemangioma/Vascular
	HB	Mesenchymal Hamartoma
	Malignant rhabdoid tumor	Focal Nodular Hyperplasia
	Malignant germ cell tumor	Teratoma
	Angiosarcoma	

Abbreviation: HB, hepatoblastoma.

Table 2
Genetic syndromes associated with pediatric liver lesions

Disease	Tumor	Chromosome	Gene
Beckwith-Wiedemann syndrome[5,6]	HB, infantile hemangioma	11p15.5	P57KiP2, WNT pathway, others
Familial adenomatous polyposis[7,8]	Adenoma, HB, HCC	5q21.22	APC
Fanconi anemia[9]	Adenoma, HCC	1q42, 3p, 20q13	FAA, FAC
Glycogen storage disease type I, III, IV[10]	Adenoma, HB, HCC	Several	GBE1, G6PC
Li-Fraumeni syndrome[11]	HB, undifferentiated sarcoma	17p13	TP53, others
Trisomy 18[12]	HB	18	—

Abbreviation: HCC, hepatocellular carcinoma.

life, the normal increased AFP levels may be significant and can easily mask increased levels from a malignant lesion. In such cases, imaging and biopsy may be needed to clarify the potential for a pediatric malignancy. Increased AFP level is almost always seen in HB.[13] Historically, AFP-negative HBs were likely to have been misdiagnosed based on less sophisticated diagnostic tools and were more likely to have been malignant rhabdoid tumors, which can now be definitively diagnosed with genetic evaluation.[14] Increased AFP levels are also seen in conventional hepatocellular carcinoma (HCC), but not the fibrolamellar subtype, and also in germ cell tumors. Increased AFP levels may also be seen in some benign lesions, including mesenchymal hamartoma, as well as in regenerating liver after surgery or after injury. The expected AFP decline has a half-life of 5 to 7 days if the tumor is completely removed. However, the rate of AFP decline may be prolonged if an AFP-secreting tumor has yet to be resected and is being treated with chemotherapy to cause shrinkage in an effort to facilitate resection. Care should be taken to determine a precise AFP value for each patient. Markedly increased AFP levels (>1 million) but even some modestly increased (>36,000) may require serial dilutions to overcome the limit of certain specific AFP testing kits and determine a precise AFP level. This determination is critical in order to be able to monitor the response to therapy and whether a tumor is responding or progressing.

Normal AFP levels essentially rule out HB and should prompt consideration of other diagnoses. The so-called hook effect, where an exceedingly high AFP level overcomes the mechanics of the specific AFP testing method and results in a falsely normal value, must also be considered and evaluated by serial dilutions to ensure an accurate and interpretable AFP level.

The initial laboratory work-up of liver lesions is straightforward and can be accomplished fairly rapidly (**Box 1, Table 3**). The laboratory work-up should typically include:

- Complete blood count
- Metabolic profile/serum chemistries
- Liver function panel
- Coagulation profile (prothrombin time/International Normalized Ratio/partial thromboplastin time/fibrinogen)
- AFP level (tumor marker)
- β-Human chorionic gonadotropin level (tumor marker)

Box 1
Pediatric tumors of the liver

Premalignant lesions
  Dysplastic nodules (low grade and high grade)

Benign
  Focal nodular hyperplasia
  Hemangioma
  Hepatocellular adenoma (adenomatosis)
  Macroregenerative nodules
  Mesenchymal hamartoma
  Bile duct adenoma (biliary cystadenoma)
  Teratoma

Malignant
  HB
    Fetal, pleomorphic
    Fetal, cholangioblastic variant
    Mixed
    Small cell component, INI+/−
    Teratoid HB
    Well-differentiated fetal/pure fetal HB
  HCC
    Fibrolamellar HCC
  Hepatocellular malignant neoplasm, not otherwise specified
  Epithelioid hemangioendothelioma
  Germ cell tumors
  Malignant rhabdoid tumor
    INI− (documented *INI* mutation)
    INI+
  Nested epithelial stromal tumor
  Angiosarcoma

Malignant: other (older)
  Embryonal sarcoma
  Rhabdomyosarcoma
  Synovial sarcoma
  Miscellaneous (including desmoplastic small round cell tumor)
    Peripheral neuroectodermal tumor
    NUT carcinoma

Malignant: metastatic
  Acute lymphoblastic leukemia
  Acute myeloid leukemia
  Hemophagocytic lymphohistiocytosis)/hemophagocytic syndrome
  Langerhans cell histiocytosis
  Neuroblastoma

Imaging

Plain radiographs may suggest a primary liver lesion with hepatomegaly and can occasionally show calcifications, but are not usually confirmatory of a specific diagnosis.

Ultrasonography[15] is usually the initial radiographic study that is obtained and can delineate solid versus cystic as well as vascular lesions. Doppler analysis is critical in providing information to surgeons about the status of vascular structures and the presence of thrombosis, which is a critical factor in resectability.

Computed tomography (CT) scans are the most reliable way to image the tumor, usually avoids sedation, and efficiently evaluates metastatic sites. MRI is often the

Table 3
Laboratory work-up of liver lesions

	Findings in Primary Liver Malignancy	Findings in Metastatic Liver Malignancy	Findings in Benign Disorders
Diagnosis Test	HB, HCC, malignant rhabdoid tumor, germ cell tumor, undifferentiated sarcoma, angiosarcoma	Neuroblastoma, leukemia, Langerhans cell histiocytosis, hemophagocytic syndromes (eg, HLH)	Hemangioma, mesenchymal hamartoma, focal nodular hyperplasia, teratoma
Complete blood count	Low hemoglobin level if patient has had bleeding into tumor or has had prolonged presentation and systemic symptoms/ malnutrition, thrombocytosis	Low white cell count, hemoglobin or platelet level in leukemia, HLH, or neuroblastoma	Low platelets in hemangioma (Kasabach/Merritt syndrome)
Metabolic profile	Usually normal	Usually normal	Usually normal
Liver function tests	Usually normal	Usually normal	Usually normal
Coagulation studies	May or may not be normal	May be abnormal in leukemia or HLH	May be abnormal in hemangioma associated Kasabach-Merritt syndrome
AFP	Increased in HB, germ cell tumors	Not increased	Not increased
β-HCG	Can be increased in HB, germ cell tumors	Not increased	Not increased

Abbreviations: HCG, human chorionic gonadotropin; HLH, hemophagocytic lymphohistiocytosis.

preferred study for malignant disorders in order to image vascular structures but there may be limited scheduling availability, it often requires sedation because of the duration of the scan, and it is not appropriate for imaging of pulmonary metastatic sites.

PET[16] has no defined role in imaging liver tumors, especially in upfront diagnoses. However, their anecdotal use is well described in patients with early suggestion of disease release in an effort to determine the occult site of metastasis.

Several liver-specific contrast agents are available for use in imaging liver tumors and their evaluation and specificity is thought to often yield a fairly definitive radiographic diagnosis.[17]

Surgery

Surgical resection is typically the critical element for curative treatment of primary malignant lesions. The PRETEXT (Pretreatment Extent of Disease) staging system was developed by SIOPEL (International Childhood Liver Tumor Strategy Group) to predict resectability.[18,19] The PRETEXT staging system (**Fig. 1**) has been adapted and codified by the international community to provide specific guidelines to identify

PRETEXT denotes Pretreatment Extent of disease. POST-TEXT denotes Post-Treatment Extent of disease. The tumor group (I, II, III, or IV) describes the intraparenchymal extent of tumor. The PRETEXT Annotation Factors (VPEFRCNM) define caudate and extraparenchymal extent of tumor.

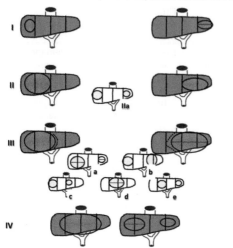

PRETEXT
*Pret*reatment *Ext*ent of Disease
Extent of liver involvement at diagnosis
POST-TEXT
*Post*treatment *Ext*ent of Disease,
extent of liver involvement after
pre-operative chemotherapy
I ... 3 contiguous sections tumor free
II ... 2 contiguous sections tumor free
III ... 1 contiguous sections tumor free
IV ...no contiguous sections tumor free

**In addition, any group
may have one or more positive
PRETEXT Annotation Factors:**
V ...ingrowth vena cava, all 3 hepatic veins
P ...ingrowth portal vein, portal bifurcation
E ...contiguous extrahepatic tumor
F ....mutifocal tumor
R ... tumor rupture prior to diagnosis
C ...caudate
N ... lymph node involvement
M ...metastasis, distant extrahepatic tumor

Fig. 1. PRETEXT classification.

appropriate timing for resection and liver transplant. The North American[20,21] approach has favored upfront resection when feasible for accurate pathologic evaluation and to minimize the amount of adjuvant chemotherapy.[22] In contrast, the international community has favored initial biopsy and neoadjuvant chemotherapy to minimize surgical morbidity.[23,24] Evaluation of surgical morbidity shows that it is very low in pediatric liver tumors. A variety of surgical resection strategies may be used to remove liver lesions; the most critical feature is that gross tumor not be left behind. Extreme surgical resections are sometimes performed in centers with established expertise in liver tumors in order to avoid liver transplant.[25] The use of liver transplant is well established for HB and is associated with excellent outcomes.[26–29] The success of liver transplant in HB suggests that its use in less chemoresponsive tumors, such as HCC, malignant rhabdoid tumor, and embryonal sarcoma, may provide dramatic improvements in survival. However, liver transplant results in the need for lifelong medical therapy. Therefore, efforts to identify novel therapies that can increase resectability and decrease transplant rates remain important clinical trial goals.

Alternative Local Therapies

Local therapies such as transarterial chemoembolization,[30–32] transarterial radioembolization,[33,34] and radiofrequency ablation[35] all have established roles in adult liver malignant processes. Their roles in pediatric patients still remain to be defined. Their potential use in infants and neonates would be expected to be challenging because of the size of the patients.

MALIGNANT LESIONS

Primary liver tumors comprise only about 1% of all pediatric cancers,[1,3,4] which makes metastatic malignant disorders the most common malignancies affecting the liver. Neuroblastoma (both stage M and MS),[36] leukemia, and histiocytic disorders (Langerhans cell histiocytosis[37] and hemophagocytic syndromes such as hemophagocytic lymphohistiocytosis) are all more likely to be associated with diffuse liver involvement as opposed to a discrete primary mass. Treatment is typically medical and not surgical for the liver involvement of these disorders, and resolution of any liver-related symptoms is typical, with no lingering liver dysfunction.

Hepatoblastoma

HB is the most common primary pediatric liver tumor (80%) observed in newly diagnosed patients and typically occurs in the first few years of life (**Fig. 2**).[1,3,4,38] The incidence of HB is increasing worldwide, primarily because of an association with prematurity and improved survival rates of premature infants.[39] The rate of HB occurrence increases with lower birth weights. Several causal events/exposures that occur during the perinatal or neonatal period have been postulated to contribute to the development of HB in premature infants; for example, oxygen exposure, blood transfusions, nutritional supplements, and medications. Although these have been extensively studied, the specific cause of HB in premature infants remains uncertain.[40,41]

HB has been associated with few/many/several underlying inherited conditions, including Beckwith-Wiedemann syndrome[5,6] and hemihyperplasia overgrowth syndrome, which both require tumor screening with abdominal ultrasonography and AFP level measurement in affected syndromic patients every 3 months for the first 8 years of life.[6] HB is also associated with familial adenomatous polyposis, and these patients should undergo routine periodic surveillance screening as well.[7,8]

The prognosis of HB, as it is for all primary liver tumors, is based on the presence of metastatic disease and the ability for the primary tumor to be completely resected.[42] Excellent results have been obtained with both primary and delayed resections, and whether or not the patient is able to undergo a conventional resection or orthotopic liver transplant.[43,44] Importantly, however, the one-third of newly diagnosed patients with HB who undergo upfront resection typically receive significantly less chemotherapy (2 vs 6+ cycles), and thus have diminished acute and long-term toxicities and morbidity.[13,45,46] Resection of the primary tumor as early as can be done safely should be the strategy. In contrast, it is not clear whether there is a difference in outcome for patients who have pulmonary metastatic lesions that resolve as a result of chemotherapy or are completely removed surgically.[45,46] Other prognostic factors include age, PRETEXT stage, AFP level, histology, and the absence of radiographic

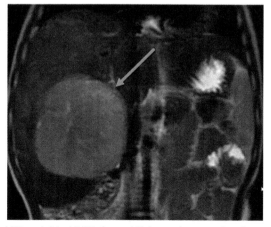

Fig. 2. HB. Coronal T2-weighted MRI shows HB (*arrow*) measuring 8 cm.

annotation factors such as proximity to portal or vena caval structures, extrahepatic tumor, multifocal tumors (20%) (which typical require transplant), ruptured tumor (preoperative or postoperative), and nodal disease.[13]

The PRETEXT staging was developed by the SIOPEL and provides predictive capacity evaluating the likelihood of achieving a complete surgical resection.[47–49] The liver is divided into 4 sectors composed of 8 Couinaud segments. Radiographic reports as the standard of care should now include both PRETEXT stage, annotation factors (V, P, E, M, C, F, R, N), and the involved segments as the standard of care (**Fig. 3**).[18] Assessment of gross vascular involvement and tumor thrombosis is important in planning surgical intervention. An international surgical algorithm (**Fig. 4**) has been established to guide decision making on surgical intervention for local surgeons who may not have frequent exposure to liver tumors because of their overall rarity. Every effort must be made to perform the correct surgery the first time in order to reduce relapse rates and outcomes. Liver transplant for recurrent disease has had a significantly lower survival rate compared with primary liver transplant.[50] Early referral for all patients whose tumors cannot be resected upfront should be made at the time of diagnosis to a liver transplant service so that appropriate planning can take place to perform surgery at the desired time point and to prevent extra chemotherapy cycles and the associated toxicities of extra chemotherapy caused by poor logistical planning. Imaging is typically performed after every 2 chemotherapy cycles until resection is feasible. Downstaging of a POSTTEXT scan (POSt Treatment EXTent of disease), which is different from RECIST[51] response, would suggest that resection may be safely performed, but the continued presence of annotation factors affect this decision. The importance of microscopic vascular invasion and positive microscopic margins has yet to be definitively studied.

Initial imaging by ultrasonography usually reveals either a single or hyperechoic mass or multifocal masses. On occasion, multifocality may only appear after

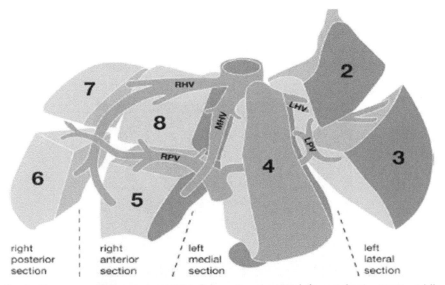

Fig. 3. Liver segmental anatomy. LHV, left hepatic vein; LPV, left portal vein; MHV, middle hepatic vein; RHV, right hepatic vein; RPV, right portal vein. (Reused with permission from Hertzberg BS, Middleton WD. Ultrasound: The Requisites (Requisites in Radiology). 3rd ed. Philadelphia: Elsevier; 2015, F3-1).

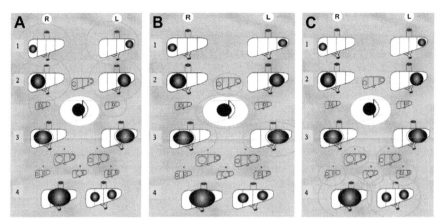

Fig. 4. (*A*) Liver tumor surgical guidelines: resectable at diagnosis. (*B*) Liver tumor surgical guidelines: unresectable at diagnosis/biopsy and chemotherapy. (*C*) Liver tumor surgical guidelines: unresectable at diagnosis/biopsy, chemotherapy, and liver transplant referral/consult.

chemotherapy has resulted in overall tumor shrinkage. Doppler studies are critical to studying the patency of vascular structures and the possibility of vascular tumor thrombus. Although MRI is the preferred method of primary tumor imaging in many centers, CT may be sufficient, and is required for evaluation of the lungs, and may be performed quickly to avoid the need for sedation/anesthesia. Certain MRI liver-specific contrast agents are thought to be able to clearly differentiate between malignant versus benign disorders. There is no clear role for PET scanning, although anecdotal reports exist concerning its use in relapsed patients to help identify the presence of an initially occult radiographic lesion in a patient with a mild increase in AFP level.

Cisplatin and doxorubicin are the two most active chemotherapeutic agents used in HB, but each has inherent dosing limitations because of associated hearing loss and cardiac dysfunction, respectively.[52] The use of chemotherapy for patients with unresectable, nonmetastatic tumors at diagnosis has been described to make 66% to 80% of these initially unresectable tumors resectable, whereas the remaining patients will ultimately require liver transplant.[53] Liver transplant has improved over the years, and the outcome of patients with nonmetastatic HB who undergo transplant is excellent. The maximal tumor shrinkage is expected to be achieved by the third or fourth cycle of chemotherapy.[54,55]

Sodium thiosulfate (STS) was used successfully in the SIOPEL6 trial to decrease cisplatin-associated hearing loss without any change in outcome; that is, STS administration does not seem to impair the antitumor effect of cisplatin. The safety and efficacy are based on 6 cycles of chemotherapy.[52] Although the potential of STS remains exciting, at this time its safe use in patients with metastatic disease is not clear. The use of dexrazoxane as a cardioprotectant in HB is now standard and viewed as safe, although the rate of anthracycline-induced cardiac toxicity in patients with HB historically is low.[53]

Radiation is not an established therapy for this disease, although anecdotal use has been reported in palliative cases.

Grossly tumors may have hemorrhage, necrosis, and calcification. Microscopically, tumors can be heterogeneous and include both epithelial and mesenchymal elements.[56,57]

Malignant Rhabdoid Tumor

Malignant rhabdoid tumor (MRT) is one of the most aggressive pediatric neoplasms and most commonly occurs in the brain or kidney, but the liver is a well-described location.[58] Regardless of the location, these tumors have a common genetic fingerprint and a mutation of the SMARCB1 (hSNF5/INI1) gene, which results histologically in the loss of INI expression.[59] Therefore, liver tumors that retain INI expression are not MRTs. Distinguishing MRTs from small cell undifferentiated HB has sometimes been challenging. The use of the *SMARCB1* genetic signature makes the diagnosis much more reliable. There is no established standard of care/curative therapy for MRTs, although ifosfamide has been described to be the most active agent. Treatment protocols have been used for central nervous system (CNS) and non-CNS locations, and patients with liver tumors have been eligible on MRT protocols from the Children's Oncology Group Wilms Tumor Committee. Curative therapy is based on a lack of metastatic disease and the ability to remove the primary lesion surgically. Consideration of the use of orthotopic liver transplant should be considered if this is the only means to remove the primary tumor in its entirety.

Angiosarcoma

Angiosarcomas are rare liver tumors and have a poor prognosis unless diagnosed early, when there is no metastatic disease and the tumor can be resected. There is no established therapeutic treatment regimen.[60]

These tumors have been described to occur in infantile hemangiomas, and the malignant transformation from a hemangioma to an angiosarcoma should be considered if the hemangioma behaves atypically with either rapid local progression or recurrence.

Germ Cell Tumors

Primary germ cell tumors are tumors that rarely occur in the liver and have an equal propensity of being benign or malignant.[61] The presence of an increased AFP level might be confusing to the final diagnosis because it could be seen in both germ cell tumors and HB and even in benign lesions, and might be difficult to interpret, especially in younger infants. The pathologic evaluation of the lesion and the presence of frankly malignant components of yolk sac, choriocarcinoma, or other germ cell layers would help make the diagnosis.

Hepatocellular Carcinoma

HCC is the second most common primary pediatric malignant liver tumor overall but is most commonly seen in the second decade of life on a background of preexisting liver disease.[62] The occurrence of HCC during the neonatal period or infancy is extremely rare.

BENIGN LESIONS
Infantile Hemangioma

Infantile hemangiomas may occur as isolated liver lesions in about two-thirds of cases and can be small and incidental, large and symptomatic, or multifocal (**Fig. 5**). Some lesions may be seen in conjunction with visible cutaneous lesions. The nomenclature of liver vascular lesions may be confusing.[63] Typical infantile liver hemangiomas can be diagnosed and followed by ultrasonography and often spontaneously regress. Increasingly medical therapy with propranolol[64] as an antiangiogenic agent often results in stabilization and eventual involution, although this often takes several years.

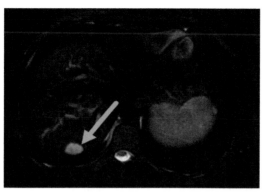

Fig. 5. Hemangioma. Axial T2-weighted MRI shows hepatic hemangioma (*arrow*) measuring 1.7 cm.

On occasion, large lesions can result in high-output cardiac failure, visceral organ compression and compromise, and/or consumptive coagulopathy, known as Kasabach-Merritt syndrome.[65] Steroids have also been used as part of therapy. Interferon is an antiangiogenic agent, but its use is contraindicated in children less than 1 year of age because of risks of irreversible spastic diplegia.[66] In extreme cases, treatment with local techniques, including embolization or excision, may be required if the lesion is causing life-threatening symptoms. Further details about neonatal vascular malformations are provided elsewhere in this issue.

Mesenchymal Hamartoma

Mesenchymal hamartoma (MH) is the second most frequent benign tumor in infancy (**Fig. 6**).[67] These tumors grow and are often identified when they become large enough to cause symptoms of either pain or organ dysfunction caused by compression of vascular, respiratory, or gastrointestinal compartments. These lesions can appear anywhere in the liver and are identified on ultrasonography as either a single echogenic mass or multiple echogenic cysts. CT scan may show a well-delineated multicystic mass separated by septae and stroma. AFP levels may be increased, making

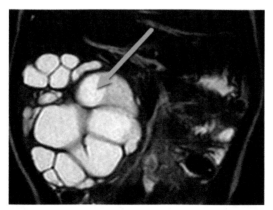

Fig. 6. MH. Coronal T2-weighted MRI shows multicystic hepatic MH (*arrow*) measuring approximately 11 cm.

the distinction between MH and HB challenging. The treatment of choice is surgical removal for not only diagnostic and clinical reasons but also because MH has been described to either hide or transform into undifferentiated sarcomas.[68]

On histology, these tumors are composed of bile ducts, liver cell cysts, and mesenchymal tissue. Elongated proliferating bile ducts are often found at the periphery of expanding lesions. Although the underlying pathogenesis is not clearly defined, DICER1 abnormalities and alterations in chromosome 19q13 have been found.[69]

Focal Nodular Hyperplasia

Focal nodular hyperplasia (FNH) can be diagnosed at any age, although it typically is seen in slightly older infants and toddlers between 2 and 5 years of age (**Fig. 7**).[70] Patients can present incidentally with an asymptomatic mass or with symptoms of abdominal pain, and can present as single or multiple nodules ranging in size from small (<1 cm) to very large (20 cm). These lesions can be diagnosed relatively confidently by MRI. The pathognomonic radiologic finding is a central stellate scar typically seen in about half of cases as well as retained contrast in the lesion on delayed phases of imaging. On ultrasonography, FNH appears as a well-delineated homogeneous, hyperechoic lesion. These findings make biopsy unnecessary in most cases and resection is therefore only needed if the patient has symptoms or if there is concern about the true diagnosis. Locoregional therapies can be used to eliminate symptoms in lieu of resection if treatment is needed and there is confidence in the diagnosis.

Benign FNH tumors can be associated with several predisposing conditions or factors, including liver trauma, exposure to chemotherapy during treatment of other pediatric cancers, the use of oral contraceptives, smoking, and congenital absence of the portal vein (Abernethy syndrome).[71] Grossly, these lesions are made of bile ducts peripherally with the central scar containing numerous blood vessels supplying the lesion. Microscopically, these lesions contain proliferating hepatocytes similar in appearance to normal liver tissue.

Teratoma

As discussed earlier, primary germ cell tumors can occur in the liver and have an equal propensity to be benign or malignant. Following increased AFP levels and confirming that they normalize is helpful to ensuring that no malignant cells were present occultly and the lesion is benign.

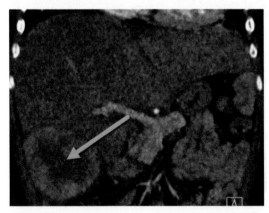

Fig. 7. FNH. Coronal CT image of biopsy-proven FNH with central stellate scar (*arrow*).

SUMMARY

Liver lesions are common in infants and neonates. These lesions can be either benign or malignant. Metastatic malignant disorder is more common than primary liver malignancies. Radiologic assessment is often helpful not only in identifying the extent of the lesion and the potential for resection but also in making a diagnosis because of specific radiographic characteristics observed on various imaging techniques. AFP is a useful laboratory marker for malignancy. Surgical resection is the foundation of curative therapy for primary liver malignancies, symptomatic benign lesions, as well as benign lesions that have the potential for transformation to a malignant lesion. Other benign lesions may sometimes be observed in lesions that are known to regress.

DISCLOSURE

The authors have no financial information to disclose.

REFERENCES

1. Darbari A, Sabin KM, Shapiro CN, et al. Epidemiology of primary hepatic malignancies in U.S. children. Hepatology 2003;38(3):560–6.
2. Halperin EC. Neonatal neoplasms. Int J Radiat Oncol Biol Phys 2000;47(1): 171–8.
3. Spector LG, Birch J. The epidemiology of hepatoblastoma. Pediatr Blood Cancer 2012;59(5):776–9.
4. Isaacs H Jr. Fetal and neonatal hepatic tumors. J Pediatr Surg 2007;42(11): 1797–803.
5. Fukuzawa R, Hata J, Hayashi Y, et al. Beckwith-Wiedemann syndrome-associated hepatoblastoma: wnt signal activation occurs later in tumorigenesis in patients with 11p15.5 uniparental disomy. Pediatr Dev Pathol 2003;6(4): 299–306.
6. Kalish JM, Doros L, Helman LJ, et al. Surveillance recommendations for children with overgrowth syndromes and predisposition to Wilms tumors and hepatoblastoma. Clin Cancer Res 2017;23(13):e115–22.
7. Achatz MI, Porter CC, Brugieres L, et al. Cancer screening recommendations and clinical management of inherited gastrointestinal cancer syndromes in childhood. Clin Cancer Res 2017;23(13):e107–14.
8. Bala S, Wunsch PH, Ballhausen WG. Childhood hepatocellular adenoma in familial adenomatous polyposis: mutations in adenomatous polyposis coli gene and p53. Gastroenterology 1997;112(3):919–22.
9. Ozenne V, Paradis V, Vullierme MP, et al. Liver tumours in patients with Fanconi anaemia: a report of three cases. Eur J Gastroenterol Hepatol 2008;20(10): 1036–9.
10. Franco LM, Krishnamurthy V, Bali D, et al. Hepatocellular carcinoma in glycogen storage disease type Ia: a case series. J Inherit Metab Dis 2005;28(2):153–62.
11. Ozawa MG, Cooney T, Rangaswami A, et al. Synchronous hepatoblastoma, neuroblastoma, and cutaneous capillary hemangiomas: a case report. Pediatr Dev Pathol 2016;19(1):74–9.
12. Inoue A, Suzuki R, Urabe K, et al. Therapeutic experience with hepatoblastoma associated with trisomy 18. Pediatr Blood Cancer 2018;65(8):e27093.
13. Meyers RL, Maibach R, Hiyama E, et al. Risk-stratified staging in paediatric hepatoblastoma: a unified analysis from the Children's Hepatic tumors International Collaboration. Lancet Oncol 2017;18(1):122–31.

14. Al Nassan A, Sughayer M, Matalka I, et al. INI1 (BAF 47) immunohistochemistry is an essential diagnostic tool for children with hepatic tumors and low alpha fetoprotein. J Pediatr Hematol Oncol 2010;32(2):e79–81.

15. Sato M, Ishida H, Konno K, et al. Liver tumors in children and young patients: sonographic and color Doppler findings. Abdom Imaging 2000;25(6):596–601.

16. Philip I, Shun A, McCowage G, et al. Positron emission tomography in recurrent hepatoblastoma. Pediatr Surg Int 2005;21(5):341–5.

17. Youk JH, Lee JM, Kim CS. MRI for detection of hepatocellular carcinoma: comparison of mangafodipir trisodium and gadopentetate dimeglumine contrast agents. AJR Am J Roentgenol 2004;183(4):1049–54.

18. Towbin AJ, Meyers RL, Woodley H, et al. 2017 PRETEXT: radiologic staging system for primary hepatic malignancies of childhood revised for the Paediatric Hepatic International Tumour Trial (PHITT). Pediatr Radiol 2018;48(4):536–54.

19. Maibach R, Roebuck D, Brugieres L, et al. Prognostic stratification for children with hepatoblastoma: the SIOPEL experience. Eur J Cancer 2012;48(10):1543–9.

20. Malogolowkin MH, Katzenstein HM, Krailo M, et al. Treatment of hepatoblastoma: the North American cooperative group experience. Front Biosci (Elite Ed) 2012;4: 1717–23.

21. Evans AE, D'Angio GJ, Sather HN, et al. A comparison of four staging systems for localized and regional neuroblastoma: a report from the Childrens Cancer Study Group. J Clin Oncol 1990;8(4):678–88.

22. Malogolowkin MH, Katzenstein HM, Meyers RL, et al. Complete surgical resection is curative for children with hepatoblastoma with pure fetal histology: a report from the Children's Oncology Group. J Clin Oncol 2011;29(24):3301–6.

23. Vigano L, Ferrero A, Sgotto E, et al. Bile leak after hepatectomy: predictive factors of spontaneous healing. Am J Surg 2008;196(2):195–200.

24. Becker K, Furch C, Schmid I, et al. Impact of postoperative complications on overall survival of patients with hepatoblastoma. Pediatr Blood Cancer 2015; 62(1):24–8.

25. Pimpalwar AP, Sharif K, Ramani P, et al. Strategy for hepatoblastoma management: transplant versus nontransplant surgery. J Pediatr Surg 2002;37(2):240–5.

26. Otte JB, Meyers RL, de Ville de Goyet J. Transplantation for liver tumors in children: time to (re)set the guidelines? Pediatr Transplant 2013;17(8):710–2.

27. Lautz TB, Ben-Ami T, Tantemsapya N, et al. Successful nontransplant resection of POST-TEXT III and IV hepatoblastoma. Cancer 2011;117(9):1976–83.

28. Otte JB, de Ville de Goyet J, Reding R. Liver transplantation for hepatoblastoma: indications and contraindications in the modern era. Pediatr Transplant 2005; 9(5):557–65.

29. Ramos-Gonzalez G, LaQuaglia M, O'Neill AF, et al. Long-term outcomes of liver transplantation for hepatoblastoma: a single-center 14-year experience. Pediatr Transplant 2018;e13250. https://doi.org/10.1111/petr.13250.

30. Malogolowkin MH, Stanley P, Steele DA, et al. Feasibility and toxicity of chemoembolization for children with liver tumors. J Clin Oncol 2000;18(6):1279–84.

31. Birn J, Williams TR, Croteau D, et al. Transarterial embolization of symptomatic focal nodular hyperplasia. J Vasc Interv Radiol 2013;24(11):1647–55.

32. Czauderna P, Zbrzezniak G, Narozanski W, et al. Preliminary experience with arterial chemoembolization for hepatoblastoma and hepatocellular carcinoma in children. Pediatr Blood Cancer 2006;46(7):825–8.

33. Aguado A, Ristagno R, Towbin AJ, et al. Transarterial radioembolization with yttrium-90 of unresectable primary hepatic malignancy in children. Pediatr Blood Cancer 2019;66(7):e27510.

34. Aguado A, Dunn SP, Averill LW, et al. Successful use of transarterial radioembolization with yttrium-90 (TARE-Y90) in two children with hepatoblastoma. Pediatr Blood Cancer 2020;67(9):e28421.

35. Curley SA, Marra P, Beaty K, et al. Early and late complications after radiofrequency ablation of malignant liver tumors in 608 patients. Ann Surg 2004; 239(4):450–8.

36. Heij HA, Verschuur AC, Kaspers GJ, et al. Is aggressive local treatment necessary for diffuse liver involvement in patients with progression of stage 4s neuroblastoma to stage 4? J Pediatr Surg 2008;43(9):1630–5.

37. Shi Y, Qiao Z, Xia C, et al. Hepatic involvement of Langerhans cell histiocytosis in children–imaging findings of computed tomography, magnetic resonance imaging and magnetic resonance cholangiopancreatography. Pediatr Radiol 2014; 44(6):713–8.

38. McAteer JP, Goldin AB, Healey PJ, et al. Surgical treatment of primary liver tumors in children: outcomes analysis of resection and transplantation in the SEER database. Pediatr Transplant 2013;17(8):744–50.

39. Hubbard AK, Spector LG, Fortuna G, et al. Trends in international incidence of pediatric cancers in children under 5 Years of age: 1988-2012. JNCI Cancer Spectr 2019;3(1):pkz007.

40. Janitz AE, Ramachandran G, Tomlinson GE, et al. Maternal and paternal occupational exposures and hepatoblastoma: results from the HOPE study through the Children's Oncology Group. J Expo Sci Environ Epidemiol 2017;27(4):359–64.

41. Turcotte LM, Georgieff MK, Ross JA, et al. Neonatal medical exposures and characteristics of low birth weight hepatoblastoma cases: a report from the Children's Oncology Group. Pediatr Blood Cancer 2014;61(11):2018–23.

42. Meyers RL, Rowland JR, Krailo M, et al. Predictive power of pretreatment prognostic factors in children with hepatoblastoma: a report from the Children's Oncology Group. Pediatr Blood Cancer 2009;53(6):1016–22.

43. Meyers RL, Tiao GM, Dunn SP, et al. Central Surgical Review Committee CsOGA-ToCwASH. Surgical management of children with locally advanced hepatoblastoma. Cancer 2012;118(16):4090–1 [author reply: 4-5].

44. Katzenstein HM, Chang KW, Krailo M, et al. Children's Oncology G. Amifostine does not prevent platinum-induced hearing loss associated with the treatment of children with hepatoblastoma: a report of the Intergroup Hepatoblastoma Study P9645 as a part of the Children's Oncology Group. Cancer 2009; 115(24):5828–35.

45. O'Neill AF, Towbin AJ, Krailo MD, et al. Characterization of pulmonary metastases in children with hepatoblastoma treated on Children's Oncology group protocol AHEP0731 (the treatment of children with all stages of hepatoblastoma): a report from the Children's Oncology group. J Clin Oncol 2017;35(30):3465–73.

46. Zsiros J, Brugieres L, Brock P, et al. International Childhood Liver Tumours Strategy G. Dose-dense cisplatin-based chemotherapy and surgery for children with high-risk hepatoblastoma (SIOPEL-4): a prospective, single-arm, feasibility study. Lancet Oncol 2013;14(9):834–42.

47. Zsiros J, Maibach R, Shafford E, et al. Successful treatment of childhood high-risk hepatoblastoma with dose-intensive multiagent chemotherapy and surgery: final results of the SIOPEL-3HR study. J Clin Oncol 2010;28(15):2584–90.

48. Perilongo G, Maibach R, Shafford E, et al. Cisplatin versus cisplatin plus doxorubicin for standard-risk hepatoblastoma. N Engl J Med 2009;361(17):1662–70.

49. Semeraro M, Branchereau S, Maibach R, et al. Relapses in hepatoblastoma patients: clinical characteristics and outcome–experience of the International Childhood Liver Tumour Strategy Group (SIOPEL). Eur J Cancer 2013;49(4):915–22.

50. Hery G, Franchi-Abella S, Habes D, et al. Initial liver transplantation for unresectable hepatoblastoma after chemotherapy. Pediatr Blood Cancer 2011;57(7): 1270–5.

51. Schwartz LH, Seymour L, Litière S, et al. RECIST 1.1 - standardisation and disease-specific adaptations: perspectives from the RECIST Working group. Eur J Cancer 2016;62:138–45.

52. Brock PR, Maibach R, Childs M, et al. Sodium thiosulfate for protection from cisplatin-induced hearing loss. N Engl J Med 2018;378(25):2376–85.

53. Malogolowkin MH, Katzenstein HM, Krailo M, et al. Redefining the role of doxorubicin for the treatment of children with hepatoblastoma. J Clin Oncol 2008;26(14): 2379–83.

54. Katzenstein HM, Langham MR, Malogolowkin MH, et al. Minimal adjuvant chemotherapy for children with hepatoblastoma resected at diagnosis (AHEP0731): a Children's Oncology Group, multicentre, phase 3 trial. Lancet Oncol 2019. https://doi.org/10.1016/s1470-2045(18)30895-7.

55. Katzenstein HM, Furman WL, Malogolowkin MH, et al. Upfront window vincristine/irinotecan treatment of high-risk hepatoblastoma: a report from the Children's Oncology Group AHEP0731 study committee. Cancer 2017;123(12):2360–7.

56. Finegold MJ, Lopez-Terrada DH, Bowen J, et al. Protocol for the examination of specimens from pediatric patients with hepatoblastoma. Arch Pathol Lab Med 2007;131(4):520–9.

57. Lopez-Terrada D, Alaggio R, de Davila MT, et al. Towards an international pediatric liver tumor consensus classification: proceedings of the Los Angeles COG liver tumors symposium. Mod Pathol 2014;27(3):472–91.

58. Trobaugh-Lotrario AD, Tomlinson GE, Finegold MJ, et al. Small cell undifferentiated variant of hepatoblastoma: adverse clinical and molecular features similar to rhabdoid tumors. Pediatr Blood Cancer 2009;52(3):328–34.

59. Russo P, Biegel JA. SMARCB1/INI1 alterations and hepatoblastoma: another extrarenal rhabdoid tumor revealed? Pediatr Blood Cancer 2009;52(3):312–3.

60. Awan S, Davenport M, Portmann B, et al. Angiosarcoma of the liver in children. J Pediatr Surg 1996;31(12):1729–32.

61. Nakashima N, Fukatsu T, Nagasaka T, et al. The frequency and histology of hepatic tissue in germ cell tumors. Am J Surg Pathol 1987;11(9):682–92.

62. Villanueva A. Hepatocellular carcinoma. N Engl J Med 2019;380(15):1450–62.

63. Christison-Lagay ER, Burrows PE, Alomari A, et al. Hepatic hemangiomas: subtype classification and development of a clinical practice algorithm and registry. J Pediatr Surg 2007;42(1):62–7 [discussion: 7–8].

64. Drolet BA, Frommelt PC, Chamlin SL, et al. Initiation and use of propranolol for infantile hemangioma: report of a consensus conference. Pediatrics 2013; 131(1):128–40.

65. Draper H, Diamond IR, Temple M, et al. Multimodal management of endangering hepatic hemangioma: impact on transplant avoidance: a descriptive case series. J Pediatr Surg 2008;43(1):120–5 [discussion: 6].

66. Michaud AP, Bauman NM, Burke DK, et al. Spastic diplegia and other motor disturbances in infants receiving interferon-alpha. Laryngoscope 2004;114(7): 1231–6.

67. Stringer MD, Alizai NK. Mesenchymal hamartoma of the liver: a systematic review. J Pediatr Surg 2005;40(11):1681–90.

68. Rajaram V, Knezevich S, Bove KE, et al. DNA sequence of the translocation breakpoints in undifferentiated embryonal sarcoma arising in mesenchymal hamartoma of the liver harboring the t(11;19)(q11;q13.4) translocation. Genes Chromosomes Cancer 2007;46(5):508–13.
69. Apellaniz-Ruiz M, Segni M, Kettwig M, et al. Mesenchymal hamartoma of the liver and DICER1 syndrome. N Engl J Med 2019;380(19):1834–42.
70. Citak EC, Karadeniz C, Oguz A, et al. Nodular regenerative hyperplasia and focal nodular hyperplasia of the liver mimicking hepatic metastasis in children with solid tumors and a review of literature. Pediatr Hematol Oncol 2007;24(4):281–9.
71. Scalori A, Tavani A, Gallus S, et al. Oral contraceptives and the risk of focal nodular hyperplasia of the liver: a case-control study. Am J Obstet Gynecol 2002;186(2):195–7.

Neonatal Neuroblastoma

Andrew M. Davidoff, MD

KEYWORDS

- Neuroblastoma • Neonatal • Observation • Regression • Hepatomegaly

KEY POINTS

- Neuroblastoma occurring in a neonate comprises 5% of the cases of neuroblastoma.
- Most cases of neonatal neuroblastoma are detected in utero by ultrasonography.
- The outcome for neonates with neuroblastoma is excellent, with greater than 90% survival.
- Because of the excellent oncologic outcome for neonatal neuroblastoma, increasingly, these neonates are simply being observed without any initial intervention or therapy.
- Neonates with extensive metastatic tumor burden in the liver fare less well and may benefit from early initiation of systemic chemotherapy.

INTRODUCTION

Neuroblastoma is the most common solid, extracranial malignant neoplasm of childhood and the most common malignant tumor in infants less than 1 year of age, with an overall incidence of 1 per 100,000 children in the United States.[1] The Children's Oncology Group (COG) Statistics and Data Center estimates that neonatal neuroblastoma, defined as neuroblastoma diagnosed prenatally or within 28 days after birth, represents 5% of all neuroblastoma cases.[2]

Neuroblastoma displays a very heterogeneous clinical phenotype, with some tumors spontaneously regressing or maturing (with or without adjuvant therapy), whereas others exhibit an aggressive clinical phenotype and respond poorly to adjuvant therapy. Overall, the 5-year survival rate for children with neuroblastoma is approximately 75%, but those younger than 18 months at presentation, including neonates, have a 5-year survival rate greater than 85%.[3,4] Therefore, the prevailing trend for treating neonates with localized neuroblastoma is to minimize or avoid therapeutic interventions altogether, including surgery and chemotherapy, except for a few specific indications. Most of the morbidity and mortality associated with neonatal neuroblastoma occurs in a subset of patients with disease that has disseminated in a specific pattern, primarily to the liver and not to the bone. This often bulky disease can result in respiratory compromise and abdominal compartment syndrome.

Department of Surgery, St. Jude Children's Research Hospital, 262 Danny Thomas Place, Memphis, TN 38105-3678, USA
E-mail address: andrew.davidoff@stjude.org

Clin Perinatol 48 (2021) 101–115
https://doi.org/10.1016/j.clp.2020.11.006
0095-5108/21/© 2020 Elsevier Inc. All rights reserved.
perinatology.theclinics.com

Approximately 1% to 2% of neuroblastomas are thought to be hereditary, most of which are related to highly penetrant, autosomal dominant germline mutations in PHOX2B (associated with neural crest disorders, including congenital central hypoventilation syndrome and Hirschsprung disease) and ALK.[5,6] As with most pediatric tumors that result from an inherited predisposition, neuroblastomas that develop in the context of these diseases typically occur earlier than sporadic ones, with 1 study identifying a mean age of diagnosis of 9 months versus 2 to 3 years, respectively.[7] Although neuroblastoma is the most common neonatal cancer diagnosis, it is detected rarely within the context of its known cancer predisposition syndromes, such as Li-Fraumeni syndrome (especially the R337H pathogenic variant of TP53), Beckwith Wiedemann syndrome with a germline CDKN1C mutation, germline RAS pathway gene mutations (most frequently Costello syndrome and Noonan syndrome), Simpson-Golabi-Behmel syndrome, or germline variants in more newly discovered genes KIF1B and GALNT14.[8]

PATHOLOGY

Neuroblastoma is an embryonal tumor of the sympathetic nervous system that arises during fetal or early postnatal life from sympathetic cells (sympathogonia) derived from the neural crest. Interestingly, small nodules of primitive neuroblasts are routinely found in the developing adrenal gland, even during the early postnatal period. Beckwith and Perrin[9] described microscopic nodules that they termed neuroblastoma in situ in autopsies of the adrenal glands of infants who died of noncancer-related causes. The incidence of this finding was more than 200-fold greater than the clinical incidence of neuroblastoma, suggesting that many neuroblastoma tumors spontaneously regress or mature into lesions that never become clinically apparent. The process of involution is well described during embryonic life, especially in the developing central and peripheral nervous systems. Although approximately 50% of all neuroblastoma tumors arise in the adrenal gland, greater than 90% of perinatally diagnosed neuroblastoma tumors arise in the adrenals, suggesting a link between perinatal tumors and the nodular collections of neuroblasts that arise during adrenal development. In addition, the cystic variant of perinatal neuroblastoma may be caused by a perturbation of the involution program of these neuroblastic nodules and is associated with excellent prognosis.[10] Although this regression was initially hypothesized to be mediated by the immune system, involution may result from the withdrawal of neurotrophic maintenance factors, such as nerve growth factor. Clinically apparent neuroblastoma can also regress or spontaneously mature, but this mechanism also remains unknown. The notion that many of these incidentally identified neuroblastoma tumors in neonates spontaneously regress and have a favorable prognosis is the premise for the current conservative management of neonatal neuroblastoma.

CLINICAL PRESENTATION

Most perinatal cases arise in the third trimester of gestation in the developing adrenal gland and are detected by fetal ultrasound during routine obstetric care as a solid, subdiaphragmatic mass, although many have a notable cystic component.[10] However, these masses can be identified at times as incidental solid or cystic masses on 20-week screening ultrasound imaging. The increased use of abdominal ultrasonography during pregnancy has led to an increase in the diagnosis of suprarenal masses.[11] In some cases, fetal MRI may be used to evaluate and better define suprarenal masses in utero.[12]

The most common adrenal masses identified in newborns are adrenal hemorrhages, with an estimated incidence of approximately 1 in 500 live births.[13] However, different incidences are reported for other entities in the differential diagnosis of a neonatal adrenal mass.[14,15] Sauvat and colleagues[16] found that approximately 60% of suprarenal masses identified by imaging comprise localized neuroblastoma tumors, although these masses can exhibit appearances similar to those of adrenal hemorrhage, extrapulmonary sequestration, bronchogenic cyst, and renal abnormalities. More recently, a pooled analysis by Schwab and colleagues[17] reported that the most common final diagnosis of prenatally detected suprarenal masses was extralobar pulmonary sequestration (33%), with neuroblastoma comprising 26.5% of 155 cases. Curtis and colleagues[18] developed an algorithm to distinguish between these 2 pathologic entities according to fetal gestational age, mass sidedness, and mass sonographic characteristics (ie, echogenic vs cystic). These masses typically do not cause symptoms either before or after birth; thus, localized neuroblastoma tumors not diagnosed by prenatal imaging usually present as asymptomatic but palpable masses on physical examination.[10]

Paravertebral tumors presenting with spinal cord compression and flaccid leg paralysis and/or bladder and bowel dysfunction were reported in less than 20% of patients with neonatal neuroblastoma.[19] Such tumors represent clinical emergencies that require urgent intervention. Neonatal patients can also present with uncommon paraneoplastic syndromes, such as opsoclonus-myoclonus ataxia, which may arise from cross-reactivity of antineuroblastoma antibodies that recognize Purkinje cells in the cerebellum.[20] The symptoms of opsoclonus-myoclonus syndrome (OMS) consist of myoclonic jerks and random eye movements or progressive cerebellar ataxia. OMS occurs in as many as 4% of patients with neuroblastoma, particularly in infants with thoracic primary tumors.

Neonates with neuroblastoma rarely exhibit standard metastatic disease at diagnosis. Metastatic neonatal neuroblastoma, when it occurs, is most often a unique variant, first described in 1971 by D'Angio and colleagues,[21] and termed stage IVS. Patients with stage IVS neuroblastoma were infants with small primary tumors restricted to 1 side of the midline but with metastases to the liver, skin nodules (ie, blueberry muffin lesions), or limited disease in the bone marrow (<10% of the mononuclear cells), and no involvement of cortical bone. The clinical course of infants with stage IVS neuroblastoma (now referred to as stage MS neuroblastoma and now including patients up to 18 months of age and with any local stage primary tumors) is quite remarkable because the large amount of disease typically undergoes spontaneous regression, even without treatment, and the infants ultimately have no evidence of disease (**Fig. 1**A, B). However, infants, most typically those under 3 months of age, with massive hepatomegaly from large tumor burdens (**Fig. 1**C, D), may suffer organ dysfunction, including respiratory compromise, abdominal compartment syndrome, and coagulopathy, leading to considerable morbidity and even mortality. Acharya and colleagues[22] reported that 5% of perinatal neuroblastoma cases had typical metastatic disease, whereas 22% had the unique pattern of metastatic MS neuroblastoma.

NEUROBLASTOMA SCREENING

Tumor stage and patient age at diagnosis are the principal clinical predictors of outcomes for patients with neuroblastoma. Therefore, early neuroblastoma detection during newborn screenings was hypothesized to reduce neuroblastoma-associated mortality. To this end, urinary vanillylmandelic acid (VMA) and homovanillic acid

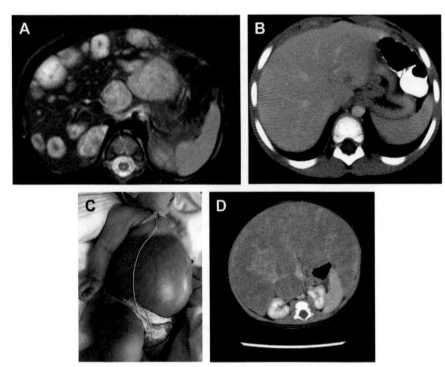

Fig. 1. (A) CT scan of an asymptomatic infant with MS neuroblastoma showing extensive liver infiltration. (B) CT scan of the same infant 3 years later. The patient had received no therapy. (C) A 1-month-old infant with respiratory compromise owing to hepatomegaly from MS neuroblastoma. (D) CT scan of the same 1-month-old infant.

(HVA) levels were assessed in neonates in Japan in the 1980s,[23] but later studies in Germany and North America revealed that these tumors are often early stage and low risk.[24,25] Indeed, the overall mortality of patients with neuroblastoma was not affected by the increased number of cases identified by such screening initiatives. Therefore, these neuroblastoma tumors most likely undergo spontaneous regression before being clinically detected, and so, currently, screening for neuroblastoma is no longer done.

WORKUP
Diagnostic Imaging

Ultrasonography is the modality most often used for fetal assessment and is, therefore, the modality by which most adrenal masses are detected in utero. Ultrasound imaging is generally repeated during the postnatal period to confirm the presence of in utero–detected adrenal masses. Computed tomography (CT) or MRI is then performed to assist in the formation of a differential diagnosis and for further anatomic definition. MRI is the preferred modality for detecting metastases to the bone (very rare in neonates) and bone marrow, in addition to intraspinal tumor extension.[26]

Metaiodobenzylguanidine (MIBG) scintiscan is the preferred imaging modality for evaluating metastatic spread of neuroblastoma. In addition, it is very useful for follow-up surveillance to identify recurrent disease. MIBG is transported to and stored in chromaffin cells in the same way as norepinephrine. Iodine 123–labeled MIBG uptake can be imaged with a scintiscan instrument. However, approximately 10% of neuroblastoma tumors do not exhibit MIBG uptake.

Laboratory Evaluations

The serologic workup for possible neuroblastoma in neonates is limited and nonspecific. Blood tests include lactate dehydrogenase (LDH) and ferritin, both of which lack specificity for neuroblastoma but have prognostic significance. Serologic LDH and ferritin tests are generally readily available, even in poorly resourced countries.[27] High-serum levels of LDH and ferritin reflect the high proliferative activity of the tumor and/or large tumor burden. LDH levels greater than 1500 IU/L and ferritin levels greater than 150 ng/mL appear to be associated with poor prognosis.[27–29] In addition, these serum markers can be used to monitor disease activity or response to therapy.

Urinary levels of catecholamine metabolites are a critical and highly specific laboratory marker for neuroblastoma. Neuroblastoma is characterized by the relatively unique capacity for secretion of catecholamine products, the metabolites of which (ie, HVA and VMA) can be detected in the urine of more than 90% of patients with neuroblastoma. Thus, urine specimens are clinically valuable for diagnosing neuroblastoma and determining response to therapy. Urinary levels of these 2 catabolites can also be used as markers of tumor progression or relapse. Random urine samples are preferable to 24-hour urine estimations for younger children.[30] Spot urine samples for VMA and HVA should be obtained in neonates with an adrenal mass suspected of being a neuroblastoma to further direct the workup and management plan.

RISK STRATIFICATION

Increasing evidence indicates that the clinical, biologic, and molecular features of neuroblastoma are highly predictive of clinical behavior. Therefore, neuroblastoma has been a paradigm for phenotypic risk assessments and treatment assignments. Patients at low risk for relapse, including most neonates, can have treatment intensity diminished to avoid therapy-associated toxicity and still achieve a high rate of cure. Patient age and extent of disease at diagnosis are important clinical variables.[31–33]

Data from London and colleagues,[32] on behalf of the COG, suggest that the prognostic contribution of age to outcome in patients with neuroblastoma is continuous in nature. They found that an age cutoff of 460 days is clinically relevant for risk stratification of high-risk disease. Additional data from Moroz and colleagues,[31] on behalf of the International Neuroblastoma Risk Group (INRG), suggest that an age-at-diagnosis cutoff of greater than 18 months is associated with high-risk disease.

Most perinatal patients with neuroblastoma (>70%) have localized tumors that arise in the adrenal gland (>90%). The current pretreatment staging system, developed by the INRG in 2009, is based on tumor imaging rather than on the extent of surgical resection.[34] In this staging system (Table 1), localized tumors are staged based on the absence (L1) or presence (L2) of 1 or more of 20 image-defined risk factors (IDRFs). Cecchetto and colleagues[35] reported that the presence of 1 or more of these surgical IDRFs was associated with a lower complete resection rate and a greater risk of surgery-related complications when attempting initial resection of localized neuroblastoma.

The IDRFs are listed in Table 2 and generally reflect encasement of vital structures, primarily vessels, and nerves, as determined by diagnostic imaging studies. In a review of 661 patients in the INRG database, Monclair and colleagues[34] found that INRG staging had prognostic value. Patients with stage L1 disease had significantly

Table 1
The International Neuroblastoma Risk Group staging system

INRG Stage	Description
L1	Localized tumor not involving vital structures as defined by IDRFs and confined to 1 body compartment (neck, chest, abdomen, pelvis)
L2	Locoregional tumor with one or more IDRFs
M	Distant metastatic disease (except MS)
MS	Metastatic disease in children younger than 18 mo with metastases confined to skin, liver, and/or bone marrow (bone marrow involvement should be limited to <10% of total nucleated cells on smears or biopsy). Primary tumor may be L1 or L2 as defined above

Table 2
Image-defined risk factors for primary resection of localized neuroblastoma

Anatomic Region	Description
Multiple body compartments	Ipsilateral tumor extension within 2 body compartments (ie, neck and chest, chest and abdomen, or abdomen and pelvis)
Neck	Tumor encasing carotid artery, vertebral artery, and/or internal jugular vein Tumor extending to skull base Tumor compressing trachea
Cervicothoracic junction	Tumor encasing brachial plexus roots Tumor encasing subclavian vessels, vertebral artery, and/or carotid artery Tumor compressing trachea
Thorax	Tumor encasing aorta and/or major branches Tumor compressing trachea and/or principal bronchi Lower mediastinal tumor infiltrating costovertebral junction between T9 and T12 (may involve the artery of Adamkiewicz supplying the lower spinal cord)
Thoracoabdominal junction	Tumor encasing aorta and/or vena cava
Abdomen and pelvis	Tumor infiltrating porta hepatis and/or hepatoduodenal ligament Tumor encasing branches of superior mesenteric artery at mesenteric root Tumor encasing origin of celiac axis and/or origin of superior mesenteric artery Tumor invading one or both renal pedicles Tumor encasing aorta and/or vena cava Tumor encasing iliac vessels Pelvic tumor crossing sciatic notch
Intraspinal tumor extension	Intraspinal tumor extension (whatever the location) provided that more than one-third of spinal canal in axial plane is invaded, the perimedullary leptomeningeal spaces are not visible, or the spinal cord signal intensity is abnormal
Infiltration of adjacent organs and structures	Pericardium, diaphragm, kidney, liver, duodenopancreatic block, and mesentery

greater 5-year event-free survival (EFS) rates than those with stage L2 disease (90% ± 3% vs 78% ± 4%, P = .001).

The most powerful biologic factors include MYCN status, DNA index (ploidy), the allelic status at chromosome 11q23, and histopathologic classification.[36–38] Overall, approximately 25% of primary neuroblastoma tumors in children display amplification of the MYCN protooncogene, with amplifications in 40% of patients with advanced disease, but in only 5% to 10% of patients with low-stage disease.[37] Amplification of MYCN is associated with rapid tumor progression and poor outcomes; therefore, it is a powerful prognostic indicator of tumor behavior.[37,39] However, MYCN amplification is rarely present in neonates with neuroblastoma.

The ploidy or DNA index of a tumor is the ratio of the number of chromosomes present to the diploid number of chromosomes (ie, 46). Patients with near-triploid (or hyperdiploid) tumors typically have favorable clinical and biologic prognostic factors, and excellent survival rates, as compared with that of patients who have near-diploid or near-tetraploid tumors.[40] Neuroblastoma tumors that are near-diploid or near-tetraploid usually have structural genetic abnormalities, most frequently chromosome 1p deletion and MYCN amplification. This association is most important for infants with advanced disease because the prognostic importance of tumor ploidy appears to be lost in patients older than 2 years.[41] Thus, ploidy is relevant only for risk group assessment of very limited subgroups of patients with neuroblastoma.

Deletion of the long arm of chromosome 11 (11q) is also common in neuroblastoma and is present in approximately 40% of cases. Unbalanced deletion of 11q (loss with either retention or gain of 11p material) is inversely related to MYCN amplification[42] yet is strongly associated with other high-risk features. Attiyeh and colleagues,[42] on behalf of the COG, showed in a large cohort of patients that unbalanced deletion of 11q is independently associated with worse outcomes in patients with neuroblastoma. Thirty percent of tumors in infants had 11p aberrations, whereas 36% of tumors in patients older than 1 year had 11p aberrations (P = .07).[42] Taken together, these clinical and biologic variables define the COG risk stratification used for current clinical trials.

Risk Classification

To establish an international consensus on pretreatment risk stratification, the INRG task force developed the INRG Classification System, in which 7 prognostic variables defined 16 different pretreatment risk groups (**Table 3**). These risk groups were then separated into 4 categories according to the expected 5-year EFS: very low (>85% EFS, 28.2% of patients), low (>75% to ≤85% EFS, 26.8% of patients), intermediate (≥50% to 75% EFS, 9.0% of patients), and high (<50% EFS, 36.1% of patients) risk.[34] The predicted overall survival for patients in each group is greater than 90% except for those in the high-risk group, whose overall survival is less than 50%. Most neonates are categorized into the very low- or low-risk groups. A small percentage of patients have stage L2 disease with 11q aberrations (or other unfavorable genetic characteristics) or metastatic disease with diploid tumors and, therefore, have intermediate-risk neuroblastoma. Because the incidence of high-risk neuroblastoma in neonates is so rare, the management of high-risk neuroblastoma is not discussed further in this review.

TREATMENT

The clinical and biologic characteristics present at diagnosis identify cohorts of patients with non–high-risk neuroblastoma. The survival rates of non–high-risk neuroblastoma approach 100%, and exposure to chemotherapy or surgery may be

Table 3
International Neuroblastoma Risk Group pretreatment classification

INRG Stage	Age (mo)	Histologic Category	Grade of Tumor Differentiation	MYCN	11q Aberration	Ploidy	Pretreatment Risk Group
L1/L2		GN maturing; GNB intermixed					A: Very low
L1		Any, except GN maturing or GNB intermixed		NA			B: Very low
				Amp			K: High
L2	<18	Any, except GN maturing or GNB intermixed		NA	No		D: Low
				NA	Yes		G: Intermediate
	>18	GNB nodular, neuroblastoma	Differentiating	NA	No		E: Low
				NA	Yes		H: Intermediate
			Poorly differentiated or undifferentiated	NA			H: Intermediate
				Amp			N: High
M	<18			NA		Hyperdiploid	F: Low
	<12			NA		Diploid	I: Intermediate
	12 to <18			NA		Diploid	J: Intermediate
	<18			Amp			O: High
	≥18						P: High
MS	<18			NA	No		C: Very low
					Yes		Q: High
							R: High

unnecessary for these patients. Small case series and recent clinical trials suggest that infants with perinatally diagnosed small primary tumors and nonmetastatic disease have excellent outcomes without intervention, including surgical biopsies or resections.[43,44] Therefore, an expectant observation study of patients with these lesions to further define their natural history was performed by the COG (ANBL00P2). This study was designed to test the hypothesis that close biochemical and sonographic observation could be safely applied in infants with small adrenal masses. Resection was reserved for rare cases with evidence of continued growth. To be eligible for the trial, infants with adrenal masses had to be younger than 6 months when the mass was first identified; the mass had to be less than 16 mL in volume for solid tumors or less than 65 mL for $\geq$25% cystic tumors, and the disease must have been limited to the adrenal gland. The results from this study confirmed that expectant observation of infants with small adrenal masses led to excellent 3-year EFS rates (97.7% $\pm$ 2.3%) and 100% overall survival, while avoiding surgical interventions in greater than 80% of patients.[45]

Currently, localized tumors without any IDRFs (stage L1) in patients younger than 1 year at the time of presentation and with tumors less than 5 cm by imaging studies are being followed in the observation-only COG study ANBL1232 in group A of this study. This trial expands upon the eligibility for the ANBL00P2 trial by increasing the age cutoff from 6 months to 12 months, increasing the tumor size from 3.1 cm to 5 cm, and permitting nonadrenal primary tumors to be observed. Patients with nonadrenal tumors must have either a positive MIBG scintiscan or elevated levels of urinary catecholamine metabolites to be eligible. Bone marrow aspirates and/or biopsies for staging are not required unless a patient has abnormal complete blood count values or demonstrates clinical symptoms suggestive of bone marrow involvement. A spine MRI is required for patients with a paraspinal mass to evaluate whether cord compression is evident.

Patients who meet the group A treatment criteria are observed without tumor biopsy or intervention for 96 weeks (approximately 2 years) with routine follow-ups. The follow-up examinations include imaging evaluations in which serial imaging by ultrasound and MRI are preferred to CT imaging to decrease the degree of radiation exposure, and ultrasound is preferred to MRI, when feasible, to avoid the risks associated with general anesthesia. The follow-up examinations also include laboratory assessments (ie, urine or serum catecholamines, HVA, and VMA) and physical examinations for evidence of progression and/or metastatic spread. If patients experience disease progression (>50% increase in the primary tumor volume or >50% increase in either VMA or HVA), surgical resection is recommended. If tumors are completely resected, as should be possible with most L1 tumors, no adjuvant therapy is administered, regardless of the tumor biologic factors. Tumors that persist after 96 weeks of observation do not need to be resected.

Patients younger than 18 months with INRG stage L2 tumors (at least 1 IDRF) are also potentially eligible for the ANBL1232 study, in group B. However, biopsies are required, and only those patients who are asymptomatic (ie, no life-threatening symptoms or impending neurologic or other organ function compromise) and whose tumors have favorable histologic and genomic features can be observed. Favorable genomics are defined as hyperdiploid tumors without segmental aberrations, including somatic copy number loss at 1p, 3p, 4p, or 11q or somatic copy number gain at 1q, 2p, or 17q. Any patient with greater than 25% increased tumor volume at any time during the 3-year observation period will receive 2 cycles of chemotherapy and/or surgical resection, if feasible. Additional cycles of chemotherapy may be administered in 2-cycle increments for a total of 4, 6, or 8 (maximum) cycles of front-line chemotherapy. The goal of this approach is to attain a partial response or better by using a combination of chemotherapy and surgical resection. Once a partial response or better is achieved, patients will be observed with routine imaging for 3 years after completing chemotherapy and/or surgery.

The study objective for very young patients with localized (stage L1 or L2) disease is to eliminate therapy as the initial approach, while maintaining an overall survival rate of greater than 99%. The main impetus for such observational protocols for managing very low- and low-risk neuroblastoma in young children is to mitigate the risks of surgery and anesthesia for neonates and infants. Because extensive surgery is often required for tumors with IDRFs, intraoperative and postoperative complications are common, including bleeding, vascular injuries, and injuries to other viscera (eg, stomach, bowel, liver, spleen, or kidney).[46,47] Considerable risks are associated with tumor resection in patients with neuroblastoma, particularly in young infants, with complication rates ranging from 10% to 18%.[48] A report from the LNESG1 study reported a 4.8% surgical complication rate in a patient population similar to that of ANBL1232 group A patients without surgical IDRFs. In addition, 2% of patients who underwent biopsy without attempted resection experienced surgical complications (ie, severe bleeding, Horner syndrome, and venous thrombosis).[35] In addition, hypertension, chylous leak, pleural effusion, infection and sepsis, diarrhea, and prolonged total parenteral nutrition requirement can occur with neuroblastoma resection.[48,49] Rarely, patients require emergency reexplorative surgeries for postoperative hemorrhages or for bowel obstructions. Wound complications and postoperative bowel obstructions occur in 1% to 5% of cases. The overall mortality for young infants receiving adrenal gland surgeries for tumor resection is approximately 2%.[48] Finally, anesthetic complications are a risk for all surgical procedures, and infants are at higher risk. Such anesthetic complications include acute airway/oxygenation issues and long-term neurologic sequelae.[50,51] Ironically, the trend for observing localized neuroblastic tumors rather than surgical resection comes at a time when considerable advances are being made in minimally invasive surgery (eg, laparoscopy and thoracoscopy). Consequently, most stage L1 lesions can be easily resected by a surgeon with experience in minimally invasive techniques with minimal morbidity, small incisions, and rapid recovery.

Stage MS Neuroblastoma

Supportive therapy only is recommended for this stage of neuroblastoma because of the high incidence of spontaneous regression and generally excellent prognosis.[52] Most of these patients have tumors with favorable biology (ie, single-copy MYCN, favorable Shimada histology, and DNA index >1). Therefore, they are assigned to the low-risk group and receive no therapy. However, despite the typically benign course of their cancer, these infants can die of complications caused by the initial bulk of their disease, and earlier initiation of treatment or modification of current therapy may be beneficial. Limited chemotherapy, local irradiation, or minimal resection can be used to treat infants with stage MS neuroblastoma and the life-threatening symptoms of hepatomegaly who have the potential for rapid clinical deterioration and may benefit from early initiation of therapy.

The age at diagnosis for stage MS neuroblastoma is an important prognostic factor for clinical deterioration owing to hepatomegaly.[52–54] Younger patients (ie, neonates) are at higher risk of death from hepatomegaly and/or related complications. Of infants who died of stage MS disease associated with hepatomegaly, greater than 90% of these deaths occurred in patients younger than 2 months at diagnosis and were attributed to respiratory compromise or disseminated intravascular coagulation/hepatic dysfunction. These data suggest that this cohort could benefit from earlier interventions and more intense treatments. Decompressive laparotomy with creation of a silastic pouch may be needed for marked hepatomegaly, causing either respiratory compromise secondary to diaphragmatic elevation or obstruction of the inferior vena cava. This procedure may prevent life-threatening events until reduction of liver size is achieved by either spontaneous regression or therapy.

As proposed in the ANBL1232 protocol (group C), patients younger than 18 months who are asymptomatic and have tumors with favorable biology are observed. If patients are symptomatic, age is the next considered criteria: patients younger than 3 months receive immediate chemotherapy (without biopsy), whereas patients 3 to 18 months old have a tumor biopsy and proceed through a response-based algorithm to determine the length of treatment. Rare cases of stage MS neuroblastoma in infants with either unfavorable Shimada histology or a DNA index of 1 (or if the biology is not known) are treated as intermediate-risk disease. The very rare neonatal stage MS tumors with *MYCN* amplifications are treated as high-risk disease. The algorithm for managing neonatal stage MS disease in the COG protocol is shown in **Table 4**. The goal for patients in group C who require treatment is to achieve a reduction in primary tumor size by at least 50% (ie, partial response) with resolution of all symptoms and any laboratory abnormalities present at therapy initiation. Patients must be asymptomatic to stop therapy. Once this has been achieved, patients will be observed with routine imaging for 3 years after completing chemotherapy and/or surgery.

Intraspinal Extension of Neuroblastoma

In a subset of patients with paraspinal neuroblastoma, tumor growth may extend into the spinal canal (ie, dumbbell tumors). If neurologic symptoms result, urgent treatment is required to prevent permanent injury caused by cord compression. Chemotherapy is generally considered most appropriate for the initial management of these tumors, given the long-term consequences of spinal surgery and radiation therapy, especially in young patients. In patients with acutely progressive symptoms, however, emergent surgical decompression of the spinal cord may be critical to yield acceptable neurologic outcomes.[55]

The appropriate approach for patients with asymptomatic intraspinal tumor extension is also uncertain. For patients with low- or intermediate-risk disease, the risks of attempting to remove the intraspinal component of a paraspinal tumor most likely outweigh its potential benefits. This situation most commonly arises in patients with

---

Table 4
Children's Oncology Group Trial ANBL1232 treatment assignment for neonates with stage MS neuroblastoma

Biology (Histology and Genomics)	Symptoms	Treatment
Any	Existing or evolving hepatomegaly	Immediate treatment with response-based chemotherapy
Favorable	Asymptomatic, without existing or evolving hepatomegaly	Observe
Unfavorable histology or unfavorable genomics or histology/ genomics unknown		Response-based chemotherapy

thoracic primary tumors. The intrathoracic component is resected, and gross residual disease remains in the spinal canal. Care should be taken to minimize operative complications, such as leakage of cerebrospinal fluid or uncontrollable intraspinal bleeding. Because residual foraminal disease rarely reaches a symptomatic size, the importance of conservative therapy in this circumstance should be emphasized.

SUMMARY

Most perinatal neuroblastoma tumors are detected by prenatal ultrasonography as solid or cystic subdiaphragmatic masses, have favorable biologic and clinical features (ie, >95% *MYCN* nonamplified, >95% favorable histology, <5% metastases [excluding stage MS tumors]), and have excellent outcomes (4-year EFS = 92%, overall survival = 96%). Therefore, patients with these tumors are increasingly being observed without any initial therapy. Neonates with stage MS disease also have excellent outcomes, although those with hepatomegaly are at risk of respiratory decompensation and abdominal compartment syndrome and will most likely benefit from early initiation of systemic chemotherapy.

ACKNOWLEDGMENTS

Thanks to Nisha Badders for editing this article.

DISCLOSURES

None.

REFERENCES

1. Brodeur GM, Hogarty MD, Mosse YP, et al. Neuroblastoma. In: Pizzo PA, Poplack DG, editors. Principles and practice of pediatric oncology. 6th edition. Philadelphia: Lippincott; 2011. p. 886–922.
2. Interiano RB, Davidoff AM. Current management of neonatal neuroblastoma. Curr Pediatr Rev 2015;11(3):179–87.
3. Gigliotti AR, Di Cataldo A, Sorrentino S, et al. Neuroblastoma in the newborn. A study of the Italian neuroblastoma registry. Eur J Cancer 2009;45(18):3220–7.
4. Zhou YLK, Zheng S, Chen L. Retrospective study of neuroblastoma in Chinese neonates from 1994 to 2011: an evaluation of diagnosis, treatments, and prognosis: a 10-year retrospective study of neonatal neuroblastoma. J Cancer Res Clin Oncol 2014;140(1):83–7.
5. Kamihara J, Bourdeaut F, Foulkes WD, et al. Retinoblastoma and neuroblastoma predisposition and surveillance. Clin Cancer Res 2017;23(13):e98–106.
6. Ritenour LE, Randall MP, Bosse KR, et al. Genetic susceptibility to neuroblastoma: current knowledge and future directions. Cell Tissue Res 2018;372(2): 287–307.
7. Park JR, Eggert A, Caron H. Neuroblastoma: biology, prognosis, and treatment. Hematol Oncol Clin North Am 2010;24(1):65–86.
8. Scollon S, Anglin AK, Thomas M, et al. A comprehensive review of pediatric tumors and associated cancer predisposition syndromes. J Genet Couns 2017; 26(3):387–434.
9. Beckwith JB, Perrin EV. In situ neuroblastomas: a contribution to the natural history of neural crest. Am J Pathol 1963;43(6):1089–104.
10. Nuchtern JG. Perinatal neuroblastoma. Semin Pediatr Surg 2006;15(1):10–6.

11. Nadler EP, Barksdale EM. Adrenal masses in the newborn. Semin Pediatr Surg 2000;9(3):156–64.

12. Flanagan SM, Rubesova E, Jaramillo D, et al. Fetal suprarenal masses–assessing the complementary role of magnetic resonance and ultrasound for diagnosis. Pediatr Radiol 2016;46(2):246–54.

13. Fang SB, Lee HC, Sheu JC, et al. Prenatal sonographic detection of adrenal hemorrhage confirmed by postnatal surgery. J Clin Ultrasound 1999;27(4):206–9.

14. Yao W, Li K, Xiao X, et al. Neonatal suprarenal mass: differential diagnosis and treatment. J Cancer Res Clin Oncol 2013;139(2):281–6.

15. Geurten C, Geurten M, Rigo V, et al. Neonatal cancer epidemiology and outcome: a retrospective study. J Pediatr Hematol Oncol 2020;42(5):e286–92.

16. Sauvat F, Sarnacki S, Brisse H, et al. Outcome of suprarenal localized masses diagnosed during the perinatal period: a retrospective multicenter study. Cancer 2002;94(9):2474–80.

17. Schwab ME, Braun HJ, Padilla BE. Imaging modalities and management of prenatally diagnosed suprarenal masses: an updated literature review and the experience at a high volume Fetal Treatment Center. J Matern Fetal Neonatal Med 2020;1–8. https://doi.org/10.1080/14767058.2020.1716719.

18. Curtis MR, Mooney DP, Vaccaro TJ, et al. Prenatal ultrasound characterization of the suprarenal mass: distinction between neuroblastoma and subdiaphragmatic extralobar pulmonary sequestration. J Ultrasound Med 1997;16(2):75–83.

19. Moppet JHI, Foot AB. Neonatal neuroblastoma. Arch Dis Child Fetal Neonatal Ed 1999;81(2):F134–7.

20. Antunes NL, Khakoo Y, Matthay KK, et al. Antineuronal antibodies in patients with neuroblastoma and paraneoplastic opsoclonus-myoclonus. J Pediatr Hematol Oncol 2000;22(4):315–20.

21. D'Angio GJ, Evans AE, Koop CE. Special pattern of widespread neuroblastoma with a favourable prognosis. Lancet 1971;1(7708):1046–9.

22. Acharya S, Jayabose S, Kogan SJ, et al. Prenatally diagnosed neuroblastoma. Cancer 1997;80(2):304–10.

23. Sawada T. Past and future of neuroblastoma screening in Japan. Am J Pediatr Hematol Oncol 1992;14(4):320–6.

24. Schilling FH, Spix C, Berthold F, et al. Neuroblastoma screening at one year of age. N Engl J Med 2002;346(14):1047–53.

25. Woods WG, Gao RN, Shuster JJ, et al. Screening of infants and mortality due to neuroblastoma. N Engl J Med 2002;346(14):1041–6.

26. Siegel MJ, Ishwaran H, Fletcher BD, et al. Staging of neuroblastoma at imaging: report of the radiology diagnostic oncology group. Radiology 2002;223(1):168–75.

27. Moroz V, Machin D, Hero B, et al. The prognostic strength of serum LDH and serum ferritin in children with neuroblastoma: a report from the International Neuroblastoma Risk Group (INRG) project. Pediatr Blood Cancer 2020;67(8):e28359.

28. Joshi VV, Cantor AB, Brodeur GM, et al. Correlation between morphologic and other prognostic markers of neuroblastoma. A study of histologic grade, DNA index, N-myc gene copy number, and lactic dehydrogenase in patients in the Pediatric Oncology Group. Cancer 1993;71(10):3173–81.

29. Silber JH, Evans AE, Fridman M. Models to predict outcome from childhood neuroblastoma: the role of serum ferritin and tumor histology. Cancer Res 1991;51(5):1426–33.

30. Fitzgibbon MC, Tormey WP. Paediatric reference ranges for urinary catechol-amines/metabolites and their relevance in neuroblastoma diagnosis. Ann Clin Biochem 1994;31(Pt 1):1–11.
31. Moroz V, Machin D, Faldum A, et al. Changes over three decades in outcome and the prognostic influence of age-at-diagnosis in young patients with neuroblastoma: a report from the International Neuroblastoma Risk Group project. Eur J Cancer 2011;47(4):561–71.
32. London WB, Castleberry RP, Matthay KK, et al. Evidence for an age cutoff greater than 365 days for neuroblastoma risk group stratification in the Children's Oncology Group. J Clin Oncol 2005;23(27):6459–65.
33. Evans AE, D'Angio GJ, Propert K, et al. Prognostic factor in neuroblastoma. Cancer 1987;59(11):1853–9.
34. Monclair T, Brodeur GM, Ambros PF, et al. The International Neuroblastoma Risk Group (INRG) staging system: an INRG task force report. J Clin Oncol 2009;27(2):298–303.
35. Cecchetto G, Mosseri V, De Bernardi B, et al. Surgical risk factors in primary surgery for localized neuroblastoma: the LNESG1 study of the European international society of pediatric oncology neuroblastoma group. J Clin Oncol 2005;23(33):8483–9.
36. Shimada H, Umehara S, Monobe Y, et al. International neuroblastoma pathology classification for prognostic evaluation of patients with peripheral neuroblastic tumors: a report from the Children's cancer group. Cancer 2001;92(9):2451–61.
37. Brodeur GM, Seeger RC, Schwab M, et al. Amplification of N-myc in untreated human neuroblastomas correlates with advanced disease stage. Science 1984;224(4653):1121–4.
38. Seeger RC, Brodeur GM, Sather H, et al. Association of multiple copies of the N-myc oncogene with rapid progression of neuroblastomas. N Engl J Med 1985;313(18):1111–6.
39. Brodeur GM, Hayes FA, Green AA, et al. Consistent N-myc copy number in simultaneous or consecutive neuroblastoma samples from sixty individual patients. Cancer Res 1987;47(16):4248–53.
40. Look AT, Hayes FA, Nitschke R, et al. Cellular DNA content as a predictor of response to chemotherapy in infants with unresectable neuroblastoma. N Engl J Med 1984;311(4):231–5.
41. Bowman LC, Castleberry RP, Cantor A, et al. Genetic staging of unresectable or metastatic neuroblastoma in infants: a Pediatric Oncology Group study. J Natl Cancer Inst 1997;89(5):373–80.
42. Attiyeh EF, London WB, Mossé YP, et al. Chromosome 1p and 11q deletions and outcome in neuroblastoma. N Engl J Med 2005;353(21):2243–53.
43. Yamamoto K, Hanada R, Kikuchi A, et al. Spontaneous regression of localized neuroblastoma detected by mass screening. J Clin Oncol 1998;16(4):1265–9.
44. Oue T, Inoue M, Yoneda A, et al. Profile of neuroblastoma detected by mass screening, resected after observation without treatment: results of the Wait and See pilot study. J Pediatr Surg 2005;40(2):359–63.
45. Nuchtern JG, London WB, Barnewolt CE, et al. A prospective study of expectant observation as primary therapy for neuroblastoma in young infants: a Children's Oncology Group study. Ann Surg 2012;256(4):573–80.
46. Azizkhan RG, Shaw A, Chandler JG. Surgical complications of neuroblastoma resection. Surgery 1985;97(5):514–7.
47. Losty P, Quinn F, Breatnach F, et al. Neuroblastoma–a surgical perspective. Eur J Surg Oncol 1993;19(1):33–6.

48. Ikeda H, Suzuki N, Takahashi A, et al. Surgical treatment of neuroblastomas in infants under 12 months of age. J Pediatr Surg 1998;33(8):1246–50.

49. Barrette S, Bernstein ML, Leclerc JM, et al. Treatment complications in children diagnosed with neuroblastoma during a screening program. J Clin Oncol 2006; 24(10):1542–5.

50. Tiret L, Nivoche Y, Hatton F, et al. Complications related to anaesthesia in infants and children. A prospective survey of 40240 anaesthetics. Br J Anaesth 1988; 61(3):263–9.

51. Sun LS, Li G, Miller TL, et al. Association between a single general anesthesia exposure before age 36 months and neurocognitive outcomes in later childhood. JAMA 2016;315(21):2312–20.

52. Nickerson HJ, Matthay KK, Seeger RC, et al. Favorable biology and outcome of stage IV-S neuroblastoma with supportive care or minimal therapy: a Children's Cancer Group study. J Clin Oncol 2000;18(3):477–86.

53. De Bernardi B, Di Cataldo A, Garaventa A, et al. Stage 4 s neuroblastoma: features, management and outcome of 268 cases from the Italian Neuroblastoma Registry. Ital J Pediatr 2019;45(1):8.

54. Twist CJ, Naranjo A, Schmidt ML, et al. Defining risk factors for chemotherapeutic intervention in infants with stage 4S neuroblastoma: a report from Children's Oncology Group study ANBL0531. J Clin Oncol 2019;37(2):115–24.

55. Katzenstein HM, Kent PM, London WB, et al. Treatment and outcome of 83 children with intraspinal neuroblastoma: the Pediatric Oncology Group experience. J Clin Oncol 2001;19(4):1047–55.

Advances in the Diagnosis and Management of Neonatal Sarcomas

Tooba Rashid, BSc[a], David H. Noyd, MD, MPH[a],
Natasha Iranzad, MD[b], Joseph T. Davis, MD[c],
Michael D. Deel, MD[a],*

KEYWORDS

- Neonatal • Sarcoma • Infantile fibrosarcoma • Rhabdomyosarcoma
- Soft tissue sarcoma

INTRODUCTION

Neonatal soft tissue sarcomas represent a heterogeneous group of malignant tumors of primitive mesenchymal tissue. Tumors occurring in the neonatal period are generally defined as those presenting prenatally or within the first few months of life. Neonatal cancers represent only a small percentage of all pediatric malignancies, and neonatal sarcomas represent only a small fraction of neoplastic disorders occurring in this population. The rarity and heterogeneity of neonatal sarcomas contribute to the paucity of understanding of their underlying biology and knowledge of the most optimal treatment approaches. Despite having overlapping histologic features, the clinical behavior and sometimes molecular profile of neonatal sarcomas can be vastly different from that of similar histologic sarcoma subtypes seen in older children and adults. Because researchers cannot extrapolate from data in older patients, the biologic differences unique to neonatal sarcomas have made studying these tumors especially difficult.

Historically, therapy for neonatal sarcomas involved aggressive surgical resections that frequently necessitated disabling or mutilating procedures. However, cooperation through collaborative clinical trials over the past few decades has led to an improved understanding of neonatal sarcoma biology and clinical behavior. Today, a multimodal approach with surgery, radiotherapy, and chemotherapy is typically used. Despite

[a] Pediatric Hematology/Oncology, Duke University School of Medicine, DUMC, Box 102382, Durham, NC 27710, USA; [b] Pediatric Hematology/Oncology, Duke University School of Medicine, DUMC, Box 3712, Durham, NC 27710, USA; [c] Pediatric Hematology/Oncology, Duke University School of Medicine, DUMC, Box 3808, Durham, NC 27710, USA
* Corresponding author. DUMC, Box 102382, Durham, NC 27710.
E-mail address: michael.deel@duke.edu

Clin Perinatol 48 (2021) 117–145
https://doi.org/10.1016/j.clp.2020.11.007
0095-5108/21/© 2020 Elsevier Inc. All rights reserved.
perinatology.theclinics.com

DIAGNOSTIC CONSIDERATIONS

The diagnostic workup for a neonatal soft tissue mass typically includes radiographic imaging and either surgical tissue sampling or excision. Radiographic findings are often nonspecific, making it difficult to distinguish benign from malignant tumors. Selecting the optimal imaging modality to evaluate a neonatal mass requires a careful consideration of both logistical and safety concerns specific to this young age group. Ultrasound examination lacks ionizing radiation and has the advantages of being readily available without the need for sedation or anesthesia. However, most neonates with a soft tissue mass will require cross-sectional imaging to better delineate the tumor involvement and staging, to determine the resectability of the tumor, and to assess for sites of metastatic disease.[7,8]

Because computed tomography (CT) scans are rapid—usually 10 seconds or less—these scans can often be performed in neonates without needing sedation. CT scans are also preferred for chest imaging when assessing for lung metastases.[9] However, despite efforts to decrease the amount of ionizing radiation exposure during the study, CT scans do carry a risk of secondary malignancies associated with radiation exposure, and this risk varies with (and is in fact inversely proportional to) age.[10] MRI offers the advantage of not using ionizing radiation. However, the study time for MRI is substantially longer and can be limited by motion artifact. Therefore, performing an MRI in a neonate may necessitate sedation or anesthesia, which carry short-term safety risks as well as well as concerns for longer term neurocognitive development. The stochastic risks of CT radiation and short-term safety and long-term neurocognitive risks of general anesthesia are both quite small and difficult to quantify.[10] It should also be noted that any loss of life expectancy from diagnostic ionizing radiation exposure is almost certainly a negligible fraction of the loss of life expectance from simply having a diagnosis of malignancy. Therefore, the choice of imaging modality should be based on which modality will offer the most helpful and actionable information.

In addition to cross-sectional imaging, completing the staging workup for malignant soft tissue sarcomas has historically included performing a bone scan. However, for some sarcomas, including Ewing sarcoma and rhabdomyosarcoma, positron emission tomography (PET) or PET/CT scanning is increasingly being accepted as the new standard, with improvement over bone scan in detecting nodal and bone cortical and marrow involvement.[11] For nonrhabdomyosarcoma soft tissue sarcoma (NRSTS), the role of the PET scan is still being prospectively evaluated.[11] In a few pediatric sarcoma studies, PET scans have been shown to be superior to conventional CT scans or MRI in detecting nodal and bone disease, but inferior to CT scans in detecting lung metastases.[12] In addition, a few smaller studies have suggested that metabolic response in fluorine-18-fluorodeoxyglucose uptake in response to therapy may have prognostic significance,[13] although this observation was not seen in a larger study.[14] Given the potential for improved staging accuracy, PET/CT scanning is now routinely being incorporated into the diagnostic workup for pediatric sarcomas, although its usefulness should be weighed against the aforementioned risks in the neonatal population. Similarly, no standardized modality for surveillance imaging exists, although a combination of a CT scan of the chest and either a CT scan or MRI of the primary tumor or a PET/CT scan is typically performed at routine intervals.

An experienced and specialized multidisciplinary approach is essential for evaluating suspected sarcoma cases in neonates. Therefore, given the rarity and complexity of diagnosing and treating neonatal sarcomas, any infant with an atypical soft tissue mass should be managed at a tertiary care pediatric cancer center. In addition to imaging, diagnostic tissue is required. Ideally, the surgeon who will be performing the resection should be involved in the initial biopsy because untrained biopsy placement can negatively impact the ability to achieve a resection with negative margins. Diagnosing a specific rare sarcoma can be challenging, so adequate diagnostic tissue to perform conventional histology and immunohistochemical analysis, as well as cytogenetic and molecular testing, is crucial.[15]

The pathologic evaluation of neonatal soft tissue tumors begins with a gross evaluation followed by the collection of representative samples. The selection of tumor sections for a morphologic evaluation is guided by macroscopic features, tumor heterogeneity, and specimen size. This process is similar to that which is performed in the evaluation of adult soft tissue tumors. One additional step taken for pediatric patients, particularly for those with small round blue cell tumors, is ideally a small piece of fresh tissue should be snap frozen at triage and put on hold to await selection of additional studies after the morphologic evaluation. Neonatal soft tissue tumors can broadly be divided into 3 morphologic categories: spindle cell tumors, vascular tumors, and small round cell tumors.[16] Within these categories, certain tumors may have characteristic features, but, in general, there tends to be considerable morphologic overlap. As such, immunohistochemical stains play a pivotal role in the diagnosis of soft tissue tumors. In addition, molecular genetic studies are increasingly being used for diagnostic, prognostic, and therapeutic purposes.

ADVANCES IN THE MANAGEMENT OF BENIGN SOFT TISSUE TUMORS

Benign soft tissue tumors constitute an important consideration within the differential diagnosis of neonatal soft tissue masses. Although benign, this group of tumors will usually also require an interdisciplinary team of sarcoma specialists for optimal management. Adequate diagnostic tissue is necessary to differentiate benign from malignant tumors, and the choice and extent of the initial surgery can impact treatment options and outcomes. Therefore, early engagement of an experienced pediatric sarcoma team is recommended.

Fibrous Hamartoma

Fibrous hamartomas typically present as a solitary nontender mass most commonly in the trunk, neck, axillary regions, upper arms, and external genital areas.[17] Approximately 25% of the cases are congenital,[18] with the majority of cases occurring in the first year of life and nearly all cases being diagnosed in the first 2 years of life.[18-20] There is a slight predilection for males, with a male to female ratio of 2:1.[17,19,20] Although a case of fibrous hamartoma has been reported in a patient with Williams syndrome, a rare developmental disorder of the cardiovascular and central nervous system, there is no clear association with syndromic or familial conditions.[19,20] Fibrous hamartomas are benign tumors of the subcutis and lower dermis and was first described by Reye[21] in 1965 as "subdermal fibromatous tumor of infancy." Histologically, they are characterized by a triphasic organoid appearance.[20,21] Various cytogenetic aberrations have been reported, but fibrous hamartomas have no recurrent translocation or karyotypic abnormalities.[17,20] Complete surgical excision is curative and is the primary means of treatment.[22] Approximately 15% of cases are associated with local recurrence, which is believed to be due to incomplete or poor excision, especially in cases with irregular borders.[19,20] Slow growth is typical of fibrous hamartoma, although rare cases showing rapid growth associated with more sarcomatous morphology have been reported.[17,20,22] In such rare cases, chemotherapy or radical surgery may be considered.[17]

Rhabdomyoma

Rhabdomyomas are rare benign tumors characterized histologically by striated skeletal muscle.[23] They can be either extracardiac, where they often present as a solid mass in the head and neck region,[23] or cardiac, which is associated with tuberous sclerosis.[24] For rhabdomyomas in tuberous sclerosis, mutations in the *TSC1* (chromosome 9q34.13) or *TSC2* (chromosome 16p13.3) tumor suppressor genes are found in 85% of cases.[25] Rhabdomyomas are often detected on prenatal ultrasound examinations and are usually asymptomatic, although they can cause arrhythmias or obstruction of the airway or cardiac ventricles.[25] In the absence of arrhythmias or obstructive symptoms, conservative management is generally favored because spontaneous regression is usually seen, particularly in rhabdomyoma cases associated with tuberous sclerosis.[25,26] For symptomatic tumors requiring therapy, complete surgical excision is curative.[27] Recurrence is rare and is believed to be associated with incomplete resection.[23] Emergent medical treatment may be necessary for inoperable hemodynamically unstable patients. Everolimus, a mammalian target of rapamycin inhibitor, has been shown to induce rapid tumor regression, but caution is warranted owing to side effects.[25,26]

Lipoma

Lipomas are common benign mesenchymal tumors composed of mature adipose tissue.[28] They most frequently occur in the subcutaneous tissue of the trunk and extremities, although rare cases involve the deep fascia and muscle.[28,29] They typically present as a painless, slow growing mass.[29] Most lipomas harbor 12q13-15 gene rearrangements resulting in dysregulated *HMGA2* expression, although about 25% of cases have *HMGA1-LLP2/1* fusions.[28,30] Complete surgical excision is usually curative, although recurrence rates ranging from 3% to 65% have been reported.[29]

Lipoblastoma and Lipoblastomatosis

Lipoblastomas are rare benign tumors arising in the adipose tissue and occur almost exclusively in infants and children. They can be rapidly growing and occur at any anatomic site containing fetal-embryonal fat tissue and most commonly occur in the extremities or retroperitoneum. Most tumors are well-circumscribed but some are more diffusely infiltrative and are termed lipoblastomatosis.[30] The histologic appearance of lipoblastoma resembles a lipoma or malignant liposarcoma, but molecular testing demonstrating characteristic rearrangements of chromosomal region 8q11-13 is diagnostic.[31] Although these tumors are frequently locally invasive, they can be cured with surgical resection.[32] In asymptomatic cases where surgery could be problematic, a cautious wait and see approach may not be unreasonable because, in rare instances, lipoblastoma may regress spontaneously.[33] The recurrence rate for lipoblastoma has been reported to be as high as 25%, although many of the recurrent cases represent lipoblastomatosis.[34]

Neurofibroma

Neurofibromas are benign peripheral neural neoplasms that occur in the skin, subcutis, and deeper soft tissues.[35] Histologic variants include solitary, plexiform, diffuse, cellular, and atypical. Most neurofibromas occur sporadically, although a small proportion are associated with type 1 neurofibromatosis.[35] Cutaneous neurofibromas can be excised surgically, although the management of neurofibromas is typically conservative. Plexiform neurofibromas are diffuse, often involve multiple nerve branches and plexi, and can be associated with significant morbidity. Conventionally, neurofibromas do not respond to chemotherapy or radiotherapy.[36] However clinical trials are underway to examine the efficacy of conventional chemotherapeutic agents as well as biological agents, such as MEK inhibitors, for plexiform neurofibromas.[37]

Fibroblastic–Myofibroblastic Tumors

Myofibroblastic tumors such as infantile myofibroma and infantile hemangiopericytoma behave as benign tumors, but can be locally invasive. Infantile myofibromas or myofibromatosis are characterized by flesh-colored myofibroblastic nodules of the skin, subcutaneous tissue, striated muscles, or rarely in bones or the visceral organs.[38] They have a broad range of presentations and can present as either solitary single or multiple lesions involving the skin and muscles, or present with skin and muscle lesions as well as visceral involvement (**Figs. 2** and **3**). Infantile myofibromatosis is often diagnosed shortly after birth, and 90% occur within the first 2 years of life.[38] Myopericytomas, which are rare benign tumors originating from pericytes that contain

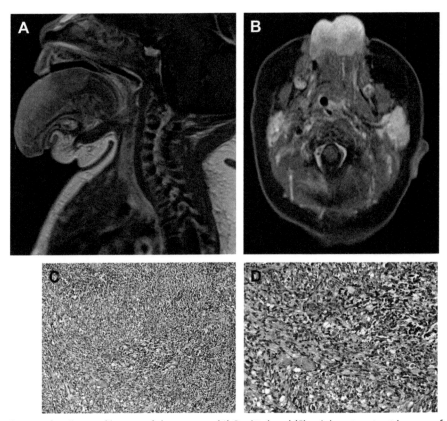

Fig. 2. Infantile myofibroma of the tongue. (*A*) Sagittal and (*B*) axial postcontrast images of the face show a mildly enhancing infiltrative lesion of the tongue causing enlargement and protrusion, consistent with infantile myofibroma of the tongue. Histologic sections show a biphasic tumor with (*C*) areas of myoid differentiation composed of cells with eosinophilic cytoplasm and oval to tapered nuclei separated by (*D*) cellular zones with hemangiopericytoma-like vasculature. (Stain: hematoxylin and eosin; original magnification ×100 [*C, D*]).

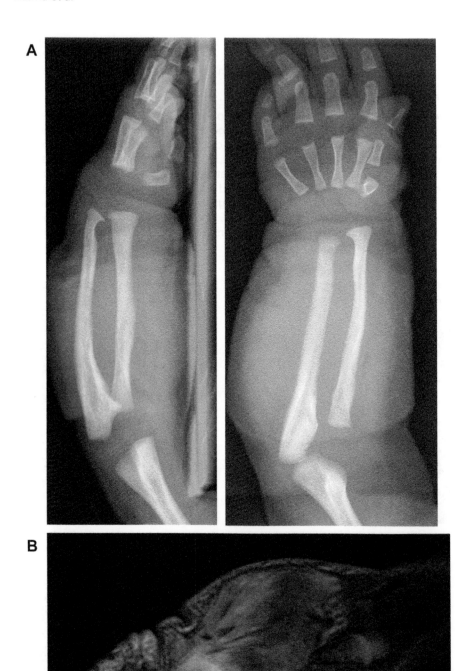

numerous thin-walled blood vessels, occur in the deep soft tissues.[39] Infantile hemangiopericytomas are rare benign tumors originating from capillary pericytes and often arise in the head and neck region.[40] Patients are often asymptomatic with occasional complications from bleeding or local compression. Unlike the adult variant that occurs in older children, infantile hemangiopericytomas rarely metastasize and have a lower rate of recurrence.[40,41] In contrast, lipofibromatosis represents a spectrum of fibroblastic tumors containing adipose as well as myofibroblastic elements that present as extremity tumors during infancy and have a high rate of local recurrence.[42]

Histologically, myofibroblastic tumors are now conceptualized as being on a continuum with hemangiopericytoma on the primitive end of the spectrum.[43] Infantile myofibroma is a biphasic tumor with cellular zones of hemangiopericytoma-like vessels and myoid nodules composed of plump, eosinophilic myofibroblasts[15] (see **Fig. 2**C–D). The proportion of each component is variable. Infantile hemangiopericytoma, composed of primitive round cells with pericytomatous vascular pattern, is morphologically indistinguishable from the cellular zones seen in infantile myofibroma. By immunohistochemistry, both tumors are typically positive for smooth muscle actin, muscle-specific actin, and calponin and negative for desmin and caldesmon. These tumors demonstrate significant morphologic overlap with infantile fibrosarcoma. Thus, detecting the t(12;15) (p13;q25) *ETV6-NTRK3* fusion characteristic of infantile fibrosarcoma is instrumental in avoiding misclassification (described elsewhere in this article).

Most cases of infantile myofibromatosis are sporadic, but rare familial cases have been described.[5] Mutations in *PDGFRB* or *NOTCH3* have been implicated in the pathogenesis.[44] When possible, a conservative approach is recommended because most lesions will spontaneously regress within a few years. Lesions isolated to the skin and muscle are associated with a low morbidity. However, visceral lesions have a guarded prognosis with an untreated mortality rate from cardiopulmonary compromise or gastrointestinal compression as high as 70%.[45] Life-threatening visceral lesions can be treated with radical surgical excision and chemotherapy with low-dose weekly methotrexate and vinblastine.[46]

DESMOID-TYPE FIBROMATOSIS

Desmoid-type fibromatosis (aggressive fibromatosis), commonly called desmoids, are also locally aggressive fibroblastic tumors. They are slow growing lesions that often present as a painless infiltrating mass.[38] Approximately 30% of desmoid tumors occur in the first year of life. Most cases are sporadic and involve mutations in the β-catenin gene *CTNNB1*.[5] However, 2% of desmoid tumors have germline loss of the *APC* gene causing familial adenomatous polyposis, which is an autosomal-dominant cancer predisposition syndrome associated with intestinal polyps and colon cancer.[38] About 10% to 20% of patients with familial adenomatous polyposis will get desmoid tumors during their lifetime, which is a rate 800- to 1000-fold higher than found in the general population.[47] Desmoid tumors associated with familial adenomatous polyposis are

Fig. 3. Infantile myofibromatosis of the distal right upper extremity. (*A*) Posteroanterior and lateral radiographs of the right forearm of a child with infantile myofibromatosis shows enlargement of the muscular tissues of the forearm from the elbow to the wrist. (*B*) Sagittal T2-weighted (fluid-sensitive) imaging of this region demonstrates increased fluid signal of the muscles of the forearm in a diffuse infiltrative pattern.

more likely to arise in the abdomen, whereas sporadic tumors are more likely to arise in the extremities, spinal area, or head and neck regions.[5]

Although these tumors do not metastasize, desmoids are frequently associated with high morbidity because they can extend along fascial planes, infiltrate adjacent structures, and compress blood vessels, nerves, and the abdominal viscera. The natural history of desmoid tumors should be considered when making treatment decisions. Desmoids usually grow slowly over years and can spontaneously stop growing or even regress without intervention. Because they can remain quiescent over a long period of time, careful observation is appropriate in many cases. However, in the developing neonate, desmoid tumors threatening limb or organ function may warrant treatment. In the past, many desmoid tumors were surgically excised. However, a decision for surgical intervention should be weighed against the morbidity of the surgery and the high rate of local recurrence, which is reported to range from 33% to 88% in pediatric patients.[38] Radiotherapy has some efficacy in treating desmoids, but its use in neonates is discouraged owing to developmental risks and the risks of secondary malignancies, including sarcoma. Newer therapies for desmoid tumors, such as cryoablation or radiofrequency ablation are now emerging, although their use in infants needs to be better studied.[48,49] There is no standard medical therapy for desmoid-type fibromatosis, although conventional chemotherapies such as doxorubicin, dacarbazine, methotrexate, vinorelbine, and vinblastine have been used. Other therapies demonstrated to be efficacious in small studies include sulindac, a nonsteroidal anti-inflammatory agent, and tamoxifen, an antihormonal agent. More recently, tyrosine kinase inhibitors such as sorafenib and pazopanib have been shown to be beneficial in decreasing or slowing desmoid tumor growth, although the availability of oral suspension formulations may limit their use in neonates. Finally, newer agents targeting β-catenin and the Notch pathway are currently being investigated in clinical trials.[50]

ADVANCES IN THE MANAGEMENT OF MALIGNANT NEONATAL SARCOMAS
Infantile Fibrosarcoma

Infantile fibrosarcomas, one of the most common soft tissue sarcomas in children less than 1 year of age, occur almost exclusively in neonates. The majority of cases occur within the first 3 months of life and approximately one-half are either diagnosed prenatally or are present at birth.[51] They commonly present as a firm, noninflammatory, rapidly growing mass in the deep soft tissues of the extremities or, less frequently, in the trunk or head and neck region.[52] The clinical presentation and radiographic findings may mimic vascular malformations, because they are highly vascularized and are sometimes ulcerated[53] (**Fig. 4**). Although histologically similar to the adult form of fibrosarcoma that arises in older children and adults,[54] infantile fibrosarcomas are less likely to metastasize, are more responsive to therapy, and are associated with better prognoses.

Histologically, infantile fibrosarcoma is a primitive tumor composed of fibroblasts. It can display a wide range of morphologic features, although classic histologic findings are those of a monomorphic spindle cell tumor with a fascicular or herringbone architecture.[15] Additional characteristic features include scattered lymphocytes and hemangiopericytoma-like vasculature. Frequent mitotic figures and areas of necrosis and/or hemorrhage are often seen. The main distinguishing features differentiating infantile and adult forms of fibrosarcoma are patient age and the characteristic t(12;15) (p13;q25) chromosomal translocations leading to *ETV6–NTRK3* fusions that are recurrent in infantile fibrosarcoma.[55] Other less common *NRTK* fusions such as *TMT1–NTRK1* have also been described in infantile fibrosarcoma,[56] and intragenic deletions

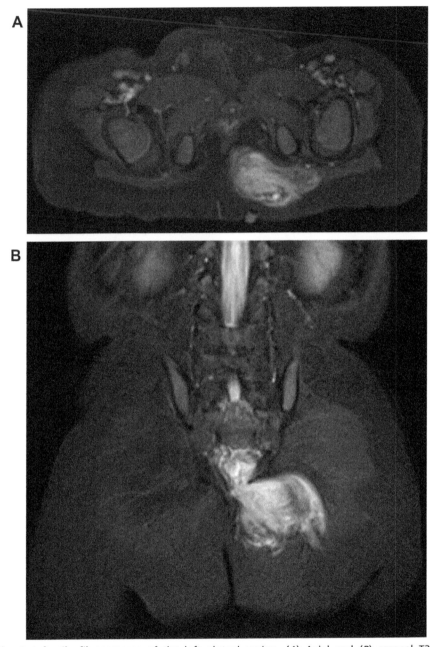

Fig. 4. Infantile fibrosarcoma of the left gluteal region. (*A*) Axial and (*B*) coronal T2-weighted (fluid-sensitive) imaging of the pelvis demonstrate a T2 hyperintense solid mass centered within the medial superficial soft tissues of the left buttock; biopsy-proven infantile fibrosarcoma.

in *BRAF* can co-occur with the *NRTK* fusions.[57,58] Rare *NTRK* fusion negative variants involving *BRAF* fusions or *TFG–MET* fusions are also found in infantile spindle cell sarcoma, but these entities seem to share similar histologic features and clinical behavior to the *NTRK* fusion tumors.[57,59]

Historically, infantile fibrosarcomas were treated and frequently cured with surgical resection alone. However, because these are typically large tumors infiltrating adjacent structures such blood vessels and nerves, amputations or other mutilating surgeries were typically necessary. Today, unless a complete resection can be achieved with minimal morbidity, the use of neoadjuvant chemotherapy to elicit tumor shrinkage before more conservative limb- or organ-sparing surgeries is recommended. Rhabdomyosarcoma-like therapy using vincristine and actinomycin D and either cyclophosphamide (VAC) or ifosfamide have been demonstrated to have excellent activity in infantile fibrosarcoma.[60] More recently, several trials aimed at reducing short- and long-term toxicities associated with alkylators have demonstrated VA alone is also highly effective.[61,62] Therefore, VA is now the standard neoadjuvant regimen and is also used as adjuvant therapy for macroscopic residual disease. In rare cases, infantile fibrosarcoma has been shown to spontaneously regress,[63,64] which indicates that, for select patients with a stable unresectable tumor in a nonthreatening location, a careful wait and see approach may be reasonable.[62]

Newer targeted therapies have shown promise in treating infantile fibrosarcoma. The ubiquitous *NTRK* fusions lead to constitutive activation of neutrotrophin tyrosine kinase receptors, which is thought to be the main oncogenic contributor responsible for tumorigenesis.[65] As such, infantile fibrosarcoma is specifically sensitive to tropomyosin receptor kinase (TRK) inhibitors. Larotrectinib and entrectinib, first-generation TRK inhibitors, received approval from the US Food and Drug Administration in 2018 and 2019, respectively, and have been demonstrated to be efficacious in *NTRK* fusion-associated malignancies.[66,67] Second-generation TRK inhibitors such as selitrectinib and repotrectinib are currently in clinical trials and may prove to be helpful in overcoming acquired resistance to TRK inhibitors.[67] Although the TRK inhibitors are well-tolerated in infants,[68,69] their routine integration into the standard VA backbone or use as a single agent needs further investigation in larger clinical trials. Long-term survival outcomes for infantile fibrosarcoma are excellent given the low likelihood of metastatic spread and chemotherapy responsiveness.[5,44] Using a multimodal approach with surgical resection and neoadjuvant and/or adjuvant chemotherapy has led to 3-year event-free and overall survival rates exceeding 80% and 90%, respectively.[61,62]

Primitive Myxoid Mesenchymal Tumor of Infancy

Primitive myxoid mesenchymal tumor of infancy represents a rare and relatively recently described tumor that has a clinical presentation overlapping with infantile fibrosarcoma. As the name suggests, primitive myxoid mesenchymal tumor of infancy morphology resembles primitive mesenchymal cells within abundant myxoid stroma, which can also mimic infantile fibrosarcoma.[70] However, key distinguishing molecular features of primitive myxoid mesenchymal tumor of infancy include the lack of *NTRK* fusions and the presence of *BCOR* internal tandem duplication, resulting in an amplified expression of and immunoreactivity for *BCOR* and/or *BCL6*.[71,72] Like infantile fibrosarcoma, these tumors rarely metastasize. However, although the long-term outcomes and optimal management of primitive myxoid mesenchymal tumor of infancy are not known, clinical courses from the few published cases of primitive myxoid mesenchymal tumor of infancy suggest that they may be less responsive to chemotherapy.[70,73]

Rhabdomyosarcoma

Rhabdomyosarcomas are the most common childhood soft tissue sarcoma and comprise about one-third of all neonatal sarcomas (see **Fig. 1B**, see **Table 2**).[74] Although it is now characterized by molecular features, rhabdomyosarcoma has classically been described by 4 distinct histologic subtypes: embryonal, alveolar, spindle cell or sclerosing, and pleomorphic.[75] Embryonal histology is the most common in young children and commonly occurs in the head and neck or retroperitoneal regions[76,77] (**Figs. 5** and **6**). Alveolar rhabdomyosarcoma is more common in older children, but can also occur in infants and commonly present as a soft tissue extremity mass. The majority of histologic alveolar tumors have characteristic t(2;13) (q35;q14) or t(1;13) (p36;q14) chromosomal translocations that lead to *PAX3-*or *PAX7–FOXO1* gene fusions, respectively, although about 20% are fusion negative.[76–78] A distinct variant of spindle cell or sclerosing rhabdomyosarcoma occurs in neonates and is characterized by *NCOA2* or *VGLL2* translocations.[75] Pleomorphic histology comprises almost one-half of rhabdomyosarcoma cases in adults, but is exceedingly rare in children.[79]

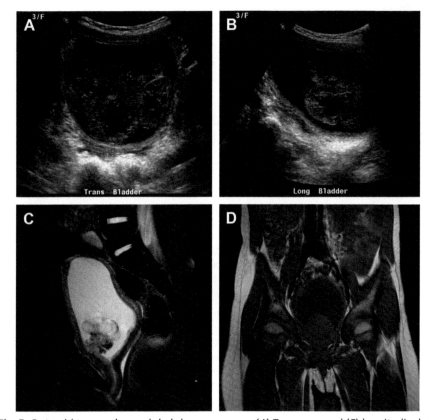

Fig. 5. Botryoid type embryonal rhabdomyosarcoma. (*A*) Transverse and (*B*) longitudinal ultrasound images of the bladder in a 3-year-old child with recurrent botryoid-type embryonal rhabdomyosarcoma show a large, lobular solid mass with areas of central cystic change/necrosis near completely filling the bladder lumen. (*C, D*) Subsequent MR images (sagittal T2/fluid sensitive and coronal T1) redemonstrate this mass and better characterize its origin from the anterior/inferior bladder just anterior to the bladder outlet.

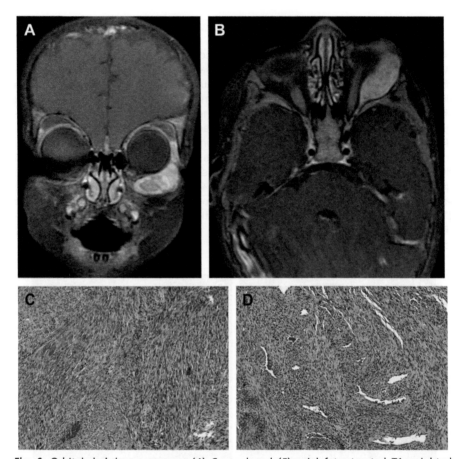

Fig. 6. Orbital rhabdomyosarcoma. (*A*) Coronal and (*B*) axial fat-saturated T1-weighted postcontrast images in a child with rhabdomyosarcoma of the left orbit show a solid enhancing mass in the expected location of the left inferior rectus muscle with mass effect on the left eye and subsequent proptosis. (*C, D*) Histologic sections show neoplastic cells with variable degrees of myogenic differentiation composed of undifferentiated mesenchymal small, round, blue cells, rhabdomyoblasts, and more well-differentiated myofibers. (Stain: hematoxylin and eosin; original magnification ×100 [*C*], ×200 [*D*]).

Rhabdomyosarcoma is derived from immature mesenchyme with evidence of myogenic differentiation by morphology, immunohistochemistry, and ancillary studies.[75] Immunohistochemical staining for myogenic markers such as myogenin and MYOD1 are both sensitive and specific for rhabdomyosarcoma.[80] Rhabdomyoblasts, primitive small cells, and more well-differentiated myofibers are seen in varying proportions by morphology[15] (see **Fig. 6**C, D). Rhabdomyoblasts may not be as obvious in alveolar or spindle cell or sclerosing subtypes, which demonstrate structures resembling alveoli, spindle cell morphology, and hyalinizing matrix, respectively. Mitotic figures are typically evident. Given the wide range of possible histologic features, the differential diagnosis is broad and includes 3 general categories: spindle cell neoplasms, myogenic neoplasms, and small round cell neoplasms.

Although most cases of rhabdmyosarcoma are sporadic, very young children are more likely to have an underlying genetic cancer predisposition, such as Li–

Fraumeni syndrome, which is caused by germline loss-of-function mutations in *TP53*, or Costello syndrome, which is an overgrowth syndrome caused by germline mutations in *HRAS*. Rhabdomyosarcoma develops in 18% to 27% of patients with Li–Fraumeni syndrome[81,82] and in about 10% of patients with Costello syndrome.[83] Other rare cancer predisposition syndromes associated with rhabdomyosarcoma include Beckwith–Wiedemann syndrome, type 1 neurofibromatosis, DICER1, Gorlin's basal cell nevus, and Rubinstein–Taybi syndrome.[84,85] Genetic testing for *TP53* and/or a referral to genetic counseling is recommended for any infant with rhabdomyosarcoma, especially when the tumor histology demonstrates anaplasia.[86]

Risk stratification for rhabdomyosarcoma incorporates presurgical (TNM) staging, which is based on the tumor's anatomic location, invasiveness, size, and nodal or metastatic sites, as well as postsurgical grouping, which is based on extent of residual local and distant tumor following initial resection.[87,88] TNM staging and clinical grouping are prognostic and stratifying patients based on this schema allows for deescalation of therapy for select low-risk tumors or intensification for patients at higher risk. Outcomes for localized low-risk tumors are excellent, with the 5-year overall survival rates exceeding 90%.[76,89] However, survival rates for high-risk metastatic rhabdomyosarcoma are less than 30%.[77] In addition to TNM staging and clinical grading, *FOXO1* fusion status, which is a poor prognostic indicator, is also now being used for risk stratification in prospective cooperative clinical trials.[90,91] Fusion-positive tumors are associated with a 5-year overall survival of 65% for localized disease and 19% for metastatic disease, compared with 88% and 58%, respectively, for fusion-negative tumors.[92]

Rhabdomyosarcoma treatment combines systemic chemotherapy with local control measures. Upfront surgery as local control is preferred when complete tumor resection with negative microscopic margins can be achieved while resulting in minimal morbidity. However, because this outcome is usually not possible in neonates, a treatment strategy incorporating neoadjuvant chemotherapy and radiotherapy, with or without a delayed surgical excision, is typically used.[93,94] Since the 1970s, first-line chemotherapy for rhabdomyosarcoma includes VA and an alkylator—either cyclophosphamide (VAC) or ifosfamide (IVA).[89] Alternating cycles of VAC with cycles of vincristine and irinotecan (VAC/VI) is also an accepted standard first-line therapy that was demonstrated to be equivalent to VAC alone, but with less toxicity for intermediate-risk rhabdomyosarcoma.[95,96] Unfortunately, for patients with metastatic disease, intensifying therapy using an interval compression regimen that includes ifosfamide, etoposide, and doxorubicin demonstrated no additional benefit, and newer targeted therapies have also not improved outcomes over VAC or VAC/VI.[97,98] There is no established standard for relapsed or refractory rhabdomyosarcoma, although potential salvage regimens were recently reviewed elsewhere by a panel of pediatric rhabdomyosarcoma experts.[95]

Rhabdomyosarcoma in neonates present several other unique challenges for clinical management. Chemotherapy dosing in very young infants less than 2 months of age is frequently decreased because of concerns for toxicity. In addition, local control is particularly challenging as complete resection is usually not feasible and radiotherapy at standard dosing (50.4 Gy) can arrest growth of the surrounding tissue.[99] Multiple clinical trials have shown that the outcomes for neonatal rhabdomyosarcoma are inferior to outcomes observed in older toddler-aged children.[1,100,101] Analyses from these trials reveal that, in an attempt to minimize toxicity, physicians treating infants with rhabdomyosarcoma are more likely to deviate from protocol-directed therapy by delaying or decreasing therapy intensity.[3,102,103] The Children's Oncology Group (COG) recently reported that radiotherapy was either delayed or omitted in

43% of infants treated on ARST0331 and ARST0531 trials. Individuals who received individualized non–protocol-directed local therapy had a 5-year event-free survival of 55.6%, compared with 77.5% of individuals who received protocol-specified therapy.[3]

Finally, although rhabdomyosarcoma during infancy is generally associated with inferior outcomes, congenital spindle cell rhabdomyosarcoma, characterized by NCOA2 or VGLL2 translocations, may represent a distinct biologic subtype with a more favorable prognosis. There are no reports of metastasis or deaths in patients with the congenital spindle cell variant. Furthermore, there have been a few cases where sustained remission was achieved without radiotherapy despite microscopic positive margins.[104] Further investigations are needed to determine if congenital spindle cell rhabdomyosarcoma can be successfully treated with a decreased intensity therapy.

The results of recent cooperative group rhabdomyosarcoma clinical trials aimed at decreasing toxicity while maintaining acceptable survival rates have been mixed. The COG low-risk trial ARST0331 demonstrated that decreasing cyclophosphamide exposure did not impact the 3-year failure-free or overall survival, which were 89% and 98%, respectively for subset I patients—those with stage 1/2 group I/II or stage 1 group III orbital tumors.[105] However, the event-free survival was only 64% in subset II patients—those with stage 1 group III nonorbital or stage 3 group I/II tumors, which was inferior to the 5-year event-free survival rates seen in the predecessor trial D8602.[106] Similarly, compared with the D9803 trial, decreasing the cumulative cyclophosphamide dosing for intermediate-risk rhabdomyosarcoma per ARST0531 was associated with worse local recurrence rates (19.4% vs 27.9%) and inferior overall survival.[96,107,108] In contrast, the European pediatric Soft tissue sarcoma Study Group trial RMS 2005 demonstrated that adding 24 weeks of maintenance therapy with vinorelbine and low-dose continuous oral cyclophosphamide for intermediate-risk rhabdomyosarcoma improves both disease-free and overall survivals, which were 72.3% and 77.4%, respectively, in the control group but 78.4% and 87.3%, respectively, in the treatment arm.[109] As a result of these recent trials, the ongoing prospective phase III intermediate-risk COG study ARST1431 is treating the previously stratified low-risk subset II cases as intermediate risk, incorporates a maintenance phase for all patients, and increases radiotherapy dosing from 50.4 Gy to 59.4 Gy for bulky tumors greater than 5 cm. This study is also investigating whether temsirolimus, an mammalian target of rapamycin inhibitor shown to be active in relapsed rhabdomyosarcoma,[90] will improve outcomes when added upfront to the standard VAC/VI backbone.

Nonrhabdomyosarcoma Soft Tissue Sarcoma

NRSTS comprise a heterogeneous group of malignant soft tissue neoplasms. Collectively, NRSTS represents about one-quarter of neonatal sarcomas (see **Fig. 1**B, see **Table 2**). However, each subtype is quite rare and includes sarcomas with complex karyotypes such as leiomyosarcoma, as well as translocation-associated sarcomas such as synovial sarcoma and Ewing sarcoma family of tumors.[6] NRSTS can present anywhere in the body, but most frequently arise in the distal extremities.[110] Any neonate with a sarcoma should raise suspicion for an underlying germline genetic mutation. Loss of RB1 or TP53 tumor suppressors are associated with an increased risk of developing NRSTS, including leiomyosarcoma.[111,112] About 4% of patients with type 1 neurofibromatosis develop malignant peripheral nerve sheath tumors,[113] and patients with adenosine deaminase-deficient severe combined immunodeficiency have a higher risk of developing multicentric dermatofibrosarcoma protuberans.[114]

Several other rare genetic syndromes, such as tuberous sclerosis complex and Werner syndrome, also are associated with increased risk of soft tissue sarcoma.[115–117] Therefore, a genetic counseling referral and evaluation is typically performed on neonates presenting with an NRSTS.

The prognosis for NRSTS largely depends on the histologic grade, staging, and recurrent cytogenetic changes. In terms of grading soft tissue sarcomas, the 2 most widely used systems were created by the National Cancer Institute and the Fédération Nationale des Centers de Lutte Contre le Cancer (FNCLCC).[118,119] The Pediatric Oncology Group system was adapted from the National Cancer Institute system for the purpose of grading pediatric NRSTS.[120] The Pediatric Oncology Group system relies on histologic type, mitotic index, and necrosis. Few entities are assigned to grade group 1 (low grade) or 3 (high grade) based on histologic type alone. The majority that remain are assigned either grade 2 (intermediate grade) or 3 (high grade) based on necrosis and mitotic index. The FNCLCC system is based on tumor differentiation, mitotic count, tumor necrosis, and histologic grade. A study comparing the Pediatric Oncology Group and FNCLCC systems found both were adequate predictors of event free survival with differences only in grading of the intermediate grade group.[121] NRSTS staging involves a complex TNM algorithm that accounts for tumor size, nodal status, histologic grade, and metastatic spread, as well as the anatomic primary site (trunk, extremities, and retroperitoneum; head and neck; or abdomen and thoracic visceral organs).[122,123]

Given the rarity and heterogeneity within NRSTS subtypes during infancy, outcomes and the optimal treatment approaches for this population is not precisely known. However, therapy-related morbidity is exacerbated in very young developing children, which necessitates caution in treatment decisions and careful short- and long-term monitoring.[124] In general, most NRSTS tumors are relatively chemoresistant. In contrast with rhabdomyosarcoma, in which even local tumors often present with micrometastatic disease,[125] complete surgical resection alone can be curative in NRSTS. However, for pediatric high-grade or unresectable sarcomas, neoadjuvant chemotherapy or chemoradiotherapy plays a significant role, especially for deep invasive or bulky tumors and those with a high burden of disease.[126,127] The prospective COG trial ARST0332 established a strategy for the risk stratification of pediatric NRSTS based on the extent of the residual tumor after resection, tumor size, and histologic grade.[128] Surgical resection is classified as R0 if completely resected with negative microscopic margins, R1 if microscopic positive margins, and R2 if macroscopic residual tumor. Low-risk tumors are defined as R0 or R1 and low grade or small R1 high grade tumors that are less than 5 cm in size, and they have a 96% overall survival rate at 5 years. Intermediate-risk tumors include any unresected tumor or high grade R0 or R1 tumors that are more than 5 cm in size, and they have a 5-year overall survival of 79%. High-risk NRSTS is any metastatic tumor, and they are associated with a dismal prognosis, with 5-year event-free and overall survivals of 21.0% and 35.5%, respectively.[128] Because the extent of residual tumor has prognostic implications, any neonate with a suspected sarcoma should be managed by an interdisciplinary team that includes a surgeon with expertise in the resection of pediatric soft tissue sarcomas.

Radiotherapy, given either preoperatively or postoperatively, can augment surgery for local control, or is sometimes given as definitive local control when surgery is not feasible.[129] Radiation is typically administered at high doses and has been shown to improve outcomes for patients with large, high-grade tumors and tumors with inadequate surgical margins.[128,130] For most NRSTS, first-line chemotherapy includes ifosfamide with doxorubicin, although alternating cycles of vincristine, doxorubicin, and

- Genetic counseling referral and evaluation is typically recommended for neonates who present with rhabdomyosarcoma or NRSTS.
- With the exception of infantile fibrosarcoma, outcomes for neonatal sarcoma remain poor. Whenever possible, participation in collaborative clinical trials should be encouraged.
- Advances in the molecular characterization of soft tissue sarcomas improves diagnostics and provides promise for improvements in targeted therapies.
- Infantile fibrosarcomas are characterized by NTRK fusions and can be specifically targeted using TRK inhibitors. Although TRK inhibitors have been demonstrated to be well-tolerated in neonates, their routine use in upfront therapy warrants prospective studies.
- Suboptimal local control measures associated with individualized non–protocol-directed therapy contribute to increased rates of local recurrence. Better adherence to protocol-directed therapy, when feasible, is recommend.
- Alternatives to conventional external beam radiation, including brachytherapy and proton radiotherapy, are promising new modalities to treat neonatal soft tissue sarcomas, although these need to be more formally studied in infants.
- Low-risk subset I rhabdomyosarcoma (stage 1/2 group I/II or stage 1 group III orbital tumors) can be managed using lower intensity regimens with decreased cumulative alkylator exposure.
- For intermediate-risk rhabdomyosarcoma, conventional alkylator dosing should be used outside of a clinical trial. Decreasing cyclophosphamide exposure was associated with worse failure-free and overall survival.
- For intermediate- and high-risk rhabdomyosarcoma, incorporating maintenance chemotherapy with vinorelbine and continuous low-dose cyclophosphamide at the end of standard therapy has been shown to improve event-free and overall survival outcomes and should now be considered the standard of care.

CONFLICTS OF INTEREST

The authors have no conflicts of interest to declare.

ETHICAL STATEMENT

The authors are accountable for all aspects of the work in ensuring that questions related to the accuracy or integrity of any part of the work are appropriately investigated and resolved.

ACKNOWLEDGMENTS

This work was supported by a V Foundation Scholar Award [V2018-028] (MDD).

DISCLOSURES

The authors have no commercial or financial conflicts of interest to declare. This work was supported by a V Foundation Scholar Award (M.D. Deel).

CLINICS CARE POINTS

- The diagnosis and treatment of an atypical neonatal soft tissue mass is complex. Optimal management includes an early evaluation by pediatric sarcoma specialists prior to an initial biopsy.

- Obtaining adequate local control with minimal morbidity remains a challenge for neonatal soft tissue tumors. Suboptimal local control is associated with inferior outcomes.
- In neonates, many benign soft tissue tumors are locally invasive and are associated with a significant morbidity.
- Sarcomas are among the most difficult to treat malignancies in the neonatal period. However, recent advances in molecular profiling is informing newer targeted therapies for select neonatal sarcoma subtypes.

REFERENCES

1. Orbach D, Rey A, Oberlin O, et al. Soft tissue sarcoma or malignant mesenchymal tumors in the first year of life: experience of the International Society of Pediatric Oncology (SIOP) malignant mesenchymal tumor committee. J Clin Oncol 2005;23(19):4363–71.
2. Alfaar AS, Hassan WM, Bakry MS, et al. Neonates with cancer and causes of death; lessons from 615 cases in the SEER databases. Cancer Med 2017; 6(7):1817–26.
3. Bradley JA, Kayton ML, Chi YY, et al. Treatment approach and outcomes in infants with localized rhabdomyosarcoma: a report from the soft tissue sarcoma committee of the Children's Oncology Group. Int J Radiat Oncol Biol Phys 2019;103(1):19–27.
4. Sultan I, Casanova M, Al-Jumaily U, et al. Soft tissue sarcomas in the first year of life. Eur J Cancer 2010;46(13):2449–56.
5. Ferrari A, Orbach D, Sultan I, et al. Neonatal soft tissue sarcomas. Semin Fetal neonatal Med 2012;17(4):231–8.
6. Surveillance, Epidemiology, and end results (SEER) program (www.seer.cancer. gov). SEER*Stat Database: Incidence - SEER Research Data, 9 Registries, Nov 2019 Sub (1975-2017) - Linked To County Attributes - Time Dependent (1990-2017) Income/Rurality, 1969-2017 Counties, National Cancer Institute, DCCPS, Surveillance Research Program, released April 2020, based on the November 2019 submission. Accessed May 2020.
7. Laffan EE, Ngan BY, Navarro OM. Pediatric soft-tissue tumors and pseudotumors: MR imaging features with pathologic correlation: part 2. Tumors of fibroblastic/myofibroblastic, so-called fibrohistiocytic, muscular, lymphomatous, neurogenic, hair matrix, and uncertain origin. Radiographics 2009;29(4):e36.
8. Navarro OM, Laffan EE, Ngan BY. Pediatric soft-tissue tumors and pseudotumors: MR imaging features with pathologic correlation: part 1. Imaging approach, pseudotumors, vascular lesions, and adipocytic tumors. Radiographics 2009;29(3):887–906.
9. Restrepo R, Francavilla ML, Mas R, et al. Up-to-date practical imaging evaluation of neonatal soft-tissue tumors: what radiologists need to know. AJR Am J Roentgenol 2017;209(1):195–204.
10. Callahan MJ, MacDougall RD, Bixby SD, et al. Ionizing radiation from computed tomography versus anesthesia for magnetic resonance imaging in infants and children: patient safety considerations. Pediatr Radiol 2018;48(1):21–30.
11. Harrison DJ, Parisi MT, Shulkin BL. The Role of (18)F-FDG-PET/CT in pediatric sarcoma. Semin Nucl Med 2017;47(3):229–41.
12. Völker T, Denecke T, Steffen I, et al. Positron emission tomography for staging of pediatric sarcoma patients: results of a prospective multicenter trial. J Clin Oncol 2007;25(34):5435–41.

13. El-Kholy E, El Nadi E, Hafez H, et al. Added predictive value of 18F-FDG PET/CT for pediatric rhabdomyosarcoma. Nucl Med Commun 2019;40(9):898–904.

14. Harrison DJ, Parisi MT, Shulkin BL, et al. 18F 2Fluoro-2deoxy-D-glucose positron emission tomography (FDG-PET) response to predict event-free survival (EFS) in intermediate risk (IR) or high risk (HR) rhabdomyosarcoma (RMS): a report from the soft tissue sarcoma committee of the Children's Oncology Group (COG). J Clin Oncol 2016;34(15_suppl):10549.

15. Goldblum J, Weiss S, Folpe AL. Enzinger and Weiss's soft tissue tumors. 7th edition. Philadelphia: Elsevier; 2019.

16. Husain AN, Stocker JT, Dehner LP. Stocker and Dehner's pediatric pathology. 4th edition. Philadelphia: Lippincott Williams & Wilkins; 2015.

17. Al-Ibraheemi A, Martinez A, Weiss SW, et al. Fibrous hamartoma of infancy: a clinicopathologic study of 145 cases, including 2 with sarcomatous features. Mod Pathol 2017;30(4):474–85.

18. Ji Y, Hu P, Zhang C, et al. Fibrous hamartoma of infancy: radiologic features and literature review. BMC Musculoskelet Disord 2019;20(1):356.

19. Dickey GE, Sotelo-Avila C. Fibrous hamartoma of infancy: current review. Pediatr Dev Pathol 1999;2(3):236–43.

20. Saab ST, McClain CM, Coffin CM. Fibrous hamartoma of infancy: a clinicopathologic analysis of 60 cases. Am J Surg Pathol 2014;38(3):394–401.

21. Reye RD. A consideration of certain subdermal fibromatous tumours of infancy. J Pathol Bacteriol 1956;72(1):149–54.

22. McGowan Jt, Smith CD, Maize J Jr, et al. Giant fibrous hamartoma of infancy: a report of two cases and review of the literature. J Am Acad Dermatol 2011;64(3):579–86.

23. Pownell PH, Brown OE, Argyle JC, et al. Rhabdomyoma of the cricopharyngeus in an infant. Int J Pediatr Otorhinolaryngol 1990;20(2):149–58.

24. Fenoglio JJ Jr, CAllister HA J M, Ferrans VJ. Cardiac rhabdomyoma: a clinicopathologic and electron microscopic study. Am J Cardiol 1976;38(2):241–51.

25. Martínez-García A, Michel-Macías C, Cordero-González G, et al. Giant left ventricular rhabdomyoma treated successfully with everolimus: case report and review of literature. Cardiol Young 2018;28(7):903–9.

26. Prabhu N, Osifodunrin N, Murphy D, et al. Innovative strategies for the management of a massive neonatal rhabdomyoma. J Pediatr Intensive Care 2018;7(2):90–3.

27. Yuan SM. Fetal primary cardiac tumors during perinatal period. Pediatr Neonatol 2017;58(3):205–10.

28. Johnson CN, Ha AS, Chen E, et al. Lipomatous soft-tissue tumors. J Am Acad Orthop Surg 2018;26(22):779–88.

29. Vincent J, Baker P, Grischkan J, et al. Subcutaneous midline nasal mass in an infant due to an intramuscular lipoma. Pediatr Dermatol 2017;34(3):e135–6.

30. Putra J, Al-Ibraheemi A. Adipocytic tumors in children: a contemporary review. Semin Diagn Pathol 2019;36(2):95–104.

31. Fallon SC, Brandt ML, Rodriguez JR, et al. Cytogenetic analysis in the diagnosis and management of lipoblastomas: results from a single institution. J Surg Res 2013;184(1):341–6.

32. McVay MR, Keller JE, Wagner CW, et al. Surgical management of lipoblastoma. J Pediatr Surg 2006;41(6):1067–71.

33. Mognato G, Cecchetto G, Carli M, et al. Is surgical treatment of lipoblastoma always necessary? J Pediatr Surg 2000;35(10):1511–3.

34. Speer AL, Schofield DE, Wang KS, et al. Contemporary management of lipo-blastoma. J Pediatr Surg 2008;43(7):1295–300.

35. Mesbah Ardakani N, Yap F, Wood BA. Cutaneous atypical neurofibroma: a case report and review of literature. Am J Dermatopathol 2018;40(11):864–7.

36. Joshi A, Lancelot M, Bhattacharjee NR, et al. Extensive plexiform neurofibroma in a premature neonate. Clin Med Res 2015;13(1):36–40.

37. MEK inhibitor for NF-1 associated plexiform neurofibroma. ClinicalTrials.gov Web site. Available at: https://clinicaltrials.gov/ct2/show/NCT03962543. Accessed May 2020.

38. Sargar KM, Sheybani EF, Shenoy A, et al. Pediatric fibroblastic and myofibro-blastic tumors: a pictorial review. Radiographics 2016;36(4):1195–214.

39. Provenzano D, Lo Bianco S, Belfiore M, et al. Foot soft tissue myopericytoma: case-report and review. Int J Surg Case Rep 2017;41:377–82.

40. Pérez A, Vigil S, Pescador I, et al. Infantile hemangiopericytoma leading to hy-povolemic shock in a neonate. Pediatr Blood Cancer 2018;65(5):e26950.

41. Hoey SA, Letts RM, Jimenez C. Infantile hemangiopericytoma of the musculo-skeletal system: case report and literature review. J Pediatr Orthop 1998; 18(3):359–62.

42. Fetsch JF, Miettinen M, Laskin WB, et al. A clinicopathologic study of 45 pediat-ric soft tissue tumors with an admixture of adipose tissue and fibroblastic ele-ments, and a proposal for classification as lipofibromatosis. Am J Surg Pathol 2000;24(11):1491–500.

43. Mentzel T, Calonje E, Nascimento AG, et al. Infantile hemangiopericytoma versus infantile myofibromatosis. Study of a series suggesting a continuous spectrum of infantile myofibroblastic lesions. Am J Surg Pathol 1994;18(9): 922–30.

44. Fernandez-Pineda I, Neel MD, Rao BN. Current management of neonatal soft-tissue sarcomas and benign tumors with local aggressiveness. Curr Pediatr Rev 2015;11(3):216–25.

45. Wiswell TE, Davis J, Cunningham BE, et al. Infantile myofibromatosis: the most common fibrous tumor of infancy. J Pediatr Surg 1988;23(4):315–8.

46. Azzam R, Abboud M, Muwakkit S, et al. First-line therapy of generalized infantile myofibromatosis with low-dose vinblastine and methotrexate. Pediatr Blood Cancer 2009;52(2):308.

47. ML DEM, Tonelli F, Quaresmini D, et al. Desmoid tumors in familial adenomatous polyposis. Anticancer Res 2017;37(7):3357–66.

48. Gómez FM, Patel PA, Stuart S, et al. Systematic review of ablation techniques for the treatment of malignant or aggressive benign lesions in children. Pediatr Ra-diol 2014;44(10):1281–9.

49. Ghanouni P, Dobrotwir A, Bazzocchi A, et al. Magnetic resonance-guided focused ultrasound treatment of extra-abdominal desmoid tumors: a retrospec-tive multicenter study. Eur Radiol 2017;27(2):732–40.

50. Aggressive fibromatosis. ClinicalTrials.gov Web site. Available at: https://clinicaltrials.gov/ct2/results?cond=Desmoid&term=fibromatosis&cntry=&state=&city=&dist=. Accessed May 2020.

51. Cecchetto G, Carli M, Alaggio R, et al. Fibrosarcoma in pediatric patients: re-sults of the Italian Cooperative Group studies (1979-1995). J Surg Oncol 2001;78(4):225–31.

52. Ferguson WS. Advances in the adjuvant treatment of infantile fibrosarcoma. Expert Rev Anticancer Ther 2003;3(2):185–91.

53. Yan AC, Chamlin SL, Liang MG, et al. Congenital infantile fibrosarcoma: a masquerader of ulcerated hemangioma. Pediatr Dermatol 2006;23(4):330–4.

54. Bahrami A, Folpe AL. Adult-type fibrosarcoma: a reevaluation of 163 putative cases diagnosed at a single institution over a 48-year period. Am J Surg Pathol 2010;34(10):1504–13.

55. Knezevich SR, McFadden DE, Tao W, et al. A novel ETV6-NTRK3 gene fusion in congenital fibrosarcoma. Nat Genet 1998;18(2):184–7.

56. Davis JL, Lockwood CM, Albert CM, et al. Infantile NTRK-associated mesenchymal tumors. Pediatr Dev Pathol 2018;21(1):68–78.

57. Kao YC, Fletcher CDM, Alaggio R, et al. Recurrent BRAF gene fusions in a subset of pediatric spindle cell sarcomas: expanding the genetic spectrum of tumors with overlapping features with infantile fibrosarcoma. Am J Surg Pathol 2018;42(1):28–38.

58. Wegert J, Vokuhl C, Collord G, et al. Recurrent intragenic rearrangements of EGFR and BRAF in soft tissue tumors of infants. Nat Commun 2018;9(1):2378.

59. Flucke U, van Noesel MM, Wijnen M, et al. TFG-MET fusion in an infantile spindle cell sarcoma with neural features. Genes Chromosomes Cancer 2017;56(9): 663–7.

60. Loh ML, Ahn P, Perez-Atayde AR, et al. Treatment of infantile fibrosarcoma with chemotherapy and surgery: results from the Dana-Farber Cancer Institute and Children's Hospital, Boston. J Pediatr Hematol Oncol 2002;24(9):722–6.

61. Parida L, Fernandez-Pineda I, Uffman JK, et al. Clinical management of infantile fibrosarcoma: a retrospective single-institution review. Pediatr Surg Int 2013; 29(7):703–8.

62. Orbach D, Brennan B, De Paoli A, et al. Conservative strategy in infantile fibrosarcoma is possible: the European paediatric Soft tissue sarcoma Study Group experience. Eur J Cancer 2016;57:1–9.

63. Miura K, Han G, Sano M, et al. Regression of congenital fibrosarcoma to hemangiomatous remnant with histological and genetic findings. Pathol Int 2002;52(9): 612–8.

64. Madden NP, Spicer RD, Allibone EB, et al. Spontaneous regression of neonatal fibrosarcoma. Br J Cancer Suppl 1992;18:S72–5.

65. Albert CM, Davis JL, Federman N, et al. TRK fusion cancers in children: a clinical review and recommendations for screening. J Clin Oncol 2019;37(6): 513–24.

66. Cocco E, Scaltriti M, Drilon A. NTRK fusion-positive cancers and TRK inhibitor therapy. Nat Rev Clin Oncol 2018;15(12):731–47.

67. Drilon A. TRK inhibitors in TRK fusion-positive cancers. Ann Oncol 2019; 30(Suppl_8):viii23–30.

68. Laetsch TW, DuBois SG, Mascarenhas L, et al. Larotrectinib for paediatric solid tumours harbouring NTRK gene fusions: phase 1 results from a multicentre, open-label, phase 1/2 study. Lancet Oncol 2018;19(5):705–14.

69. DuBois SG, Laetsch TW, Federman N, et al. The use of neoadjuvant larotrectinib in the management of children with locally advanced TRK fusion sarcomas. Cancer 2018;124(21):4241–7.

70. Alaggio R, Ninfo V, Rosolen A, et al. Primitive myxoid mesenchymal tumor of infancy: a clinicopathologic report of 6 cases. Am J Surg Pathol 2006;30(3): 388–94.

71. Santiago T, Clay MR, Allen SJ, et al. Recurrent BCOR internal tandem duplication and BCOR or BCL6 expression distinguish primitive myxoid mesenchymal

tumor of infancy from congenital infantile fibrosarcoma. Mod Pathol 2017;30(6): 884–91.

72. Suurmeijer AJH, Kao YC, Antonescu CR. New advances in the molecular classification of pediatric mesenchymal tumors. Genes Chromosomes Cancer 2019; 58(2):100–10.

73. Cipriani NA, Ryan DP, Nielsen GP. Primitive myxoid mesenchymal tumor of infancy with rosettes: a new finding and literature review. Int J Surg Pathol 2014;22(7):647–51.

74. Ognjanovic S, Linabery AM, Charbonneau B, et al. Trends in childhood rhabdomyosarcoma incidence and survival in the United States, 1975-2005. Cancer 2009;115(18):4218–26.

75. Rudzinski ER, Anderson JR, Hawkins DS, et al. The world health organization classification of skeletal muscle tumors in pediatric rhabdomyosarcoma: a report from the Children's Oncology Group. Arch Pathol Lab Med 2015; 139(10):1281–7.

76. Meza JL, Anderson J, Pappo AS, et al. Analysis of prognostic factors in patients with nonmetastatic rhabdomyosarcoma treated on intergroup rhabdomyosarcoma studies III and IV: the Children's Oncology Group. J Clin Oncol 2006; 24(24):3844–51.

77. Oberlin O, Rey A, Lyden E, et al. Prognostic factors in metastatic rhabdomyosarcomas: results of a pooled analysis from United States and European cooperative groups. J Clin Oncol 2008;26(14):2384–9.

78. Missiaglia E, Williamson D, Chisholm J, et al. PAX3/FOXO1 fusion gene status is the key prognostic molecular marker in rhabdomyosarcoma and significantly improves current risk stratification. J Clin Oncol 2012;30(14):1670–7.

79. Little DJ, Ballo MT, Zagars GK, et al. Adult rhabdomyosarcoma: outcome following multimodality treatment. Cancer 2002;95(2):377–88.

80. Sebire NJ, Malone M. Myogenin and MyoD1 expression in paediatric rhabdomyosarcomas. J Clin Pathol 2003;56(6):412–6.

81. Bougeard G, Renaux-Petel M, Flaman JM, et al. Revisiting Li-Fraumeni syndrome from TP53 mutation carriers. J Clin Oncol 2015;33(21):2345–52.

82. Palmero EI, Achatz MI, Ashton-Prolla P, et al. Tumor protein 53 mutations and inherited cancer: beyond Li-Fraumeni syndrome. Curr Opin Oncol 2010; 22(1):64–9.

83. Kerr B, Delrue MA, Sigaudy S, et al. Genotype-phenotype correlation in Costello syndrome: HRAS mutation analysis in 43 cases. J Med Genet 2006;43(5):401–5.

84. Zangari A, Zaini J, Gulia C. Genetics of bladder malignant tumors in childhood. Curr Genomics 2016;17(1):14–32.

85. Stewart DR, Best AF, Williams GM, et al. Neoplasm risk among individuals with a pathogenic germline variant in DICER1. J Clin Oncol 2019;37(8):668–76.

86. Kesserwan C, Friedman Ross L, Bradbury AR, et al. The advantages and challenges of testing children for heritable predisposition to cancer. Am Soc Clin Oncol Educ Book 2016;35:251–69.

87. Lawrence W Jr, Anderson JR, Gehan EA, et al. Pretreatment TNM staging of childhood rhabdomyosarcoma: a report of the intergroup rhabdomyosarcoma study group. Children's cancer study group. Pediatric oncology group. Cancer 1997;80(6):1165–70.

88. Maurer HM, Beltangady M, Gehan EA, et al. The intergroup rhabdomyosarcoma study-I. A final report. Cancer 1988;61(2):209–20.

89. Crist WM, Anderson JR, Meza JL, et al. Intergroup rhabdomyosarcoma study-IV: results for patients with nonmetastatic disease. J Clin Oncol 2001;19(12): 3091–102.

90. Mascarenhas L, Chi YY, Hingorani P, et al. Randomized Phase II Trial of bevacizumab or temsirolimus in combination with chemotherapy for first relapse rhabdomyosarcoma: a report from the Children's Oncology Group. J Clin Oncol 2019;37(31):2866–74.

91. Gallego S, Zanetti I, Orbach D, et al. Fusion status in patients with lymph node-positive (N1) alveolar rhabdomyosarcoma is a powerful predictor of prognosis: experience of the European Paediatric Soft Tissue Sarcoma Study Group (EpSSG). Cancer 2018;124(15):3201–9.

92. Hibbitts E, Chi YY, Hawkins DS, et al. Refinement of risk stratification for childhood rhabdomyosarcoma using FOXO1 fusion status in addition to established clinical outcome predictors: a report from the Children's Oncology Group. Cancer Med 2019;8(14):6437–48.

93. Rodeberg DA, Anderson JR, Arndt CA, et al. Comparison of outcomes based on treatment algorithms for rhabdomyosarcoma of the bladder/prostate: combined results from the Children's oncology group, German cooperative soft tissue sarcoma study, Italian cooperative group, and international society of pediatric oncology malignant mesenchymal tumors committee. Int J Cancer 2011; 128(5):1232–9.

94. Seitz G, Fuchs J, Sparber-Sauer M, et al. Improvements in the treatment of patients suffering from bladder-prostate rhabdomyosarcoma: a report from the CWS-2002P Trial. Ann Surg Oncol 2016;23(12):4067–72.

95. Borinstein SC, Steppan D, Hayashi M, et al. Consensus and controversies regarding the treatment of rhabdomyosarcoma. Pediatr Blood Cancer 2018;65(2).

96. Hawkins DS, Chi YY, Anderson JR, et al. Addition of vincristine and irinotecan to vincristine, dactinomycin, and cyclophosphamide does not improve outcome for intermediate-risk rhabdomyosarcoma: a report from the Children's Oncology Group. J Clin Oncol 2018;36(27):2770–7.

97. Weigel BJ, Lyden E, Anderson JR, et al. Intensive multiagent therapy, including dose-compressed cycles of ifosfamide/etoposide and vincristine/doxorubicin/cyclophosphamide, irinotecan, and radiation, in patients with high-risk rhabdomyosarcoma: a report from the Children's Oncology Group. J Clin Oncol 2016; 34(2):117–22.

98. Malempati S, Weigel BJ, Chi YY, et al. The addition of cixutumumab or temozolomide to intensive multiagent chemotherapy is feasible but does not improve outcome for patients with metastatic rhabdomyosarcoma: a report from the Children's Oncology Group. Cancer 2019;125(2):290–7.

99. Pintér AB, Hock A, Kajtár P, et al. Long-term follow-up of cancer in neonates and infants: a national survey of 142 patients. Pediatr Surg Int 2003;19(4):233–9.

100. Sparber-Sauer M, Stegmaier S, Vokuhl C, et al. Rhabdomyosarcoma diagnosed in the first year of life: localized, metastatic, and relapsed disease. Outcome data from five trials and one registry of the Cooperative Weichteilsarkom Studiengruppe (CWS). Pediatr Blood Cancer 2019;66(6):e27652.

101. Malempati S, Rodeberg DA, Donaldson SS, et al. Rhabdomyosarcoma in infants younger than 1 year: a report from the Children's Oncology Group. Cancer 2011; 117(15):3493–501.

102. Ferrari A, Casanova M, Bisogno G, et al. Rhabdomyosarcoma in infants younger than one year old: a report from the Italian cooperative group. Cancer 2003; 97(10):2597–604.
103. Million L, Anderson J, Breneman J, et al. Influence of noncompliance with radiation therapy protocol guidelines and operative bed recurrences for children with rhabdomyosarcoma and microscopic residual disease: a report from the Children's Oncology Group. Int J Radiat Oncol Biol Phys 2011;80(2):333–8.
104. Whittle SB, Hicks MJ, Roy A, et al. Congenital spindle cell rhabdomyosarcoma. Pediatr Blood Cancer 2019;66(11):e27935.
105. Walterhouse DO, Pappo AS, Meza JL, et al. Shorter-duration therapy using vincristine, dactinomycin, and lower-dose cyclophosphamide with or without radiotherapy for patients with newly diagnosed low-risk rhabdomyosarcoma: a report from the soft tissue sarcoma committee of the Children's Oncology Group. J Clin Oncol 2014;32(31):3547–52.
106. Walterhouse DO, Pappo AS, Meza JL, et al. Reduction of cyclophosphamide dose for patients with subset 2 low-risk rhabdomyosarcoma is associated with an increased risk of recurrence: a report from the soft tissue sarcoma committee of the Children's Oncology Group. Cancer 2017;123(12):2368–75.
107. Casey DL, Chi YY, Donaldson SS, et al. Increased local failure for patients with intermediate-risk rhabdomyosarcoma on ARST0531: a report from the Children's Oncology Group. Cancer 2019;125(18):3242–8.
108. Wolden SL, Lyden ER, Arndt CA, et al. Local control for intermediate-risk rhabdomyosarcoma: results from D9803 according to histology, group, site, and size: a report from the Children's Oncology Group. Int J Radiat Oncol Biol Phys 2015;93(5):1071–6.
109. Bisogno G, De Salvo GL, Bergeron C, et al. Vinorelbine and continuous low-dose cyclophosphamide as maintenance chemotherapy in patients with high-risk rhabdomyosarcoma (RMS 2005): a multicentre, open-label, randomised, phase 3 trial. Lancet Oncol 2019;20(11):1566–75.
110. Dillon P, Maurer H, Jenkins J, et al. A prospective study of nonrhabdomyosarcoma soft tissue sarcomas in the pediatric age group. J Pediatr Surg 1992; 27(2):241–4 [discussion 244–45].
111. Kleinerman RA, Tucker MA, Abramson DH, et al. Risk of soft tissue sarcomas by individual subtype in survivors of hereditary retinoblastoma. J Natl Cancer Inst 2007;99(1):24–31.
112. Chang F, Syrjänen S, Syrjänen K. Implications of the p53 tumor-suppressor gene in clinical oncology. J Clin Oncol 1995;13(4):1009–22.
113. deCou JM, Rao BN, Parham DM, et al. Malignant peripheral nerve sheath tumors: the St. Jude children's research hospital experience. Ann Surg Oncol 1995;2(6):524–9.
114. Kesserwan C, Sokolic R, Cowen EW, et al. Multicentric dermatofibrosarcoma protuberans in patients with adenosine deaminase-deficient severe combined immune deficiency. J Allergy Clin Immunol 2012;129(3):762–9.e761.
115. Fricke BL, Donnelly LF, Casper KA, et al. Frequency and imaging appearance of hepatic angiomyolipomas in pediatric and adult patients with tuberous sclerosis. AJR Am J Roentgenol 2004;182(4):1027–30.
116. Goto M, Miller RW, Ishikawa Y, et al. Excess of rare cancers in Werner syndrome (adult progeria). Cancer Epidemiol Biomarkers Prev 1996;5(4):239–46.
117. Hornick JL, Fletcher CD. PEComa: what do we know so far? Histopathology 2006;48(1):75–82.

118. Trojani M, Contesso G, Coindre JM, et al. Soft-tissue sarcomas of adults; study of pathological prognostic variables and definition of a histopathological grading system. Int J Cancer 1984;33(1):37–42.

119. Costa J, Wesley RA, Glatstein E, et al. The grading of soft tissue sarcomas. Results of a clinicohistopathologic correlation in a series of 163 cases. Cancer 1984;53(3):530–41.

120. Parham DM, Webber BL, Jenkins JJ 3rd, et al. Nonrhabdomyosarcomatous soft tissue sarcomas of childhood: formulation of a simplified system for grading. Mod Pathol 1995;8(7):705–10.

121. Khoury JD, Coffin CM, Spunt SL, et al. Grading of nonrhabdomyosarcoma soft tissue sarcoma in children and adolescents: a comparison of parameters used for the Fédération Nationale des Centers de Lutte Contre le cancer and pediatric oncology group systems. Cancer 2010;116(9):2266–74.

122. Callegaro D, Miceli R, Mariani L, et al. Soft tissue sarcoma nomograms and their incorporation into practice. Cancer 2017;123(15):2802–20.

123. Tanaka K, Ozaki T. New TNM classification (AJCC eighth edition) of bone and soft tissue sarcomas: JCOG bone and soft tissue tumor study group. Jpn J Clin Oncol 2019;49(2):103–7.

124. Suit H, Spiro I. Radiation as a therapeutic modality in sarcomas of the soft tissue. Hematol Oncol Clin North Am 1995;9(4):733–46.

125. Gallego S, Llort A, Roma J, et al. Detection of bone marrow micrometastasis and microcirculating disease in rhabdomyosarcoma by a real-time RT-PCR assay. J Cancer Res Clin Oncol 2006;132(6):356–62.

126. Brooks AD, Heslin MJ, Leung DH, et al. Superficial extremity soft tissue sarcoma: an analysis of prognostic factors. Ann Surg Oncol 1998;5(1):41–7.

127. Ferrari A, Miceli R, Meazza C, et al. Soft tissue sarcomas of childhood and adolescence: the prognostic role of tumor size in relation to patient body size. J Clin Oncol 2009;27(3):371–6.

128. Spunt SL, Million L, Chi YY, et al. A risk-based treatment strategy for nonrhabdomyosarcoma soft-tissue sarcomas in patients younger than 30 years (ARST0332): a Children's Oncology Group prospective study. Lancet Oncol 2020;21(1):145–61.

129. Haas RL, Gronchi A, van de Sande MAJ, et al. Perioperative management of extremity soft tissue sarcomas. J Clin Oncol 2018;36(2):118–24.

130. Nussbaum DP, Rushing CN, Lane WO, et al. Preoperative or postoperative radiotherapy versus surgery alone for retroperitoneal sarcoma: a case-control, propensity score-matched analysis of a nationwide clinical oncology database. Lancet Oncol 2016;17(7):966–75.

131. Geoerger B, Chisholm J, Le Deley MC, et al. Phase II study of gemcitabine combined with oxaliplatin in relapsed or refractory paediatric solid malignancies: an Innovative Therapy for Children with Cancer European Consortium Study. Eur J Cancer 2011;47(2):230–8.

132. Minard-Colin V, Ichante JL, Nguyen L, et al. Phase II study of vinorelbine and continuous low doses cyclophosphamide in children and young adults with a relapsed or refractory malignant solid tumour: good tolerance profile and efficacy in rhabdomyosarcoma–a report from the Societe Francaise des Cancers et leucemies de l'Enfant et de l'adolescent (SFCE). Eur J Cancer 2012;48(15): 2409–16.

133. Kuttesch JF Jr, Krailo MD, Madden T, et al. Phase II evaluation of intravenous vinorelbine (navelbine) in recurrent or refractory pediatric malignancies: a Children's Oncology Group study. Pediatr Blood Cancer 2009;53(4):590–3.

134. Geller JI, Fox E, Turpin BK, et al. A study of axitinib, a VEGF receptor tyrosine kinase inhibitor, in children and adolescents with recurrent or refractory solid tumors: a Children's Oncology Group phase 1 and pilot consortium trial (ADVL1315). Cancer 2018;124(23):4548–55.
135. Bromodomain (BRD) and extra-terminal domain (BET) inhibitor. ClinicalTrials.gov web site. Available at: https://clinicaltrials.gov/ct2/show/NCT03936465. Accessed May 2020.
136. Pazopanib in pediatric solid tumors. ClinicalTrialsgov. Web site. Available at: https://clinicaltrials.gov/ct2/show/NCT01956669. Accessed May 2020.
137. Oda Y, Tsuneyoshi M. Extrarenal rhabdoid tumors of soft tissue: clinicopathological and molecular genetic review and distinction from other soft-tissue sarcomas with rhabdoid features. Pathol Int 2006;56(6):287–95.
138. Brennan B, Stiller C, Bourdeaut F. Extracranial rhabdoid tumours: what we have learned so far and future directions. Lancet Oncol 2013;14(8):e329–36.
139. Schneppenheim R, Frühwald MC, Gesk S, et al. Germline nonsense mutation and somatic inactivation of SMARCA4/BRG1 in a family with rhabdoid tumor predisposition syndrome. Am J Hum Genet 2010;86(2):279–84.
140. Eaton KW, Tooke LS, Wainwright LM, et al. Spectrum of SMARCB1/INI1 mutations in familial and sporadic rhabdoid tumors. Pediatr Blood Cancer 2011; 56(1):7–15.
141. Judkins AR. Immunohistochemistry of INI1 expression: a new tool for old challenges in CNS and soft tissue pathology. Adv Anat Pathol 2007;14(5):335–9.
142. Madigan CE, Armenian SH, Malogolowkin MH, et al. Extracranial malignant rhabdoid tumors in childhood: the Childrens Hospital Los Angeles experience. Cancer 2007;110(9):2061–6.
143. Isaacs H Jr. Fetal and neonatal rhabdoid tumor. J Pediatr Surg 2010;45(3): 619–26.
144. Sultan I, Qaddoumi I, Rodríguez-Galindo C, et al. Age, stage, and radiotherapy, but not primary tumor site, affects the outcome of patients with malignant rhabdoid tumors. Pediatr Blood Cancer 2010;54(1):35–40.
145. Bourdeaut F, Fréneaux P, Thuille B, et al. Extra-renal non-cerebral rhabdoid tumours. Pediatr Blood Cancer 2008;51(3):363–8.
146. Puri DR, Meyers PA, Kraus DH, et al. Radiotherapy in the multimodal treatment of extrarenal extracranial malignant rhabdoid tumors. Pediatr Blood Cancer 2008;50(1):167–9.
147. Nemes K, Clément N, Kachanov D, et al. The extraordinary challenge of treating patients with congenital rhabdoid tumors-a collaborative European effort. Pediatr Blood Cancer 2018;65(6):e26999.
148. Venkatramani R, Shoureshi P, Malvar J, et al. High dose alkylator therapy for extracranial malignant rhabdoid tumors in children. Pediatr Blood Cancer 2014;61(8):1357–61.
149. Lawell MP, Indelicato DJ, Paulino AC, et al. An open invitation to join the pediatric proton/photon consortium registry to standardize data collection in pediatric radiation oncology. Br J Radiol 2020;93(1107). 20190673.
150. Leroy R, Benahmed N, Hulstaert F, et al. Proton therapy in children: a systematic review of clinical effectiveness in 15 pediatric cancers. Int J Radiat Oncol Biol Phys 2016;95(1):267–78.
151. Jain S, Xu R, Prieto VG, et al. Molecular classification of soft tissue sarcomas and its clinical applications. Int J Clin Exp Pathol 2010;3(4):416–28.

Neonatal Malignant
Disorders: Germ Cell Tumors

Check for updates

Rachana Shah, MD, MS[a],*, Brent R. Weil, MD, MPH[b,c],
Christopher B. Weldon, MD, PhD[b,c], James F. Amatruda, MD, PhD[a],
A. Lindsay Frazier, MD, ScM[c]

KEYWORDS

- Germ cell tumor • Fetal • Neonatal • Molecular genetics • Teratoma
- Yolk sac tumor • Choriocarcinoma • Fetus-in-fetu

KEY POINTS

- Teratomas (mature or immature) account for a vast majority of the neonatal germ cell tumors, approximately 5% of which contain a malignant component that is predominantly yolk sac tumor.
- Most neonatal germ cell tumors are curable with surgery alone.
- In the rare instance of a neonate with metastatic malignant disease or malignant disease for which upfront surgical resection is not feasible without significant morbidity, an initial biopsy followed by neoadjuvant chemotherapy and delayed surgical resection is recommended.
- If chemotherapy is indicated, a carboplatin-based regimen should be considered to minimize treatment-related toxicity.

INTRODUCTION

Germ cell tumors (GCTs) are a wide spectrum of biologically diverse and histologically heterogenous tumors that can arise in gonadal or extragonadal sites. In the neonatal period, GCTs rank as the fifth most frequent malignant neoplasm, after neuroblastoma, leukemia, sarcoma, Wilms tumor, and retinoblastoma.[1] Benign mature or immature teratomas account for a vast majority of the neonatal GCTs, roughly 5% to 10% of which contain a malignant component that is predominantly yolk sac tumor (YST).[1,2]

[a] Division of Oncology, Department of Pediatrics, Cancer and Blood Disease Institute, Children's Hospital Los Angeles, University of Southern California, Keck School of Medicine, 4650 Sunset Boulevard, MS#54, Los Angeles, CA 90027, USA; [b] Department of Surgery, Boston Children's Hospital, Harvard Medical School, Boston, MA, USA; [c] Department of Pediatric Oncology, Children's Cancer and Blood Disorders Center, Children's Hospital Dana-Farber Cancer Center, Harvard Medical School, 450 Brookline Avenue, Boston, MA 02215, USA
* Corresponding author.
E-mail address: rshah@chla.usc.edu

Clin Perinatol 48 (2021) 147–165
https://doi.org/10.1016/j.clp.2020.11.010
0095-5108/21/© 2020 Elsevier Inc. All rights reserved.
perinatology.theclinics.com

PATHOGENESIS

Germ cells are set aside from somatic cells very early in the fetal period, and germline development proceeds in a programmatic series of steps. Defects in this developmental program can give rise to GCTs in the fetus and neonate (**Fig. 1**).

Specification and Migration of Primordial Germ Cells

At the time of blastocyst implantation, the extraembryonic ectoderm and the visceral endoderm send signals to the embryonic ectoderm, resulting in expression of the transcriptional repressor *BLIMP1/PRDM14* in a few cells in the epiblast.[3] These cells, in which expression of somatic genes, such as *Hoxb1*, *T/brachyury*, and *Snail*, is repressed, will become the primordial germ cells (PGCs). Unlike other epiblast-derived cells, PGCs regain or maintain expression of pluripotency associated genes, such as *LIN28A*, *SOX2*, *OCT3/4 (POU5F1)*, and *NANOG*.[4,5] Certain pluripotency genes can be reactivated in GCTs and may contribute to malignant potential.[6] In humans, PGCs can be identified in the wall of the yolk sac beginning around day 24.[7] The PGCs begin to proliferate as they migrate out of the yolk sac into the embryo.[8] Proper PGC migration is critical to survival of the germ cells and formation of the gonad. Failure of this migration can result in ectopic germ cells, persistence of which is one possible mechanism by which extragonadal GCTs are thought to arise. Toward the end of gastrulation, morphogenetic movements in the developing embryo bring the PGCs in proximity to the hindgut. Invading the endoderm, the PGCs colonize the hindgut and begin migration, a process dependent on the receptor tyrosine kinase *c-KIT*, expressed in PGCs, and its ligand, *KITL*, expressed in somatic cells.[9] Knockdown of *CXCR4* and its ligand *CXCL12* results in PGC mismigration and failure to reach the gonadal ridge after PGCs reach the dorsal wall.[10] At 5 to 6 weeks' after fertilization, the PGCs exit the hindgut to colonize the gonadal ridge primordia; PGCs failing to reach the gonadal ridge are eliminated by *BAX*-dependent apoptosis.[11] Once they have entered the gonadal ridges, PGCs become much less motile but

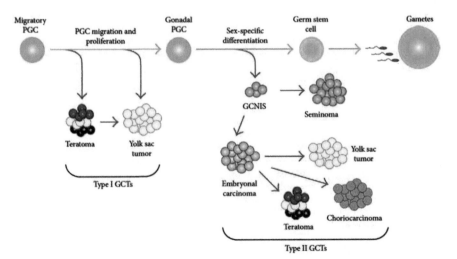

Fig. 1. Germline development and histologic subtypes of GCTs. GCNIS, germ cell neoplasia in situ. (*From* Pierce, J. L., Frazier, A. L. & Amatruda, J. F. Pediatric Germ Cell Tumors: A Developmental Perspective. Adv Urol 2018, (2018); with permission).

continue several more rounds of division. This proliferation depends on continued *KITL/c-KIT* signaling.

Erasure of Imprinting

"Imprinting" refers to the epigenetic modification of certain genes (typically by cytosine methylation) such that only the maternal or paternal allele of the gene is expressed. Lineage-specific patterns of imprinting are established in different tissues, including the germline, around the time of gastrulation. Upon entering the gonadal ridges, PGCs actively erase these genomic methylation patterns. This erasure is necessary in order to allow the maternal and paternal imprinting patterns to be established in the oocytes and sperm, respectively. Prepubertal (type I) GCTs show only partial erasure of parental imprinting, indicating that prepubertal tumors likely arise from an earlier stage of embryonic germ cell development than do the postpubertal (type II) tumors.[12] A similar pattern of imprinting is seen in gonadal and extragonadal pediatric GCTs, suggesting that gonadal and nongonadal tumors share a common pathogenesis and cell of origin.

Gonadogenesis

Beginning shortly before the arrival of the PGCs in the gonadal ridges, the coelomic epithelium begins to proliferate and invade the underlying mesenchyme, forming the primitive sex cords. Migrating PGCs entering the gonad are surrounded by the cords. Subsequently, changes occur in both the germ cells and the gonadal somatic cells, according to the genetic sex of the embryo.

In summary, the complex process of gonadal organogenesis is subject to both genetic and environmental influences. Abnormal development of the gonads during the embryonic and fetal periods leads to defects, such as cryptorchidism and gonadal dysgenesis, which are strongly associated with the risk of developing GCTs.[13,14]

MOLECULAR GENETICS

The most common chromosomal aberration seen in adolescent/adult malignant GCTs is chromosome 12p gain, typically because of isochromosome 12p,[15] regardless of histologic subtype and primary site. The genomic aberrations seen in malignant GCTs of infants and children (prepubertal) are generally distinct from those occurring in postpubertal tumors. In the prepubertal period, pure teratomas of the testis or extragonadal sites almost always exhibit a normal profile in genomic analyses, including cytogenetics, fluorescence in situ hybridization, loss of heterozygosity (LOH) analysis, and array comparative genomic hybridization. These data contrast sharply with the universally abnormal cytogenetic profile of postpubertal teratomas arising as a component of a mixed malignant GCT. Unlike teratomas, cytogenetic and other genomic aberrations are consistently reported in analyses of YSTs in infants and children. The most common imbalances reported are gains at chromosomes 1p, 3p, and 20q, and losses at chromosome 1p and chromosome 6q.[16–18] Loss of chromosomes 1p and 6q correlates with LOH analysis, indicating true allelic loss in these regions in pediatric GCTs.

MicroRNAs are short, non-protein-coding RNAs that regulate the stability and translation of target messenger RNAs. Individual microRNAs from 2 clusters, miR-371-373 and miR-302-367, are overexpressed in all malignant GCTs, regardless of patient age, tumor site, and subtype ($P \leq .00005$).[19] A panel of 4 circulating microRNAs (miR-371a-3p, miR-372-3p, miR-373-3p, miR-367-3p) is highly sensitive and specific for the diagnosis of malignant GCT, including seminoma. In contrast, microRNAs are not overexpressed in teratomas. Clinically, this may be valuable in distinguishing a recurrent teratoma from a malignant recurrence. The current Children's Oncology Group (COG) trial, AGCT1531, aims at prospective validation of serum microRNA as a candidate biomarker for early detection of relapse in malignant GCTs, especially in tumor marker negative disease.

EPIDEMIOLOGY

In the United States, GCTs occur at a rate of 5.4 per million children, representing approximately 3.5% of cancer diagnoses for children under 15 years of age.[20] The age-adjusted incidence of GCT is characterized by a bimodal pattern: there is an initial peak between birth and 4 years of age, followed by a second peak coinciding with the onset of puberty that continues into the third and fourth decades of young adult life. In male children, the incidence of testicular and extracranial extragonadal GCTs is similar between birth and 4 years of age, followed by a dramatic increase in incidence of testicular GCTs between ages 15 and 19 years (**Fig. 2**). In female children, the incidence of extracranial extragonadal GCTs accounts for a vast majority of the cases between birth and 4 years of age with a trend toward an increase in the incidence of ovarian GCTs at 8 to 9 years of age, peaking at 18 years of age (**Fig. 3**).

In newborns, the vast majority of GCTs are extragonadal as compared with gonadal predominance in children and adolescents. Neonatal GCTs are more frequent in female than male newborns (female:male, 3:1) at sacrococcygeal, gastric, orbital, and facial sites. Intracranial, head, and neck (ie, cervical and oro-nasopharyngeal), cardiac, mediastinal teratomas, and fetus-in-fetu (FIF) are equally distributed between female and male newborns.[2]

Overall, black children have a lower incidence of GCTs than white children (7.0 vs 10.7 per million).[20] Analysis of the National Cancer Institute Surveillance, Epidemiology, and End Results Program (SEER) data from 18 registries (2000–2015) demonstrated that there were no significant racial/ethnic survival differences among female children, whereas male survival differed by race/ethnicity ($P<.0001$), with non-Hispanic white male children having the best survival.[21] When adjusted for age and year at diagnosis, tumor histology, location, and stage, Asian, Pacific Islander, and Hispanic male children had significantly higher risks of death compared with non-Hispanic white male children. This association was not influenced by stage of disease, except for gonadal tumors in Hispanic male children. The investigators concluded that unidentified factors, such as differences in exposures, tumor biology, or treatment received, may be driving the observed disparity.

RISK FACTORS
Family History

In a population-based Childhood Cancer Research Network (CCRN) study evaluating the family history of GCTs and other cancers in relatives of pediatric GCT, probands demonstrated familial aggregation of GCTs, suggesting an underlying genetic cause. Male and female relatives of probands had a higher number of GCTs than expected when compared with incidence data from the SEER program, although this reached statistical significance only among male relatives. Notably, most reported GCTs occurred in relatives of probands with an intracranial tumor. The investigators observed an elevated risk of melanoma in male relatives of probands and an elevated, but nonsignificant risk of melanoma in female relatives of probands.[22]

Average annual rate per million

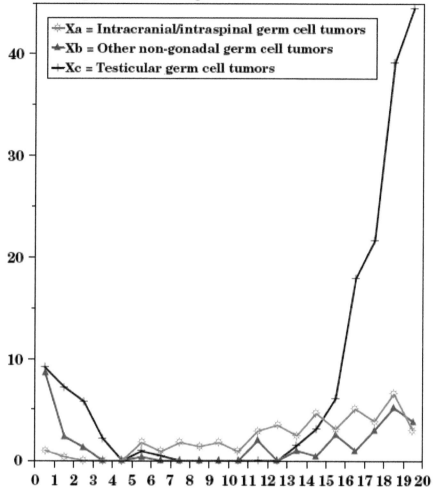

Age (in years) at diagnosis

Fig. 2. Age-specific incidence rates by selected International Classification of Childhood Cancer subgroups, male children all races, SEER, 1986 to 1994. GCTOG, germ cell, tropho-blastic and other gonadal. (*From* Figure X.2: GCTOG age-specific incidence rates by sex, all races, SEER, 1986-94. Page: 130. SEER monograph: Bernstein L, Smith MA, Liu L, Deapen D, and Friedman DL, *Germ Cell Trophoblastic and other Gonadal Neoplasms ICCC X*, in *SEER Cancer Statistics Review, 1975-2004*, Ries L, Melbert D, Krapcho M, Mariotto A, Miller BA, Feuer EJ, Clegg L, Horner MJ, Howlader N, Eisner MP, Reichman M, and Edwards BK, Editors. 2007, National Cancer Institute: Bethesda, MD p. 125-137; with permission.)

Congenital Abnormalities

Maternally reported congenital abnormalities were examined in a case-control study of 278 pediatric patients with GCTs and 423 controls. GCTs were significantly associated with cryptorchidism in male pediatric patients (odds ratio = 10.8, 95% confidence interval [CI] = 2.1 to 55.1), but not with any other specific congenital abnormality in either sex.[14]

Average annual rate per million

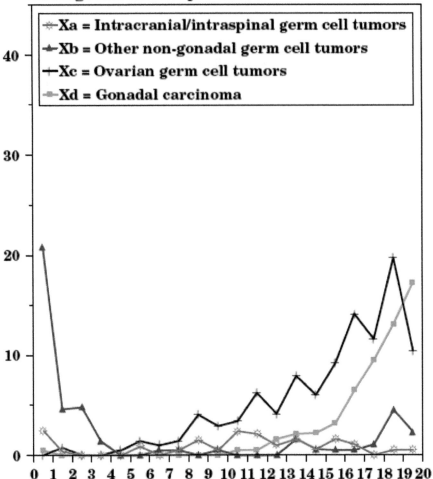

Fig. 3. Age-specific incidence rates by selected International Classification of Childhood Cancer subgroups, female children all races, SEER, 1986 to 1994. GCTOG, germ cell, trophoblastic and other gonadal. (*From* Figure X.3: GCTOG age-specific incidence rates by selected ICCC subgroups females, all races, SEER, 1986-94. Page 130: SEER monograph: Bernstein L, Smith MA, Liu L, Deapen D, and Friedman DL, *Germ Cell Trophoblastic and other Gonadal Neoplasms ICCC X*, in *SEER Cancer Statistics Review, 1975-2004*, Ries L, Melbert D, Krapcho M, Mariotto A, Miller BA, Feuer EJ, Clegg L, Horner MJ, Howlader N, Eisner MP, Reichman M, and Edwards BK, Editors. 2007, National Cancer Institute: Bethesda, MD p. 125-137; with permission.)

Virilization Syndrome

Patients with hypervirilization syndromes are not at an increased risk for development of GCTs. In contrast, patients with undervirilization syndromes, such as androgen insensitivity syndrome, have a 5.5% calculated prevalence of GCTs, which dramatically increases after puberty to reach 33% at the age of 50 years. Although the data are limited, the risk seems to be markedly higher in the partial than in the complete variant.[13] In patients with androgen biosynthetic defects, gonadectomy should be performed before puberty.[23]

Disorders of Sex Development

Disorders of sex development or intersex disorders, including patients with Y chromosome or Y-derived sequence, exhibit a significant risk of gonadal GCTs. Ovarian dysgerminoma and testicular seminoma are the most prevalent GCTs arising in dysgenetic gonads and are almost always preceded by the presence of an in situ neoplastic lesion—either germ cell neoplasia in situ or gonadoblastoma. Patients with 46,XY pure gonadal dysgenesis have the highest tumor incidence and malignancy risk.[13,24] In contrast to patients with undervirilization syndromes, GCTs in patients with gonadal dysgenesis are frequently found at a very young age (eg, in the first year of life or may even be present at birth).[13]

Analysis of pediatric patients with malignant ovarian (MO)GCT in the COG trial AGCT0132 highlighted that patients with nonseminomatous MOGCT in the context of dysgenetic gonads had higher rates of event and death (estimated 3-year event-free survival [EFS_3] and overall survival [OS_3] were 66.7% and 87.5%, respectively) compared with patients with normal gonadal development (EFS_3 = 88.8%, OS_3 = 97.6%).[25] These results emphasize the importance of noting a contralateral streak ovary or gonadoblastoma at histology for any ovarian GCT and support the recommendation for early bilateral gonadectomy in patients known to have gonadal dysgenesis with Y-chromosome material.[23]

Klinefelter Syndrome

Based on analysis of array genotyping data from a COG CCRN epidemiology study of 433 male children aged birth to 19 years, male childrenwith Klinefelter syndrome (47,XXY) were significantly more likely to be diagnosed with a mediastinal GCT compared with male children without chromosomal abnormalities (risk ratio = 18.8, 95% CI = 11.7–30, $P<.01$). Therefore, screening of male children with mediastinal GCTs for Klinefelter syndrome is warranted.[26]

CLINICAL PRESENTATION

The most common initial presentation of neonatal GCTs is a mass, detected by antenatal imaging and/or postnatally by physical examination. Signs and symptoms typically correspond to the site of origin. The sacrococcygeal region (40%) is the most common site of neonatal GCTs; other sites include intracranial (13%), cardiac (7.5%), FIF (5%), mediastinal (3%), gastric (3%), and head and neck, including cervical (13%), oropharynx and nasopharynx (8%), orbital (3%), and facial (1.5%).[2] Additional miscellaneous sites (3%) reported include tongue, tonsil, liver, retroperitoneum, mesentery, ileum, testis, vulva, and the anorectal region.

Polyhydramnios, respiratory distress, and still birth are more common findings than hydrops fetalis, prematurity, malpresentations, and dystocia.[2] Most patients with intracerebral teratoma present with macrocephaly and hydrocephalus, whereas most patients with cardiac teratoma have pericardial effusion and tamponade. Patients with sacrococcygeal teratomas (SCT, 15%) have the largest number of congenital anomalies followed by those with oronasopharyngeal (12%) and cervical teratomas (6%).[2] Common associated congenital anomalies reported include hydrocephalus, absence of septum pellucidum, congenital heart defects, Potter sequence, genitourinary malformations, shoulder dystocia, and congenital hip dislocation. Screening and/or consideration of these conditions should be a part of the initial diagnostic workup for patients with these particular teratomas.

HISTOLOGY

Histologic subtypes of GCTs include teratoma (mature or immature), YST (also known as endodermal sinus tumor), choriocarcinoma, embryonal carcinoma, and germinoma (dysgerminoma or seminoma).[6] The predominant histology in neonates is either mature (51%) or immature (49%) teratoma, with YST being the second most common. An extremely rare entity in the newborn period is FIF (see later discussion).[2]

Teratoma

The most common histologic subtype of neonatal GCTs is typically composed of tissues derived from all 3 embryonic layers, that is, ectoderm, endoderm, and mesoderm. Occasionally, teratomas may be monodermal or bidermal. The histologic composition of mature teratomas includes well-differentiated tissues, such as cartilage, bone, skin, and skin appendages. In contrast, immature teratomas contain varying degrees of immature fetal tissue, usually neuroectodermal. Teratomas are histologically graded according to the proportion of tissue containing immature neuroepithelial elements.[27] Mature teratomas containing only mature tissue are considered grade 0. Immature teratomas may be grade 1 (presence of <10% immature neuroepithelium) to grade 3 (presence of >50% immature neuroepithelium).

The Malignant Germ Cell International Consortium (MaGIC) merged data from the GCT clinical trials, conducted between 1983 to 2009, by the COG (US), which used cisplatin-based regimens, and by Children's Cancer and Leukaemia Group (CCLG, UK), which used carboplatin-based regimens. A pooled MaGIC analysis of ovarian immature teratomas in children, adolescents, and young adults demonstrated that histologic grade was the most important risk factor for relapse. Among histologic grade 3 tumors, the stage (see later discussion) was significantly associated with relapse. However, adjuvant chemotherapy did not decrease the risk of relapse in the pediatric cohort regardless of the grade or stage of the immature teratoma.[28] Surgical resection remains the mainstay of treatment in teratomas, either mature or immature.[29] A Pediatric Oncology Group (POG) study in children demonstrated that surgery alone is curative for most children and adolescents with completely resected stage I immature teratomas of any grade, even when associated with elevated levels of serum alpha-fetoprotein (AFP) or microscopic foci of YST.[30,31]

Yolk Sac Tumor

Prepubertal children predominantly present with a pure YST. In contrast, only 5% of all neonatal teratomas have a yolk sac component; the incidence is higher in neonatal SCT (10%).[2] The differentiation of tumor cells in YSTs is predominantly endodermal and can take the form of both intraembryonic (primitive gut and liver) and extraembryonic (allantois and yolk sac) derivatives. Serum AFP is generally elevated in patients with YST; however, low levels of AFP can be detected in the setting of an immature teratoma with microscopic foci of YST.

Macroscopically, YSTs are generally well-circumscribed and nonencapsulated and consist of friable, yellow, mucoid tissue with frequent areas of hemorrhage, necrosis, and liquefaction. Microscopically, they display a loose, myxoid stroma containing a reticulated pattern of microcystic spaces that are lined by a flattened, periodic acid–Schiff stain–positive, diastase-resistant epithelium. Approximately 20% of YSTs exhibit characteristic Schiller-Duval bodies, which are a clustering of cells around a small central blood vessel. In addition to the microcystic/reticular pattern, several variant histologies of YST have been described, including the solid, polyvesicular, and parietal types (corresponding to primitive endoderm and extraembryonic structures) and the glandular and hepatic types (corresponding to the intraembryonic endodermal derivatives). Chemotherapy is reserved for YSTs presenting with advanced stage or relapse.

Infantile Choriocarcinoma

Infantile choriocarcinoma was first described as a distinct clinicopathologic syndrome in 1968.[32] Choriocarcinoma is composed of cytotrophoblast, syncytiotrophoblast, and extravillous trophoblast, often mixed in random fashion, surrounding areas of hemorrhage and necrosis. Vascular invasion is a common feature.

The median age at presentation is typically 1 month (range, 0 days to 5 months).[33] Classic symptoms at diagnosis include severe anemia, failure to thrive, and hepatomegaly. Infrequently, infants can also present with hemoptysis, respiratory failure, seizures, or signs of precocious puberty.[33,34] Multiorgan involvement is fairly common, with liver (77%), lung (67%), brain (27%), or skin (10%) being the most common involved sites.[33] Beta-human chorionic gonadotropin (βhCG) is typically markedly elevated at the time of diagnosis. The natural progression of choriocarcinoma can be rapidly progressive and fatal without prompt and appropriate treatment.[33] Treatment should not be delayed for definitive histologic confirmation in an infant who presents with a markedly elevated β-hCG and a clinical presentation consistent with infantile choriocarcinoma.[33] Optimal treatment of infantile choriocarcinoma is multiagent chemotherapy with either carboplatin- or cisplatin-based regimens.[33–37] Upfront surgical resection of tumor is not recommended in these patients because of tumor friability, risk of uncontrolled bleeding, as well as clinical fragility of the infant at diagnosis.[33–37] Surgical resection of residual masses may not be necessary in a patient in whom the β-hCG has normalized.

Infantile choriocarcinoma is thought to represent a metastatic focus from primary maternal or placental gestational trophoblastic tumor; hence, maternal screening with β-hCG is recommended.[33] A history of maternal choriocarcinoma or hydatidiform molar pregnancy is associated with a higher risk of infantile choriocarcinoma in subsequent pregnancies.[37]

Fetus-In-Fetu

The term "FIF" was coined by Meckel in the eighteenth century to describe a rare congenital fetiform anomaly. The embryogenesis remains controversial, and it is unclear if FIF is a monochorionic, monozygotic, diamniotic twin of the host, or a well-differentiated teratoma (fetiform teratoma).[38,39] FIF is typically diagnosed antenatally or in infancy as a slow-growing asymptomatic mass. It occurs predominantly in the upper retroperitoneum (80%), but other reported sites of FIF include intracranial, oropharynx, neck, mediastinum, liver, kidney, sacrococcygeal, pelvis, ovary, and scrotum or undescended testicle.[40] Karyotype of the FIF is identical to that of the host.[41] The recommended treatment of FIF is complete surgical resection. Incomplete surgical resection merits postoperative surveillance for early detection of recurrences. Only 2 malignant recurrences have been reported to date.[42,43]

SERUM TUMOR MARKERS

Serum tumor markers, such as AFP and β-hCG, aid in the diagnosis, risk stratification, or prognostication, assessing response to therapy and detection of relapse of GCTs. AFP is the predominant serum-binding glycoprotein in the fetus, with peak concentration at 12 to 14 weeks of gestation. In early embryogenesis, AFP is produced in the yolk sac and subsequently in hepatocytes and the gastrointestinal tract. Over the course of the first 2 years of life, AFP gradually declines to a normal adult level as synthesis in the liver ceases, corresponding with albumin becoming the principal serum-binding protein. The interpretation of AFP levels is complex because of this age-related variability in the reference range.[44,45] Values of AFP obtained in children less than 2 years of age can be plotted on the nomogram developed by Blohm and colleagues[44] or Wu and colleagues[45] to determine whether the value falls within the normal range (**Table 1**).

AFP is generally elevated in patients with YST; however, low levels can be detected in the setting of an immature teratoma with microscopic foci of YST. Differential diagnoses for an elevated AFP may include benign liver conditions, including hepatic dysfunction, viral hepatitis (hepatitis B or C and human immunodeficiency virus-associated hepatitis) and cirrhosis, hepatoblastoma, hepatocellular carcinoma, pancreatic and gastrointestinal malignancies, cystic fibrosis, lung cancer, congenital heart defects, hypothyroidism, folate deficiencies, or platelet aggregation disorders. It is important to note that AFP is elevated in all infants at birth.

β-hCG, a peptide hormone normally elevated in pregnancy, is produced by the embryo soon after conception and later by the syncytiotrophoblast in the placenta to prevent disintegration of the corpus luteum of the ovary and thereby maintain progesterone production. β-hCG is generally significantly elevated in tumors that originate from extraembryonic tissue, such as choriocarcinoma. The serum half-life $(t_{1/2})$ of AFP and β-hCG is 5 to 7 days and 24 to 36 hours, respectively.

Table 1			
Normal range of serum alpha-fetoprotein (ng/mL) in infants			
Wu et al,[45] 1981		Blohm et al,[44] 1998	
Age	Mean ± Standard Deviation	Age	Mean (95% CI)
Premature	134,734 ± 41,444	Premature	158,125 (31,261–799,834)
Newborn	48,406 ± 34,718	Newborn	41,687 (9120–190,546)
0–2 wk	33,113 ± 32,503	Day 8–14	9333 (1480–58,887)
2 wk to 1 mo	9452 ± 12,610	Day 22–28	1396 (316–6310)
2 mo	323 ± 278	Day 46–60	178 (16–1045)
3 mo	88 ± 87	Day 61–90	80 (6–1045)
4 mo	74 + 56	Day 91–120	36 (3–417)
5 mo	47 ± 19	Day 121–150	20 (2–216)
6 mo	13 ± 10	Day 151–180	13 (1–129)
7 mo	10 ± 7	Day 181–720	8 (1–87)

Adapted from, Wu, J.T., Book, L., Sudar, K., 1981. Serum Alpha Fetoprotein (AFP) Levels in Normal Infants. Pediatric Research 15, 50 to 52. Blohm MEG, Vesterling-Horner D, Calaminus G, Gobel U. Alpha₁-Fetoprotein (AFP) reference values in infants up to 2 years of age. Pediatric Hematology & Oncology Journal 1998 15:135 to 142; with permission.

STAGING AND REVISED RISK STRATIFICATION

The POG and Children's Cancer Group devised a pediatric staging system for the intergroup studies that was subsequently adapted in the COG trials (**Table 2**). A recent MaGIC analysis of data merged from 7 GCT trials conducted by the COG (US) or the CCLG (UK) established an evidence-based clinical risk stratification for malignant extracranial pediatric GCTs.[46]

SURGICAL MANAGEMENT
General Principles

In the neonatal period, surgical resection is the mainstay of GCT treatment, regardless of site. Despite the presence of microscopic residual disease owing to positive margins, recurrence rates and mortality are low, even in tumors with malignant elements.[47] Hence, morbid procedures in order to achieve negative margins are not justified in a fetus or neonate. A fetus with a large, rapidly growing and highly vascular teratoma is at risk for developing hydrops fetalis because of high-output cardiac failure and anemia. Fetal interventions, such as laser vessel ablation, alcohol sclerosis, cyst drainage, amniodrainage, vesicoamniotic shunt insertion, or preoperative embolization, are advocated in the setting of impending hydrops in a fetus who cannot yet be delivered. Detailed cross-sectional imaging is necessary in order to delineate critical neurovascular structures in relation to these often large and vascular tumors before operative intervention. Site-specific considerations in the surgical management of extracranial GCTs are discussed herein.

Sacrococcygeal Germ Cell Tumors

The principles of resection for SCT are largely unchanged since the early description.[48] The anatomic classification of SCT, developed by Altman and colleagues,[49] relies on the amount of the tumor that is exophytic versus endophytic (**Fig. 4**). Preoperative cross-sectional imaging is critical to determine the internal extent of the tumor, and hence, the operative approach. Most presacral lesions are initially approached through a posterior, transsacral incision. If the peritoneal cavity is entered, a sample of fluid or washings should be obtained for cytology. Appropriate surgical intervention involves complete tumor resection, removal of the coccyx, and preservation of muscle and neurovascular structures. In neonates with malignant GCT, if complete excision cannot be accomplished without significant risk to adjacent structures, biopsy followed by neoadjuvant chemotherapy should be pursued. Prior studies have demonstrated no difference in survival in patients treated with initial biopsy, neoadjuvant chemotherapy, and a delayed resection compared with upfront resection.[50,51] Gastrointestinal and genitourinary dysfunction are common following neonatal SCT resection.[52] Long-term follow-up is mandatory in these children to ensure that normal bowel, bladder, and sensory-motor function is preserved.[53] Recurrence is more likely among patients with immature teratoma than mature teratoma; approximately 50% recur with a malignant component.[47]

Cervicofacial Germ Cell Tumors

Cervicofacial GCTs most commonly present during the prenatal or perinatal period. Lesions can encompass, compress, or emanate from the nasopharynx, oropharynx, hypopharynx, larynx, anterior mediastinum, or other areas. Involvement of the thyroid gland is common, and preoperative and postoperative monitoring is mandatory to assess for normal thyroid function and the need for thyroid hormone replacement. The lesions often cause esophageal and tracheal obstruction leading to

Table 2
The Children's Oncology Group pediatric staging system for germ cell tumors

Stage	Extragonadal	Ovarian	Gonadal	
			Testicular	
I	Complete resection at any site, including coccygectomy for sacrococcygeal site	Complete resection		Complete resection by high inguinal orchiectomy
	Tumor capsule intact	Tumor limited to ovary		Tumor limited to testis
	Negative margins and lymph nodes	Tumor capsule intact		Tumor capsule intact
		Negative margins, cytology, and lymph nodes		Negative margins and lymph nodes
II	Microscopic residual	Microscopic residual		Microscopic residual
	Tumor capsule intact or disrupted	Tumor capsule intact or disrupted		Transcrotal orchiectomy
	Negative lymph nodes	Negative cytology and lymph nodes		Tumor capsule intact or disrupted
		Failure of tumor markers to normalize or decrease with an appropriate half-life		Negative lymph nodes
				Failure of tumor markers to normalize or decrease with an appropriate half-life
III	Gross residual or biopsy only	Gross residual or biopsy only		Gross residual or biopsy only
	Regional lymph nodes negative or positive	Positive cytology		No visceral or extraabdominal involvement
		Contiguous visceral involvement (omentum, intestine, bladder)		Regional lymph node negative or positive
		Regional lymph nodes negative or positive		
IV	Distant metastases, including liver, lung, bone, brain	Distant metastases, including liver, lung, bone, brain		Distant metastases, including liver, lung, bone, brain

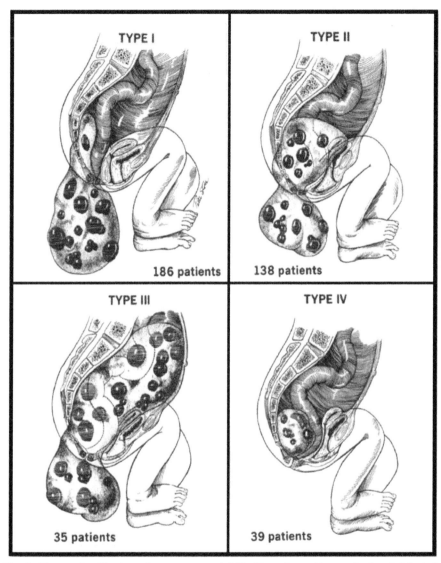

Fig. 4. Altman classification of sacrococcygeal GCTs. (*From* Peter Altman, R., Randolph, J. G. & Lilly, J. R. Sacrococcygeal teratoma: American Academy of Pediatrics Surgical Section survey—1973. Journal of Pediatric Surgery 9, 389–398 (1974); with permission).

polyhydramnios on antenatal imaging. Appropriate prenatal imaging (fetal MRI) is critical to assess the degree of involvement of surrounding structures and the possible need for emergent perinatal intervention to secure adequate airway access for oxygenation and ventilation. These interventions may entail ex utero intrapartum treatment whereby the fetus remains on the placental circulation while secure tracheal access is procured (intubation or tracheostomy) or the patient is placed on extracorporeal membrane oxygenation. Once stabilized physiologically and adequate imaging has been obtained, treatment requires removal without compromising major neurovascular structures. Achieving microscopically negative margins is often impossible without significant functional morbidity, and therefore, not necessary. If required, staged procedures to ensure complete removal of the entire tumor burden without rendering significant morbidity should be entertained by the treating physicians.[54] Outcomes are generally excellent with early surgical intervention and perinatal stabilization of the affected infants.

Abdominal Germ Cell Tumors

Abdominal GCT can be both intraperitoneal and retroperitoneal. Complete surgical resection is the procedure of choice, but resection with the intent of acquiring negative margins is often not possible or necessary. Although most tumors in this site are either mature or immature teratoma, when tumors at this site contain a malignant element, they can be challenging to treat.[55]

Thoracic Germ Cell Tumors

Most thoracic GCTs are located in the anterior mediastinum and originate in the thymus, although they can be found to rise from the posterior or middle mediastinum, heart, or epicardial structures. The tumors can be found on routine antenatal screening using standard fetal ultrasound, and the discovery of these lesions warrants further imaging with a dedicated fetal echocardiogram and MRI to document the extent of the tumor and involvement or compression of adjacent structures. Symptoms are related to the size of the tumor, and large lesions can cause fetal hydrops or airway compromise that may necessitate perinatal intervention.[56] Initial treatment consists of complete resection when possible, but gaining microscopically negative margins, again, is not necessary. Major neurovascular structures (great vessels, phrenic and recurrent laryngeal nerves) must be identified and preserved whenever possible, so as not to impair postoperative cardiorespiratory function and result in significant lifelong morbidity.[57]

CHEMOTHERAPY FOR MALIGNANT GERM CELL TUMORS

Chemotherapy is rarely indicated for neonatal GCTs. The advent of cisplatin-based chemotherapy in the treatment of advanced-stage malignant GCTs has led to excellent cure rates[46]; however, its success has been offset by the emergence of considerable long-term treatment-related morbidity and mortality affecting the quality of survivorship.[58,59] Over the last 25 years, the UK CCLG has used a carboplatin-based strategy in clinical trial design in an attempt to specifically minimize cisplatin-related toxicities.[60] A MaGIC database analysis comparing the outcomes of children and adolescents with extracranial malignant GCT treated with either carboplatin- or cisplatin-based regimens did not demonstrate a statistically significant difference in survival outcomes between the 2 regimens, even in analyses stratified by age, site, or stage.[61] The current COG trial, AGCT1531, aims to minimize toxicity by reducing therapy while maintaining current survival rates in patients with low- and standard-risk GCT. The trial will eliminate chemotherapy for low-risk patients who are likely cured with surgery and will observe the salvage rates among those who recur. Among standard-risk patients, the trial will evaluate whether cisplatin can be replaced with carboplatin.

SUMMARY

GCTs are derived from PGCs, which are destined to become either the egg or the sperm. Their intrinsic pluripotency results in a wide spectrum of benign and malignant tumors, most of which are diagnosed antenatally. The clinical spectrum of GCTs is narrower in the neonatal period, predominantly comprising teratoma (mature and immature). Given the size, location, and complexity of these tumors, optimal management requires a multidisciplinary team. Surgical resection is the mainstay of therapy. Negative surgical margins are often difficult to obtain and should not be attempted if significant mortality or morbidity would be encountered. Relapse is an infrequent occurrence even in the setting of microscopic residual disease. In the rare instance of a newborn with malignant metastatic disease or unresectable malignant disease, neoadjuvant chemotherapy after a diagnostic biopsy is the preferred management, with demonstrated better survival outcomes with a delayed resection. The chemosensitivity of GCTs to cisplatin- or carboplatin-based regimens has contributed to excellent cure rates in malignant histologies, which in neonates is usually YST. If chemotherapy is indicated, a carboplatin-based regimen should be considered to minimize short- and long-term treatment-related toxicity.

CLINICS CARE POINTS

- Teratomas (mature or immature) account for a vast majority of the neonatal germ cell tumors, approximately 5% of which contain a malignant component that is predominantly yolk sac tumor.

- Given the size, location, and complexity of these tumors, optimal management requires multidisciplinary care with both surgical and oncologic input.

- Most neonatal germ cell tumors are curable with surgery alone.

- In the rare instance of a neonate with metastatic malignant disease or malignant disease for which upfront surgical resection is not feasible without significant morbidity, an initial biopsy followed by neoadjuvant chemotherapy and delayed surgical resection is recommended.

- If chemotherapy is indicated, a carboplatin-based regimen should be considered to minimize treatment-related toxicity.

DISCLOSURE

R. Shah: The author has nothing to disclose. B.R. Weil: The author has nothing to disclose. C.B. Weldon: The author has nothing to disclose. J.F. Amatruda: The author has nothing to disclose. A.L. Frazier: Clinical advisory board, Decibel Therapeutics.

REFERENCES

1. Isaacs HJMD. Congenital and neonatal malignant tumors: a 28-year experience at Children's Hospital of Los Angeles. Am J Pediatr Hematol Oncol 1987;9(2): 121–9.
2. Isaacs H. Perinatal (fetal and neonatal) germ cell tumors. J Pediatr Surg 2004; 39(7):1003–13.
3. Tang WWC, Kobayashi T, Irie N, et al. Specification and epigenetic programming of the human germ line. Nat Rev Genet 2016;17(10):585–600.
4. Pierce JL, Frazier AL, Amatruda JF. Pediatric germ cell tumors: a developmental perspective. Adv Urol 2018;2018:9059382.

5. Looijenga LHJ, Stoop H, de Leeuw HPJC, et al. POU5F1 (OCT3/4) identifies cells with pluripotent potential in human germ cell tumors. Cancer Res 2003;63(9): 2244–50.

6. Rakheja D, Teot LA. Pathology of Germ Cell Tumors. In: Frazier A, Amatruda J, editors. Pediatric Germ Cell Tumors. Pediatric Oncology, volume 1, 2014, Springer, Berlin, Heidelberg. https://doi-org.libproxy1.usc.edu/10.1007/978-3-642-38971-9_3   https://link-springer-com.libproxy1.usc.edu/chapter/10.1007/978-3-642-38971-9_3.

7. Aeckerle N, Drummer C, Debowski K, et al. Primordial germ cell development in the marmoset monkey as revealed by pluripotency factor expression: suggestion of a novel model of embryonic germ cell translocation. Mol Hum Reprod 2015; 21(1):66–80.

8. Mamsen LS, Brøchner CB, Byskov AG, et al. The migration and loss of human primordial germ stem cells from the hind gut epithelium towards the gonadal ridge. Int J Dev Biol 2012;56(10–12):771–8.

9. Poynter JN, Hooten AJ, Frazier AL, et al. Associations between variants in KITLG, SPRY4, BAK1, and DMRT1 and pediatric germ cell tumors. Genes Chromosomes Cancer 2012;51(3):266–71.

10. Doitsidou M, Reichman-Fried M, Stebler J, et al. Guidance of primordial germ cell migration by the chemokine SDF-1. Cell 2002;111(5):647–59.

11. Runyan C, Gu Y, Shoemaker A, et al. The distribution and behavior of extragonadal primordial germ cells in Bax mutant mice suggest a novel origin for sacrococcygeal germ cell tumors. Int J Dev Biol 2008;52(4):333–44.

12. Ross JA, Schmidt PT, Perentesis JP, et al. Genomic imprinting of H19 and insulin-like growth factor-2 in pediatric germ cell tumors. Cancer 1999;85(6):1389–94.

13. Cools M, Drop SLS, Wolffenbuttel KP, et al. Germ cell tumors in the intersex gonad: old paths, new directions, moving frontiers. Endocr Rev 2006;27(5): 468–84.

14. Johnson KJ, Ross JA, Poynter JN, et al. Paediatric germ cell tumours and congenital abnormalities: a Children's Oncology Group study. Br J Cancer 2009;101(3):518–21.

15. Atkin NB, Baker MC. Specific chromosome change, i(12p), in testicular tumours? Lancet 1982;2(8311):1349.

16. Summersgill B, Goker H, Weber-Hall S, et al. Molecular cytogenetic analysis of adult testicular germ cell tumours and identification of regions of consensus copy number change. Br J Cancer 1998;77(2):305–13.

17. Veltman I, Veltman J, Janssen I, et al. Identification of recurrent chromosomal aberrations in germ cell tumors of neonates and infants using genomewide array-based comparative genomic hybridization. Genes Chromosomes Cancer 2005; 43(4):367–76.

18. Palmer RD, Foster NA, Vowler SL, et al. Malignant germ cell tumours of childhood: new associations of genomic imbalance. Br J Cancer 2007;96(4):667–76.

19. Palmer RD, Murray MJ, Saini HK, et al. Malignant germ cell tumors display common microRNA profiles resulting in global changes in expression of messenger RNA targets. Cancer Res 2010;70(7):2911–23.

20. Cancer incidence and survival among children and adolescents - pediatric monograph - SEER Publications 1975-1995. Available at: http://seer.cancer.gov/archive/publications/childhood/. Accessed March 16, 2016.

21. Williams LA, Frazier AL, Poynter JN. Survival differences by race/ethnicity among children and adolescents diagnosed with germ cell tumors. Int J Cancer 2020; 146(9):2433–41.

22. Poynter JN, Richardson M, Roesler M, et al. Family history of cancer in children and adolescents with germ cell tumours: a report from the Children's Oncology Group. Br J Cancer 2018;118(1):121–6.
23. Lee PA, Houk CP, Ahmed SF, et al. Consensus statement on management of intersex disorders. Pediatrics 2006;118(2):e488–500.
24. Huang H, Wang C, Tian Q. Gonadal tumour risk in 292 phenotypic female patients with disorders of sex development containing Y chromosome or Y-derived sequence. Clin Endocrinol (Oxf) 2017;86(4):621–7.
25. Dicken BJ, Billmire DF, Krailo M, et al. Gonadal dysgenesis is associated with worse outcomes in patients with ovarian nondysgerminomatous tumors: a report of the Children's Oncology Group AGCT 0132 study. Pediatr Blood Cancer 2018; 65(4):e26913.
26. Williams LA, Pankratz N, Lane J, et al. Klinefelter syndrome in males with germ cell tumors: a report from the Children's Oncology Group. Cancer 2018; 124(19):3900–8.
27. Thurlbeck WM, Scully RE. Solid teratoma of the ovary. A clinicopathological analysis of 9 cases. Cancer 1960;13(4):804–11.
28. Pashankar F, Hale JP, Dang H, et al. Is adjuvant chemotherapy indicated in ovarian immature teratomas? A combined data analysis from the Malignant Germ Cell Tumor International Collaborative. Cancer 2016;122(2):230–7.
29. Mann JR, Gray ES, Thornton C, et al. Mature and immature extracranial teratomas in children: the UK children's cancer study group experience. J Clin Oncol 2008; 26(21):3590–7.
30. Cushing B, Giller R, Ablin A, et al. Surgical resection alone is effective treatment for ovarian immature teratoma in children and adolescents: a report of the Pediatric Oncology Group and the Children's Cancer Group. Am J Obstet Gynecol 1999;181(2):353–8.
31. Marina NM, Cushing B, Giller R, et al. Complete surgical excision is effective treatment for children with immature teratomas with or without malignant elements: a Pediatric Oncology Group/Children's Cancer Group Intergroup Study. J Clin Oncol 1999;17(7):2137.
32. Witzleben CL, Bruninga G. Infantile choriocarcinoma: a characteristic syndrome. J Pediatr 1968;73(3):374–8.
33. Blohm MEG, Göbel U. Unexplained anaemia and failure to thrive as initial symptoms of infantile choriocarcinoma: a review. Eur J Pediatr 2004;163(1):1–6.
34. Johnson EJ, Crofton PM, O'Neill JMD, et al. Infantile choriocarcinoma treated with chemotherapy alone. Med Pediatr Oncol 2003;41(6):550–7.
35. Szavay PO, Wermes C, Fuchs J, et al. Effective treatment of infantile choriocarcinoma in the liver with chemotherapy and surgical resection: a case report. J Pediatr Surg 2000;35(7):1134–5.
36. Heath JA, Tiedemann K. Successful management of neonatal choriocarcinoma. Med Pediatr Oncol 2001;36(4):497–9.
37. Yoon JM, Burns RC, Malogolowkin MH, et al. Treatment of infantile choriocarcinoma of the liver. Pediatr Blood Cancer 2007;49(1):99–102.
38. Willis RA. The structure of teratomata. J Pathol Bacteriol 1935;40(1):1–36.
39. Spencer R. Parasitic conjoined twins: external, internal (fetuses in fetu and teratomas), and detached (acardiacs). Clin Anat 2001;14(6):428–44.
40. Ji Y, Song B, Chen S, et al. Fetus in fetu in the scrotal sac: case report and literature review. Medicine 2015;94(32):e1322.
41. Hing A, Corteville J, Foglia RP, et al. Fetus in fetu: molecular analysis of a fetiform mass. Am J Med Genet 1993;47(3):333–41.

42. Hopkins KL, Dickson PK, Ball TI, et al. Fetus-in-fetu with malignant recurrence. J Pediatr Surg 1997;32(10):1476–9.

43. Chen Y-H, Chang C-H, Chen K-C, et al. Malignant transformation of a well-organized sacrococcygeal fetiform teratoma in a newborn male. J Formos Med Assoc 2007;106(5):400–2.

44. Blohm MEG, Vesterling-Hörner D, Calaminus G, et al. Alpha1-fetoprotein (AFP) reference values in infants up to 2 years of age. Pediatr Hematol Oncol 1998; 15(2):135–42.

45. Wu JT, Book L, Sudar K. Serum alpha fetoprotein (AFP) levels in normal infants. Pediatr Res 1981;15(1):50–2.

46. Frazier AL, Hale JP, Rodriguez-Galindo C, et al. Revised risk classification for pediatric extracranial germ cell tumors based on 25 years of clinical trial data from the United Kingdom and United States. J Clin Oncol 2015;33(2): 195–201.

47. De Backer A, Madern GC, Hakvoort-Cammel FGAJ, et al. Study of the factors associated with recurrence in children with sacrococcygeal teratoma. J Pediatr Surg 2006;41(1):173–81.

48. Gross RW, Clatworthy HW, Meeker IA. Sacrococcygeal teratomas in infants and children; a report of 40 cases. Surg Gynecol Obstet 1951;92(3):341–54.

49. Altman RP, Randolph JG, Lilly JR. Sacrococcygeal teratoma: American Academy of Pediatrics Surgical Section Survey—1973. J Pediatr Surg 1974;9(3):389–98.

50. Rescorla F, Billmire D, Stolar C, et al. The effect of cisplatin dose and surgical resection in children with malignant germ cell tumors at the sacrococcygeal region: a Pediatric Intergroup Trial (POG 9049/CCG 8882). J Pediatr Surg 2001; 36(1):12–7.

51. Göbel U, Schneider DT, Calaminus G, et al. Multimodal treatment of malignant sacrococcygeal germ cell tumors: a prospective analysis of 66 patients of the German Cooperative Protocols MAKEI 83/86 and 89. J Clin Oncol 2001;19(7): 1943–50.

52. Malone PS, Spitz L, Kiely EM, et al. The functional sequelae of sacrococcygeal teratoma. J Pediatr Surg 1990;25(6):679–80.

53. Schmidt B, Haberlik A, Uray E, et al. Sacrococcygeal teratoma: clinical course and prognosis with a special view to long-term functional results. Pediatr Surg Int 1999;15(8):573–6.

54. Azizkhan RG, Haase GM, Applebaum H, et al. Diagnosis, management, and outcome of cervicofacial teratomas in neonates: a Childrens Cancer Group study. J Pediatr Surg 1995;30(2):312–6.

55. Billmire D, Vinocur C, Rescorla F, et al. Malignant retroperitoneal and abdominal germ cell tumors: an intergroup study. J Pediatr Surg 2003;38(3):315–8.

56. Merchant AM, Hedrick HL, Johnson MP, et al. Management of fetal mediastinal teratoma. J Pediatr Surg 2005;40(1):228–31.

57. Billmire D, Vinocur C, Rescorla F, et al. Malignant mediastinal germ cell tumors: an intergroup study. J Pediatr Surg 2001;36(1):18–24.

58. Travis LB, Fosså SD, Schonfeld SJ, et al. Second cancers among 40,576 testicular cancer patients: focus on long-term survivors. J Natl Cancer Inst 2005; 97(18):1354–65.

59. Travis LB, Beard C, Allan JM, et al. Testicular cancer survivorship: research strategies and recommendations. J Natl Cancer Inst 2010;102(15):1114–30.

60. Mann JR, Raafat F, Robinson K, et al. The United Kingdom Children's Cancer Study Group's second germ cell tumor study: carboplatin, etoposide, and

bleomycin are effective treatment for children with malignant extracranial germ cell tumors, with acceptable toxicity. J Clin Oncol 2000;18(22):3809–18.
61. Frazier AL, Stoneham S, Rodriguez-Galindo C, et al. Comparison of carboplatin versus cisplatin in the treatment of paediatric extracranial malignant germ cell tumours: a report of the Malignant Germ Cell International Consortium. Eur J Cancer 2018;98:30–7.

Histiocytic Diseases of Neonates

Langerhans Cell Histiocytosis, Rosai-Dorfman Disease, and Juvenile Xanthogranuloma

Kenneth L. McClain, MD, PhD

KEYWORDS

- Langerhans cell histiocytosis • Rosai-Dorfman-Destombes disease
- Juvenile xanthogranuloma

KEY POINTS

- Mutations of the MAP kinase pathway occur almost universally in LCH, but less so in RDD and JXG.
- There is often a delay in diagnosis because of confusing overlap with more common neonatal diseases.
- Proper staging of these patients is necessary as for any malignancy.
- Treatments include: observation, chemotherapy, and MAPK inhibitors.

LANGERHANS CELL HISTIOCYTOSIS
Introduction

Langerhans cell histiocytosis (LCH) is caused by pathologic myeloid dendritic cells that originate in the bone marrow.[1] LCH may present at birth or anytime in the neonatal period, most often with skin rashes (100%), hepatomegaly (16%), splenomegaly (13%), lymphadenopathy (10%), diarrhea (8%), and respiratory distress (7%); and less frequently with thrombocytopenia, still birth, jaundice, or protein-losing enteropathy.[2,3] The most affected organs are skin (100%), lung (24%), liver (24%), spleen (22%), lymph nodes (18%), bone (19%), gastrointestinal tract (14%), bone marrow (13%), oral mucosa (13%), thymus (8%), pituitary (5%), and ear and nose (5% each).[2] Less frequent sites include brain, skeletal muscle, eye, kidney, pancreas, and heart. A biopsy is necessary to make the diagnosis. Patients are divided into low-risk and high-risk (of death) categories by the organ systems involved.[4] When the spleen, liver, and/or bone marrow are involved, these patients are at higher risk

Baylor College of Medicine, Texas Children's Cancer and Hematology Centers, 6701 Fannin Street, Suite 1510, Houston, TX 77030, USA
E-mail address: klmcclai@txch.org

Clin Perinatol 48 (2021) 167–179
https://doi.org/10.1016/j.clp.2020.11.008   perinatology.theclinics.com

of fatal outcome, but with modern therapy they have a much better prognosis than even a decade ago. Low-risk patients are those with one or more of the other non-high-risk organs. Either the low- or high-risk patients may have multiple relapses, which is dictated by therapy choices and whether or not they have the BRAF mutation in the pathologic cells.[5] Because all patients with LCH have abnormal activation of phopho-ERK, LCH is considered an inflammatory myeloid neoplasm, not an immunologic disease.[1,6]

Epidemiology

The incidence of LCH in neonates is 15.3 per million[7] and is more frequent in persons of Hispanic origin, lower socioeconomic groups, and those living in crowded conditions.[8] African Americans rarely have LCH. A genome-wide association study found a variant in *SMAD6* was associated with an increased susceptibility for LCH, especially in patients with Hispanic ancestry.[9]

Cell of Origin

LCH originates from a bone marrow–derived myeloid dendritic cell, some of which are resident in tissues, whereas others circulate in the peripheral blood.[10,11] The normal function of these cells is to present antigens to T lymphocytes, but in LCH the aberrant myeloid dendritic cells are not as efficient at this function and take on new activities leading to signs and symptoms of the disease.

Pathophysiology

Nearly two-thirds of patients with LCH have a mutation in the *BRAF* gene leading to constitutive activation of phospho-*ERK*, which promotes clonal growth of the myeloid dendritic cells.[6,12] BRAF is a member of the MAPK pathway, which relays signals from a cell surface receptor to ultimately affect transcription of genes effecting growth and differentiation. Besides the $BRAF^{V600E}$ mutation, there are others including *MAP2K1* fusions and internal deletions and others, which amount to 85% of patients with LCH having identified mutations.[13] These mutations cause the LCH cells to acquire a senescent growth pattern and lack the ability to migrate out of a tissue site.[14] The pathologic cells are not dividing rapidly, but slowly accumulate at a disease site. They produce a variety of cytokines and chemokines that attract other immune cells, including lymphocytes and macrophages.[1,15] The sites and extent of LCH in an individual patient seems to be related to the state of differentiation of the myeloid dendritic cell when it acquires the $BRAF^{V600E}$ mutation.[16]

History

There is no known association of LCH with prenatal medications that a mother may have taken, diet, or the environment, other than living in crowded conditions. Familial cases are vanishingly rare. A family history of thyroid disease has been found, but the biology of this association is unknown.[3] One of the frequent historical points is that the patient was born with a rash that did not resolve with the most common types of treatments, such as steroid creams or antibiotics. Although cradle cap is a common finding in many normal neonates, it is not normal if lasting more than 2 months or reappearing after apparent resolution. Prolonged jaundice and neonatal ascites are associated with hepatic LCH. Pallor and petechiae may be signs of bone marrow involvement. Dyspnea may present in patients with diffuse pulmonary involvement with or without pneumothoraces. Natal teeth are almost pathognomonic of mandibular or maxillary LCH bone lesions. Chronic otitis externa unresponsive to antibiotics is often a sign of LCH in the external auditory canal and/or mastoids.

Clinical Presentations and Differential Diagnoses

Skin

Neonates may have isolated or extensive purple or brown papules that mimic the "blueberry muffin" appearance of patients with neuroblastoma or myeloid leukemia (**Fig. 1**A). Often they have a dense scaly, seborrheic accumulation on their scalp much the same as cradle cap. If cradle cap lasts beyond 2 months of age one should think of another diagnosis, including LCH. Other rashes have the maculopapular, multicolored appearances of congenital virus infections. Extensive whole-body rashes often look like extraordinary psoriasis (**Fig. 1**B). Extensive perineal and perianal LCH lesions often lead to deep ulcers.

Bone

Any bone may be affected, but the skull, vertebrae, ribs, and pelvis seem particularly targeted in neonatal patients with LCH (**Fig. 1**C). Lytic bone lesions in neonates could also be caused by Rosai-Dorfman disease (RDD), osteomyelitis, malignant bone tumors, or fibrous dysplasia. Unlike older children in whom bone involvement occurs in 70%, neonates and infants have around a 20% incidence.[2] A soft swelling of the skull may rapidly enlarge if there is hemorrhage into the area. Proptosis from periorbital LCH may mimic the presentations of neuroblastoma, myeloid leukemia, or rhabdomyosarcoma. Natal tooth eruption is found in patients with diffuse LCH involvement of the maxilla or mandible (**Fig. 1**D).

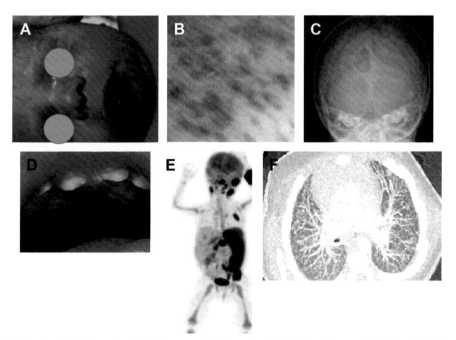

Fig. 1. (*A*) LCH skin rash, "blueberry muffin" type. (*B*) LCH skin rash, psoriatic-like. (*C*) Lytic skull lesion of LCH. (*D*) Natal teeth and gingival hypertrophy from LCH. (*E*) PET scan with abnormal fluorodeoxyglucose uptake in skull base, occiput, left fifth rib, left iliac bone, and left hemisacrum and hypermetabolic splenomegaly and bilateral cervical/upper abdominal lymphadenopathy. (*F*) Chest computed tomography showing mosaic attenuation pattern of the lungs bilaterally with innumerable reticulonodular airspace opacities bilaterally.

Lymph nodes
Bilateral enlarged cervical nodes are more frequently involved in patients with LCH than nodes in other areas, but any location is possible.

Lungs
Tachypnea and dyspnea may be presenting signs in a neonate with diffuse pulmonary LCH. Sudden onset of respiratory distress could signal the occurrence of a pneumothorax. Also massive enlargement of the thymus could cause any of these symptoms.

Liver and spleen
Subtle or massive enlargement of the spleen and liver may be detected by physical examination. Additional information obtained from radiographic and laboratory studies may be needed.

Diagnostic Modalities

Initial laboratory studies for all patients should include a complete blood count; liver panel with bilirubin, serum albumin, and total protein; complete metabolic panel; and prothrombin time/partial thromboplastin time. Screening radiographic studies should include a skull series (four views), skeletal survey, chest radiograph, and abdominal ultrasound. Although PET scans are done on patients older than 6 months of age (**Fig. 1**E), a bone scan may be more appropriate for those younger than 6 months. Because diagnosing pulmonary LCH from a plain chest radiograph in a neonate is difficult, our practice is to do a chest computed tomography on all patients younger than a year of age (**Fig. 1**F). If orbital, temporal bone, mastoid, maxillary, or mandibular involvement is a consideration, then a maxillofacial computed tomography should be done. If vertebral lesions are seen on plain films, a computed tomography or MRI of the spine is indicated to more precisely define the extent of lesions. An abdominal ultrasound or MRI may be performed to define suspected hepatic involvement. Hypoechoic areas around the biliary tracts and disturbance of hepatic architecture or mass lesions are the classic findings.

Pathology

All neonates should have a bone marrow aspirate and biopsy performed, with analysis for LCH cells by staining with CD1a and CD207 to identify the pathologic dendritic cells, and polymerase chain reaction testing for the $BRAF^{V600E}$ mutation or immunohistochemistry staining with the VE-1 antibody, which detects the BRAFV600E protein. Likewise, skin, bone, or other tissue biopsies should be evaluated with the same reagents. Our practice is to also evaluate all biopsies with stains for juvenile xanthogranuloma (JXG)-type dendritic cells, which stain with factor XIIIa and fascin.[17]

A liver biopsy is indicated for all patients with hepatic function abnormalities to document the presence of LCH and establish a baseline of whether or not there is sclerosis (see later discussion on sclerosing cholangitis).

Treatment

The current treatment standard, as established by the LCH-III study, includes vinblastine and prednisone for a year (**Table 1**).[4] There is an ongoing study comparing vinblastine and prednisone with cytarabine as initial therapy (NCT02670707) and the LCH-IV study (NCT02205762) is testing treatment for 2 years versus 1 year. Nearly 65% of patients with LCH have the $BRAF^{V600E}$ mutation, thus making them eligible for one of the BRAF-inhibitor drugs (vemurafenib or dabrafenib); those without the $BRAF^{V600E}$ mutation may be candidates for treatment with the MEK inhibitors trametinib or cobimetinib (**Table 2**). There are little published data on use of these drugs in

Table 1 Initial treatment of patients with LCH			
LCH-III			
High-risk LCH			
Induction: Weeks 1–6	Vinblastine 6 mg/m^2/wk	Prednisone 40 mg/m^2 daily	
Second induction (if poor response): Weeks 6–12	Vinblastine 6 mg/m^2/wk	Prednisone 20 mg/m^2 twice daily, 3 d/wk	
Continuation: Weeks 6–52 or 12–52	Vinblastine 6 mg/m^2 every 3 wk	Prednisone 20 mg/m^2 twice daily for 5 d	Mercaptopurine 50 mg/m^2/d
Low-risk LCH	Same as high risk	Same as high risk	No mercaptopurine
Under Investigation (All Patients)			
Cytarabine Months 1–12		100 mg/m^2 × 5 d, monthly	

neonates, but the drugs seem to have been well-tolerated in patients less than a year of age.

Clinical Outcomes

The LCH-III study using vinblastine/prednisone/mercaptopurine for high risk had a progression-free survival rate of 33% at 8 years, although the overall survival was more than 80% because of successful salvage therapy with the regimens described in **Table 2**.[4] The overall survival for pediatric LCH patients of any age treated with cladribine was 22/46 for high-risk and 36/37 low-risk individuals.[18] The combined results from two centers using clofarabine were progression-free survival in 4/7 high-risk and 9/10 low-risk patients.[19,20] Two case series described use of the BRAF and MEK inhibitors in pediatric patients from neonates to teenagers with more than 80% responses, but a high rate of relapse (50%–75%) when taken off the inhibitors because they continue to have circulating BRAF-mutated cells in their blood.[21,22] Most patients respond when the inhibitors are reintroduced. The question remains how to successfully extinguish the malignant clone. Although a few patients require a stem cell transplant, this is not being done as frequently because of the success of various salvage therapies.[23]

Table 2 Treatment of progressive/relapsed LCH	
Cladribine IV Monthly for 6 mo	5 mg/m^2/d × 5 d
Clofarabine IV Monthly for 12 mo	25 mg/m^2 × 5 d When in CR decrease to 2 d/mo
Dabrafenib oral	50 mg/m^2 twice daily
Trametinib oral	0.025–0.04 mg/kg
Cobimetinib oral	20 mg/m^2 daily for 21 d then off for 7 d

Abbreviation: IV, intravenous.

The overall survival of low-risk patients is nearly 100% and up to 80% for those with high-risk disease. Long-term complications relate to organ damage from LCH. Hepatic involvement can lead to sclerosing cholangitis, which has historically been poorly responsive to chemotherapy, leading to the need for hepatic transplantation for cure.[24] Current use of the BRAF-inhibitor drugs may provide better initial therapy, with the hope that this complication will be less prevalent. Some infants with pulmonary LCH have multiple cysts leading to potentially life-threatening pneumothoraces; these patients may be treated with multiple chest tubes, pleurodesis, and intensive care support.[25] Others have diffuse nodules (see **Fig. 1**F). Involvement of the mastoid, temporal, orbital, sphenoid, and maxillary bone have historically led to a higher incidence of diabetes insipidus.[26] However, with current treatments the frequency of this complication is around 10%. The long-term issue is that 50% of patients with LCH with diabetes insipidus develop anterior pituitary deficiencies, which lead to retardation of growth and sexual development, hypothyroidism, and hypoadrenalism.[27] Mastoid involvement can damage the hearing apparatus leading to deafness. Severe mandibular or maxillary LCH may destroy early tooth buds, resulting in significant dental issues.

Clinical Care Points

- Prompt biopsy of neonatal rashes is important in diagnosing LCH. One may prevent the neonate from developing severe ulcerative lesions.
- Cradle cap lasting beyond 2 months is likely not cradle cap and should be biopsied.
- Natal teeth are never normal.
- If a patient responds poorly to initial vinblastine/prednisone therapy promptly switch to a salvage regimen.

ROSAI-DORFMAN DISEASE
Introduction

First described by Destombes and later by Rosai and Dorfman, these patients present with markedly enlarged lymph nodes, usually cervical.[28,29] This entity has been known as Destombes-Rosai-Dorfman disease and RDD. The lymph node sinuses are filled with large histiocytes having a pale cytoplasm with occasional lymphocytes trafficking through (but not hemophagocytosis), a finding known as emperipolesis, which is needed to make the RDD diagnosis. Otherwise, these cells stain positively with macrophage markers anti-CD68 or -CD163, but not CD1a or CD207. Biopsies may also show prominent plasma cell infiltrates. There are no data on clonality of these cells in children, and pediatric cases have not been found to have mutations causing the disease. There is no consistent evidence of an infectious or environmental cause for RDD.

Epidemiology

No studies have rigorously examined the epidemiology of RDD, but unlike LCH, the disease is often found in African Americans.

Clinical Presentation

Most pediatric patients present with massively enlarged cervical lymph nodes or proptosis from retro-orbital tumors. RDD is rare in neonates and only a few case reports of true neonatal presentation are available. In a review of 221 fetal and neonatal cases of histiocytic diseases, there were none with RDD.[2] Among the few case reports is a newborn who presented with anemia, thrombocytopenia, and hepatomegaly and who was diagnosed with RDD by liver biopsy and had a spontaneous remission.[30] Nodular skin RDD lesions were found in a 6 day old with cervical and inguinal lymphadenopathy.[31] The cervical adenopathy became massively enlarged and required intermittent steroid therapy for years.

Differential Diagnosis

The list of possible diagnoses causing lymphadenopathy includes infectious diseases, malignancies, autoimmune lymphoproliferative disease, LCH, and Kikuchi lymphadenitis among others.[32]

Treatment

In some cases of RDD, lymphadenopathy spontaneously resolves. Steroid treatment may be transiently successful, but once stopped the RDD usually relapses. In others, treatment with a variety of chemotherapy regimens including vinblastine/prednisone, cladribine, and clofarabine have been used with success.[19,33,34]

Clinical Outcomes

Most patients with lymph node or cutaneous RDD have resolution of their disease over several years, perhaps more quickly with some chemotherapy. Cure for patients with extensive disease is often only possible with more aggressive chemotherapy regimens, such as clofarabine or cladribine.

Clinical Care Points

- RDD should be included in the differential diagnosis for lymphadenopathy.
- Proptosis secondary to an orbital RDD tumor mimics neuroblastoma, rhabdomyosarcoma, and LCH.
- Patients with isolated cervical adenopathy may not need treatment and steroids alone are rarely curative.
- RDD in sites other than lymph nodes may require prolonged chemotherapy to cure.

JUVENILE XANTHOGRANULOMA

Introduction

JXG most often presents with flesh-colored, yellow-orange, brown or purple macules or papules, which may occur anywhere on the body (**Fig. 2A**). Some patients have isolated or few lesions, whereas others have literally hundreds distributed over their skin. Occasionally large papules occur. JXG is present in one or two sites in 75% of patients.[35] Other sites include the liver (22%), lung (16%), soft tissue (16%), spleen (11%), eye (9%), lymph nodes (7%), brain (7%) (**Fig. 2B**), adrenal (7%), gastrointestinal tract (7%), bone marrow (7%), and heart (4%).[2]

Epidemiology

Data from the Kiel Tumor Registry suggest that JXG occurs at a frequency of approximately 1 per million children.[36] The male/female ratio is 1.4:1 with 35% having lesions at birth and 71% developing lesions within the first year of life, although there is a 3:1

predominance of females among patients with JXG with disseminated lesions.[2] There are no published data on cause.

Cell of Origin

Myeloid dendritic cells derived from bone marrow precursors of the macrophage lineage become dermal dendrocytes, which accumulate in the aberrant formations of JXG.

Pathophysiology

Whole exome or targeted DNA and/or RNA sequencing on 44 pediatric JXG cases found the following mutations: six with *MAP2K1*; six *NTRK1* fusions; five with *CSF1R* including twin siblings; four *KRAS*; three *NRAS*; and smaller numbers of mutations in *KIT*, *JAK3*, *ALK*, *MET*, and others.[37]

Clinical Presentation and Outcome

Most patients with one or a few lesions have spontaneous resolution. The Kiel study reported single lesions in 81% and Isaacs found 67%.[2,34] In some cases complete excision is curative and few have recurrences. Patients in the neonatal age group have a 27% incidence of systemic involvement as opposed to 3.9% in children of all ages.[2] In a series of 45 neonatal JXG cases, nearly a quarter of patients with systemic JXG did not have skin lesions.[2] Lesions were seen on the head and neck (41%), trunk (41%), upper extremity (7.9%), and lower extremity (10.3%). Some patients have multiple lesions around their eyes and others may have intraocular lesions. Ocular JXG

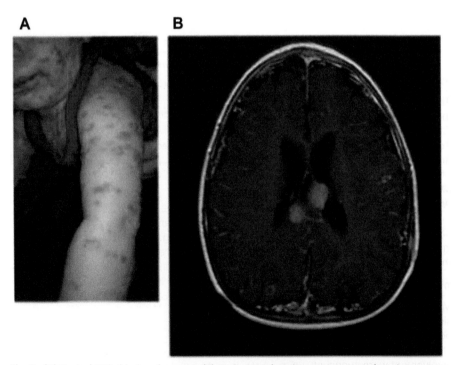

A   **B**

Fig. 2. (*A*) Typical JXG skin involvement. (*B*) Brain MRI showing numerous enhancing masses with low T2 signal and marked restricted diffusion throughout the brain parenchyma.

is most often an isolated site.[38] Patients present with redness of the eyes, tearing, hyphema, and visible lesions on the cornea or eyelids. JXG has been reported on the gingiva, buccal mucosa, tongue, and subglottic areas.[39,40] Involvement of other organs include the brain, heart, liver, spleen, kidneys, lung, bone marrow, intestines, and bone. Some patients with systemic involvement do not have skin lesions.[35] Neonates with brain lesions may have seizures, cranial nerve signs, and/or developmental delay. Cardiac involvement can cause dysrhythmias or heart failure from decreased pumping capacity. Pancytopenia is a presenting sign of infants with bone marrow infiltration by JXG and has been reported to precede the appearance of cutaneous lesions.[41,42] Liver involvement may be heralded by hepatomegaly and hyperbilirubinemia. A unique group of infants with spleen, liver, and bone marrow infiltration with histiocytes staining for ALK and the other classic stains for JXG has been reported (discussed later).[43]

Differential Diagnosis

JXG lesions may be mistaken for atheromas or lipomas, but also LCH. Urticaria pigmentosa, neurofibromatosis type I, and myelogenous leukemia have also been associated with JXG.[44] Patients with NF1 and JXG may have a 20- to 30-fold increased risk of developing juvenile myelomonocytic leukemia.[45]

Diagnostic Evaluations

For infants with only a few cutaneous lesions and no systemic symptoms or signs, evaluation should include a complete blood count, liver enzyme panel, basic metabolic panel, and ophthalmologic examination. Patients with a large number of lesions and/or systemic symptoms or abnormalities of the laboratory tests mentioned previously should undergo an MRI of the brain and abdomen. If cardiac dysfunction is evident, a cardiac MRI and echocardiogram are indicated. When cytopenias are present, bone marrow aspirates and biopsies with flow cytometry, cytogenetic analysis, and whole-exome sequencing should be done.

Histopathology

The classic JXG cells are large with a vacuolated cytoplasm and a small round or indented nucleus. These cells stain with CD68, fascin, factor XIIIa, and CD4, but not CD1a or CD207.[17] Also found are large cells with centrally grouped nuclei known as Touton giant cells. Sometimes emperipolesis is identified. Two other variants of JXG are the early and late forms of JXG. The early type has dense monomorphic groups of histiocytes without the lipid vacuoles seen in the classic type. The late form of JXG has whorls of spindle-shaped cells with foci of foamy histiocytes and giant cells. An admixture of lymphocytes and eosinophils is also found.

The newly described ALK-positive histiocytosis has foamy cells similar to classic JXG, but irregularly folded nuclei, and some multinucleated cells that stain by ALK immunohistochemistry. Patients with this finding should have molecular analysis for the *TPM3-ALK* and *KIF5B-ALK* fusion genes.

Treatment

Most lesions involute spontaneously, but excision of single or a limited number of lesions may be indicated in some cases. Patients with involvement of brain, spleen, and bone marrow have been treated by a variety of regimens used for histiocytic diseases. Three patients with brain lesions and one with diffuse bone marrow and spleen involvement were successfully treated with clofarabine, 25 mg/m^2, for 5 days monthly for a year.[19] One patient with brain, skin, spleen, and liver involvement was cured using the Japanese LCH Study Group 96 protocol.[46] Other successful treatments for patients with JXG with liver and bone marrow involvement include etoposide/vinblastine/prednisolone[42] and 2CdA-AraC.[41] A liver transplant was required for one child because of cholestasis and portal hypertension.[47] Patients with ALK-histiocytosis are cured by treatment with the ALK-inhibitor crizotinib, although one patient had a spontaneous recovery.[43]

Clinical Outcomes

Most neonates with a few JXG lesions have spontaneous resolution and never recur. Others with more extensive disease may need to undergo aggressive chemotherapy protocols, but most patients can now be cured.

CLINICAL CARE POINTS

- Isolated skin JXG lesions may resolve spontaneously.
- Ophthalmologic screening for intraocular lesions is important.
- Infants with multiple JXG lesions should have an MRI of the brain and abdomen looking for internal involvement.

SUMMARY

The histiocytic diseases have historically been recognized by their varying clinical presentations and apparent different histologies. However, it is now known that LCH, JXG, and RDD all develop from bone marrow–derived myeloid precursors, which undergo different developmental changes that result in the myeloid dendritic cell morphology of LCH and more macrophage-like cells of RDD and JXG. Mutations of the MAP2K pathway are found in most patients with LCH and a variable proportion of RDD and JXG. Clinical presentations most frequently include the skin in LCH and JXG, and bone in LCH and RDD, but pituitary and sometimes brain involvement in all three. Many treatment regimens have been applied to these diseases, but those more directed at myeloid cells, such as cytarabine and clofarabine or mutation-targeting inhibitors, are gaining favor.

DISCLOSURE

Dr. K.L. McClain is on the medical advisory board of the SOBI Corporation and the HistioCure Foundation.

REFERENCE

1. Allen CE, Li L, Peters TL, et al. Cell-specific gene expression in Langerhans cell histiocytosis lesions reveals a distinct profile compared with epidermal Langerhans cells. J Immunol 2010;184(8):4557–67.
2. Isaacs H Jr. Fetal and neonatal histiocytoses. Pediatr Blood Cancer 2006;47(2): 123–9.
3. Allen CE, Merad M, McClain KL. Langerhans-cell histiocytosis. N Engl J Med 2018;379(9):856–68.
4. Gadner H, Minkov M, Grois N, et al. Therapy prolongation improves outcome in multisystem Langerhans cell histiocytosis. Blood 2013;121(25):5006–14.

5. Heritier S, Emile JF, Barkaoui M, et al. BRAF mutation correlates with high-risk Langerhans cell histiocytosis and increased resistance to first line therapy. J Clin Oncol 2016;34(25):3023–30.

6. Badalian-Very G, Vergilio JA, Degar BA, et al. Recurrent BRAF mutations in Langerhans cell histiocytosis. Blood 2010;116(11):1919–23.

7. Guyot-Goubin A, Donadieu J, Barkaoui M, et al. Descriptive epidemiology of childhood Langerhans cell histiocytosis in France, 2000-2004. Pediatr Blood Cancer 2008;51(1):71–5.

8. Ribeiro KB, Degar B, Antoneli CB, et al. Ethnicity, race, and socioeconomic status influence incidence of Langerhans cell histiocytosis. Pediatr Blood Cancer 2015; 62(6):982–7.

9. Peckham-Gregory EC, Chakraborty R, Scheurer ME, et al. A genome-wide association study of LCH identifies a variant in SMAD6 associated with susceptibility. Blood 2017;130(20):2229–32.

10. Ginhoux F, Collin MP, Bogunovic M, et al. Blood-derived dermal langerin+ dendritic cells survey the skin in the steady state. J Exp Med 2007;204(13):3133–46.

11. Berres ML, Allen CE, Merad M. Pathological consequence of misguided dendritic cell differentiation in histiocytic diseases. Adv Immunol 2013;120:127–61.

12. Willman CL, Busque L, Griffith BB, et al. Langerhans'-cell histiocytosis (histiocytosis X): a clonal proliferative disease. N Engl J Med 1994;331(3):154–60.

13. Chakraborty R, Hampton OA, Shen X, et al. Mutually exclusive recurrent somatic mutations in MAP2K1 and BRAF support a central role for ERK activation in LCH pathogenesis. Blood 2014;124(19):3007–15.

14. Hogstad B, Berres ML, Chakraborty R, et al. RAF/MEK/extracellular signal-related kinase pathway suppresses dendritic cell migration and traps dendritic cells in Langerhans cell histiocytosis lesions. J Exp Med 2018;215(1):319–36.

15. Senechal B, Elain G, Jeziorski E, et al. Expansion of regulatory T cells in patients with Langerhans cell histiocytosis. PLoS Med 2007;4(8):e253.

16. Berres ML, Lim KP, Peters T, et al. BRAF-V600E expression in precursor versus differentiated dendritic cells defines clinically distinct LCH risk groups. J Exp Med 2014;211(4):669–83.

17. Picarsic J, Jaffe R. Nosology and pathology of Langerhans cell histiocytosis. Hematol Oncol Clin North Am 2015;29(5):799–823.

18. Weitzman S, Braier J, Donadieu J, et al. 2'-Chlorodeoxyadenosine (2-CdA) as salvage therapy for Langerhans cell histiocytosis (LCH). Results of the LCH-S-98 protocol of the Histiocyte Society. Pediatr Blood Cancer 2009;53(7):1271–6.

19. Simko SJ, Tran HD, Jones J, et al. Clofarabine salvage therapy in refractory multifocal histiocytic disorders, including Langerhans cell histiocytosis, juvenile xanthogranuloma and Rosai-Dorfman disease. Pediatr Blood Cancer 2014;61(3): 479–87.

20. Abraham A, Alsultan A, Jeng M, et al. Clofarabine salvage therapy for refractory high-risk Langerhans cell histiocytosis. Pediatr Blood Cancer 2013;60(6):E19–22.

21. Eckstein OS, Visser J, Rodriguez-Galindo C, et al. Clinical responses and persistent BRAF V600E(+) blood cells in children with LCH treated with MAPK pathway inhibition. Blood 2019;133(15):1691–4.

22. Donadieu J, Larabi IA, Tardieu M, et al. Vemurafenib for refractory multisystem Langerhans cell histiocytosis in children: an international observational study. J Clin Oncol 2019;37(31):2857–65.

23. Veys PA, Nanduri V, Baker KS, et al. Haematopoietic stem cell transplantation for refractory Langerhans cell histiocytosis: outcome by intensity of conditioning. Br J Haematol 2015;169(5):711–8.

24. Braier J, Ciocca M, Latella A, et al. Cholestasis, sclerosing cholangitis, and liver transplantation in Langerhans cell histiocytosis. Med Pediatr Oncol 2002;38: 178–82.

25. Eckstein OS, Nuchtern JG, Mallory GB, Guillerman RP, et al. Management of severe pulmonary Langerhans cell histiocytosis in children. Pediatr Pulmonol 2020; 55(8):2074–81.

26. Grois N, Pötschger U, Prosch H, et al. Risk factors for diabetes insipidus in Langerhans cell histiocytosis. Pediatr Blood Cancer 2006;46(2):228–33.

27. Donadieu J, Rolon MA, Thomas C, et al. Endocrine involvement in pediatric-onset Langerhans' cell histiocytosis: a population-based study. J Pediatr 2004;144(3): 344–50.

28. Destombes P. Adenitis with lipid excess, in children or young adults, seen in the Antilles and in Mali. (4 cases). Bull Soc Pathol Exot Filiales 1965;58(6):1169–75 [in French].

29. Rosai J, Dorfman RF. Sinus histiocytosis with massive lymphadenopathy. A newly recognized benign clinicopathological entity. Arch Pathol 1969;87(1):63–70.

30. Chow CP, Ho HK, Chan GC, et al. Congenital Rosai-Dorfman disease presenting with anemia, thrombocytopenia, and hepatomegaly. Pediatr Blood Cancer 2009; 52(3):415–7.

31. Antonius JI, Farid SM, Baez-Giangreco A. Steroid-responsive Rosai-Dorfman disease. Pediatr Hematol Oncol 1996;13(6):563–70.

32. McClain K. Peripheral lymphadenopathy in children: evaluation and diagnostic approach. In: Kaplan SL, Mahoney D, Drutz J, editors. Philadelphia: Wolters Kluwer; 2020.

33. Abla O, Jacobsen E, Picarsic J, et al. Consensus recommendations for the diagnosis and clinical management of Rosai-Dorfman-Destombes disease. Blood 2018;131(26):2877–90.

34. Konca C, Ozkurt ZN, Deger M, et al. Extranodal multifocal Rosai-Dorfman disease: response to 2-chlorodeoxyadenosine treatment. Int J Hematol 2009; 89(1):58–62.

35. Freyer DR, Kennedy R, Bostrom BC, et al. Juvenile xanthogranuloma: forms of systemic disease and their clinical implications. J Pediatr 1996;129(2):227–37.

36. Janssen D, Harms D. Juvenile xanthogranuloma in childhood and adolescence: a clinicopathologic study of 129 patients from the Kiel pediatric tumor registry. Am J Surg Pathol 2005;29(1):21–8.

37. Durham BH, Lopez Rodrigo E, Picarsic J, et al. Activating mutations in CSF1R and additional receptor tyrosine kinases in histiocytic neoplasms. Nat Med 2019;25(12):1839–42.

38. Collum LM, Power WJ, Mullaney J, et al. Limbal xanthogranuloma. J Pediatr Ophthalmol Strabismus 1991;28(3):157–9.

39. Flaitz C, Allen C, Neville B, et al. Juvenile xanthogranuloma of the oral cavity in children: a clinicopathologic study. Oral Surg Oral Med Oral Pathol Oral Radiol Endod 2002;94(3):345–52.

40. Somorai M, Goldstein NA, Alexis R, et al. Managing isolated subglottic juvenile xanthogranuloma without tracheostomy: case report and review of literature. Pediatr Pulmonol 2007;42(2):181–5.

41. Blouin P, Yvert M, Arbion F, et al. Juvenile xanthogranuloma with hematological dysfunction treated with 2CDA-AraC. Pediatr Blood Cancer 2010;55(4):757–60.

42. Hara T, Ohga S, Hattori S, et al. Prolonged severe pancytopenia preceding the cutaneous lesions of juvenile xanthogranuloma. Pediatr Blood Cancer 2006; 47(1):103–6.

43. Chang KTE, Tay AZE, Kuick CH, et al. ALK-positive histiocytosis: an expanded clinicopathologic spectrum and frequent presence of KIF5B-ALK fusion. Mod Pathol 2019;32(5):598–608.
44. Morier P, Merot Y, Paccaud D, et al. Juvenile xanthogranuloma and urticaria pigmentosa. Arch Dermatol 1975;111:365–6.
45. Zvulunov A, Barak Y, Metzker A. Juvenile xanthogranuloma, neurofibromatosis, and juvenile chronic myelogenous leukemia. World statistical analysis. Arch Dermatol 1995;131(8):904–8.
46. Nakatani T, Morimoto A, Kato R, et al. Successful treatment of congenital systemic juvenile xanthogranuloma with Langerhans cell histiocytosis-based chemotherapy. J Pediatr Hematol Oncol 2004;26(6):371–4.
47. Haughton AM, Horii KA, Shao L, et al. Disseminated juvenile xanthogranulomatosis in a newborn resulting in liver transplantation. J Am Acad Dermatol 2008;58(2 Suppl):S12–5.

Neonatal Vascular Tumors

Michael Briones, DO[a],*, Denise Adams, MD[b]

KEYWORDS

- Neonate • Vascular tumors • Multidisciplinary • Congenital • Vascular anomaly

KEY POINTS

- Pediatric vascular tumors are a heterogenous group of disorders and diagnosis and common terminology is crucial for appropriate evaluation and management.
- This process requires multidisciplinary specialists and a dedicated pediatric vascular anomaly multidisciplinary approach.
- Neonatal vascular anomalies are divided into 2 major categories: vascular tumors, which are proliferative endothelial lesions, and vascular malformations, which are developmental aberrations of arterial, venous, or lymphatic vessels.
- Most lesions are benign and single lesions and may not need therapy.
- For lesions that are locally aggressive tumors such as Kaposiform hemangioendothelioma requires multidisciplinary approach requiring chemotherapy.

INTRODUCTION

Vascular anomalies (vascular tumors and vascular malformations) represent a broad spectrum of disorders from a simple "storkbite" to life-threatening entities, which can present in the neonatal period. Neonatal vascular anomalies are divided into 2 major categories: (1) vascular tumors, which are proliferative endothelial lesions, such as hemangiomas or Kaposiform hemangioendothelioma (KHE), and (2) vascular malformations, which are developmental aberrations of arterial, venous, or lymphatic vessels (**Fig. 1**). The field of vascular anomalies is rapidly expanding with new information available on phenotype and genotype. The correct classification of these disorders is crucial for appropriate evaluation and management, which often requires a multidisciplinary team of specialists. The International Society for the Study of Vascular Anomalies first devised a simple classification system that has since been updated and now includes new diagnosis and the linkage of phenotypes to genotypes[1] (**Table 1**). Vascular malformations are distinguished from vascular tumors by their low cell turnover and lack of invasiveness. They tend to grow in proportion to the child, are

[a] Pediatric Hematology and Oncology, Aflac Cancer and Blood Disorders Center, Emory University School of Medicine, Atlanta, GA, USA; [b] Complex Vascular Anomalies Frontier Program, Children's Hospital of Philadelphia, Philadelphia, PA, USA
* Corresponding author. 5461 meridian mark road Northeast, Atlanta, GA 30322.
E-mail address: michael.briones@choa.org

Clin Perinatol 48 (2021) 181–198
https://doi.org/10.1016/j.clp.2020.11.011
0095-5108/21/© 2020 Elsevier Inc. All rights reserved.
perinatology.theclinics.com

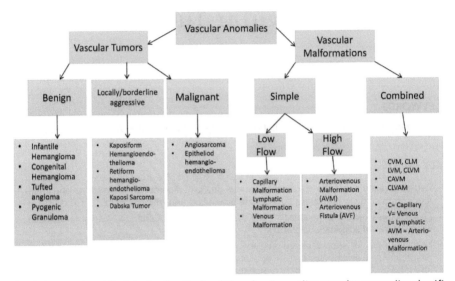

Fig. 1. International Society for the Study of Vascular Anomalies vascular anomalies classification. (Approved at the 20th ISSVA Workshop, Melbourne, April 2014, last revision May 2018)

generally stable in adulthood, and are not covered in this review. In this article, we review the most frequent vascular tumors seen in the neonatal period and their presentation, epidemiology, and genetics. We also discuss the diagnosis and management of these complex lesions.

INFANTILE HEMANGIOMA

Infantile hemangiomas (IH) are the most common soft tissue tumors of infancy and are first noted in the first few weeks of life followed by a period of active growth and then spontaneous involution. The majority of IHs do not require therapy and regress spontaneously. Of IHs, 10% to 15% require treatment secondary to complications, such as potential disfigurement, functional impairment, obstruction of vital structures, and ulceration. IHs occur in 1% to 5% of infants and up to 10% of Caucasian infants. IHs are 2 to 3 times more common in females and more common in preterm or low birth weight infants, occurring in approximately 23% of premature babies smaller than 1000 g.[2] Most IHs occur sporadically. However, they may rarely be caused by an abnormality of chromosome 5 and present in an autosomal-dominant pattern.[3] In a study that evaluated inheritance patterns of IHs, 34% of patients had a family history of IH, most commonly in a first-degree relative.[4]

Pathogenesis

The development of IHs is thought to be an interplay between vasculogenesis and angiogenesis, with dysregulation of these cell processes driving clonal proliferations of endothelial cells[5,6] resulting from vasculogenesis rather than angiogenesis. One hypothesis is that the involvement of the vascular endothelial growth factor (VEGF) signaling pathway along with hypoxic stress as a triggering signal[5] induces overexpression of angiogenic factors such as VEGF via the hypoxia inducible factor α pathway.[6,7] During the rapid growth in the first few months of life, the growth phase

Table 1 Classification system of vascular anomalies	
Category	**Vascular Tumor Type (Causal Genes)**

Benign (type 1b)	Infantile hemangioma/hemangioma of infancy
	Congenital hemangioma (GNAQ/GNA11)
	   Rapidly involuting congenital hemangioma (RICH)
	   Noninvoluting congenital hemangioma (NICH)
	   Partially involuting congenital hemangioma (PICH)
	Tufted angioma
	Spindle cell hemangioma (IDH1/IDH2)
	Epithelioid hemangioma (FOS)
	Pyogenic granuloma (also known as lobular
	   capillary hemangioma) (BRAF/RAS/GNA14)
	Others

Locally aggressive or borderline	Kaposiform hemangioendothelioma (KHE) (GNA14) Retiform hemangioendothelioma Papillary intralymphatic angioendothelioma (PILA), Dabska tumor Composite hemangioendothelioma Pseudomyogenic hemangioendothelioma (FOSB) Polymorphous hemangioendothelioma Hemangioendothelioma not otherwise specified Kaposi sarcoma Others
Malignant	Angiosarcoma (MYC: postradiation therapy) Epithelioid hemangioendothelioma (EHE) (CAMTA1/TFE3) Others

Adapted from ISSVA Classification of Vascular Anomalies. ©2018 International Society for the Study of Vascular Anomalies. Available at "issva.org/classification." Accessed June 2018.[1]

of IH, endothelial cells predominate, with formation of syncytial masses without a defined vascular architecture. The hemangioma endothelial cells are plump and metabolically active, resembling fetal endothelial cells. Evaluation of IH endothelial cells suggest that they are clonal in nature.[5,8,9] During the involution phase, there are increased mast cells and levels of metalloproteinase, as well as an upregulation of interferon and decreased basic fibroblast growth factor. Endothelial cells in IH express a particular phenotype showing positive staining for the glucose transporter protein-1 (GLUT1) glucose transporter. GLUT1 is also expressed on placental endothelial cells but is absent in other tumors and in vascular malformations. Lesions positive for GLUT1 and placenta-associated antigens suggest that they share a common genetic etiology in which both are driven by response to hypoxia.[10,11] Hypoxia seems to play a critical role in the pathogenesis of hemangiomas. There is an association of hemangiomas with placental hypoxia, which is increased in prematurity, multiple pregnancies, and placental anomalies.[10,12] Multiple targets of hypoxia[11,13] are demonstrated in proliferating hemangiomas, including VEGF-A, GLUT1, and insulin-like growth factor-2.[11,14,15] This hypothesis suggests that a proliferating hemangioma is an attempt to normalize hypoxic tissue that occurred in utero.

Clinical Presentation

In the neonatal period, most hemangiomas may not be clinically evident at birth, but become apparent within the first days to months of life. Newborns may initially present with an inconspicuous cutaneous mark, such as a patch of telangiectasias with surrounding pallor (secondary to vasoconstriction) at the hemangioma site. Less commonly, a hemangioma may appear initially as a bright red patch resembling a port-wine stain. The majority of lesions are solitary, but multiple lesions occur in up to 20% to 30% of infants, and are especially common among multiple births. Hemangiomas have a predilection for the head and neck (60%), trunk (25%), and extremities (15%), although they can occur anywhere in the skin, mucous membranes, or internal organs. Hemangiomas range in size from a few millimeters to many centimeters in diameter. Hemangioma lesions proliferate for an average of 5 months, stabilize, and then involute over several years (**Fig. 2**).[16] IHs can be classified as superficial, involving the superficial dermis and appearing as bright red lesions; deep, involving the deep dermis and subcutis and appearing bluish to skin colored; or combined (compound), and may also be subtyped into focal or segmental (**Fig. 3**). Visceral lesions are more common in patients with multifocal IH (defined as >5 lesions) and should prompt abdominal ultrasound to evaluate for visceral hemangiomas. Liver IHs can be multiple or diffuse.[17,18] Focal, solitary hepatic hemangiomas occur most often without cutaneous involvement and are usually congenital. Multifocal and diffuse involvement of the liver with hemangiomas are termed IHs and are also associated with cutaneous IH.[18] In a patient with liver hemangiomas, there can be associated hypothyroidism owing to the expression of iodothyronine deiodinase.[19] Both diffuse hepatic IH or large solitary hepatic hemangiomas are at an increased risk of developing high-output cardiac failure (**Fig. 4**).[17–19] IHs are usually diagnosed by history, clinical presentation, and examination and rarely need imaging and/or biopsy. If any concerns arise clinically or radiologically, histologic confirmation should be considered. The differential diagnosis includes other vascular tumors as well as malignant tumors (**Table 2**).

Complications

Ulceration can occur and is associated with pain (10%) and discomfort (25%) and is a common complication of IH. Common areas for ulceration are the lip, the head and neck area, and the intertriginous regions, and ulceration is more common with segmental and combined deep and superficial lesions. Anatomic issues and functional impairment with obstruction and/or visual impairment usually occurs during the early proliferation phase within the first 2 to 3 months of life. Respiratory compromise can

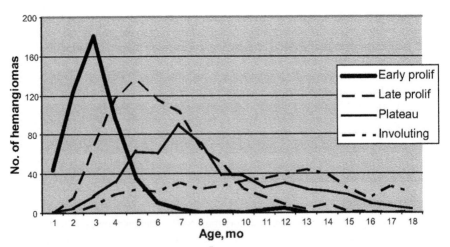

Fig. 2. Vascular tumor: IH, natural history.[7]

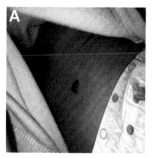
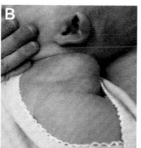
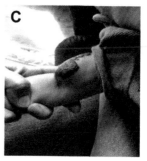

Fig. 3. Types of IHs. (*A*) Bright red superficial hemangioma. (*B*) Bluish, deep hemangioma. (*C*) Mixed type.

present with stridor with airway lesions in the paraglottic or intratracheal region and are associated with bearded distribution hemangiomas (see **Fig. 4**B). IHs located near the eyelid or on the eyelid can lead to visual obstruction causing permanent amblyopia, astigmatism, or strabismus[20] (see **Fig. 4**A).

Syndromes

Segmental IH of the face and lumbosacral regions can be associated with syndromes. Segmental distribution facial hemangiomas and large (>5 cm) facial IHs can be associated with various anomalies (**Fig. 5**A–C), which are summarized by the acronym PHACE, which includes (P) posterior fossa malformations, (H) hemangiomas, (A) arterial anomalies both intracranial and cardiac, (C) cardiac anomalies such as coarctation of aorta, and (E) eye and endocrine anomalies (**Fig. 5**) (**Table 3**).[21] Lumbar syndrome is associated with midline IH in the lumbosacral or perineal region (see **Fig. 5**D) and is associated with urogenital (hypospadias, bladder extrophy, renal anomalies), anorectal (imperforate anus), and vascular anomalies (persistent sciatic artery, hypoplastic ileofemoral artery), as well as spinal defects (tethered cord, spinal dysraphism, lipomeningocele, anomalies of the os sacrum, and scoliosis).[22]

Evaluation

The majority of IHs do not need imaging evaluation. Imaging depends on the location and morphology of the hemangioma. Infants with large (>5 cm in diameter), segmental hemangiomas, particularly when located on the face, scalp, or posterior head or neck, are at risk for PHACE syndrome. These infants should undergo careful cutaneous, ophthalmologic, cardiac, and neurologic evaluations (**Table 4**). Neonates with beard

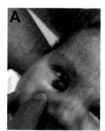
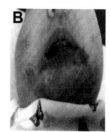
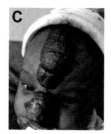
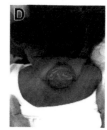

Fig. 4. Complications of IHs. (*A*) Visual obstruction. (*B*) Bearded distribution-concerning for airway obstruction. (*C*) Disfiguring facial hemangioma. (*D*) Ulcerated hemangioma.

Table 2
Differential diagnosis of neonatal vascular tumors

Vascular Tumors	Nonvascular Tumors
IH	Infantile fibrosarcoma
Congenital hemangioma	Rhabdomyosarcoma
Tufted angioma	Neuroblastoma
Pyogenic granuloma	Hepatoblastoma
KHE	Hemangiopericytomas
Angiosarcoma	Lymphomas

distribution hemangiomas (segmental cervicofacial or mandibular hemangiomas in a beard distribution) (see **Fig. 4**B) should be clinically monitored for signs of airway involvement (eg, progressive hoarseness, stridor). The possibility of PHACE syndrome should also be considered in these patients. Segmental hemangiomas over the midline lumbosacral spine and midline genitourinary distribution (see **Fig. 5**D) may be associated with lumbosacral syndrome, and ultrasound imaging can be performed instead of MRI in infants younger than 4 months of age if expertise in pediatric ultrasound examination is available. However, MRI is the most sensitive means of definitive diagnosis of spinal anomalies and should be performed in all infants or older children with a hemangioma over the lumbosacral spine. MRI is the gold standard for evaluating patients with lumbosacral hemangiomas for underlying spinal disorders.[23–25]

Periorbital hemangiomas may compromise normal visual development (see **Fig. 4**A). In concerning cases where hemangiomas are or potentially can obstruct vision, early examination by an ophthalmologist is required. Multifocal cutaneous hemangiomas at-risk for concomitant visceral hemangiomas and are defined as 5 or more small, localized lesions. The liver is the most frequently involved extracutaneous site, whereas involvement of other sites, such as the gastrointestinal tract or the brain, is rare; thus, an abdominal ultrasound examination is recommended. This recommendation is supported by a prospective study in which 16% of infants with 5 or more hemangiomas had solitary or multiple hepatic hemangiomas and 1.3% had airway or gastrointestinal hemangiomas.[17–19] None of the children with 4 or fewer cutaneous hemangiomas had visceral lesions. Infants with hepatic hemangiomas should also be screened for hypothyroidism. Hepatic hemangiomas can cause consumption hypothyroidism through the production of type 3 iodothyronine deiodinase, which is a thyroid-deactivating enzyme[19,26]

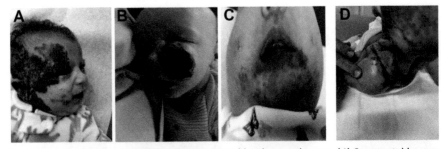

Fig. 5. Hemangiomas associated with PHACE and lumbar syndromes. (*A*) Segmental hemangioma. (*B*) Hemangiomas greater than 5 cm. (*C*) Bearded distribution. (*D*) Hemangioma in the lumbosacral or perineal region.

Table 3
Diagnostic criteria

Organ System	Major Criteria	MINOR Criteria
Cerebrovascular	Anomaly of major cerebral arteries Anomaly of the major cerebral arteries Dysplasia of the large cerebral arteries Arterial stenosis or occlusion with or without moyamoya collaterals Absence of or moderate to severe hypoplasia of the large cerebral arteries Aberrant origin or course of the large cerebral arteries Persistent trigeminal artery Saccular aneurysms of any cerebral arteries	Persistent embryonic artery other than trigeminal artery Proatlantal intersegmental artery Primitive hypoglossal artery Primitive otic artery
Structural brain	Posterior fossa anomaly Dandy–Walker complex or unilateral/bilateral cerebellar hypoplasia/dysplasia	Enhancing extra-axial lesion with features consistent with intracranial hemangioma Midline anomaly Neuronal migration disorder
Cardiovascular	Aortic arch anomaly Coarctation of the aorta dysplasia Aneurysm Aberrant origin of the subclavian artery with or without a vascular ring	Ventricular septal defect Right aortic arch (double aortic arch)
Ocular	Posterior segment abnormality Persistent fetal vasculature Retinal vascular anomalies Morning Glory disc anomaly Optic nerve hypoplasia Peripapillary staphyloma Coloboma	Anterior segment abnormality Sclerocornea Cataract Coloboma Microphthalmia
Ventral or midline	Sternal defect Sternal cleft Suparumbilical raphe	Hypopituitarism Ectopic thyroid

PHACE.[12] PHACE syndrome: facial hemangioma greater than 5 cm plus 1 major criterion or 2 minor criteria; possible PHACE syndrome: facial hemangioma >5 cm plus 1 minor criteria hemangioma of the neck or upper torso plus 1 major criterion or 2 minor criteria, no hemangioma plus 2 major criteria.

Management

Most patients do not require therapy and may be observed until spontaneous involution occurs. The management of IHs depends on whether intervention is necessary. The indications for immediate intervention include the following[1]: emergency treatment of potentially life-threatening complications[2] and urgent treatment of existing or imminent functional impairment, pain, or bleeding.[27] Elective treatment is considered to decrease the likelihood of long-term or permanent disfigurement. Life-threatening lesions include obstructing IHs of the airway; hemangiomas affecting the eye with functional impairment including loss of visual axis leading to deprivation

Table 4
Recommended minimal imaging evaluation for infants at risk for PHACE syndrome[12]

Associated Anomaly	Testing Required

Brain—posterior fossa	MRI of the brain
	  Axial spin-echo T2 volumetric gradient-echo T1 (preferred)
	  or axial spin-echo T1 axial diffusion-weighted imaging
	  (this includes ADC mapping)
	  Gadolinium-enhanced T1 in 2 planes with fat suppression

Arterial malformation	Intracranial and cervical angiography
	  Intracranial axial TOF MRA
	  Contrast-enhanced MRA (preferred) or TOF MRA of the
	  cervical vessels

Cardiac anomaly	Transthoracic echocardiography
Eye anomaly	Ophthalmology consultation and examination

Abbreviations: ADC, apparent diffusion coefficient; MRA, MR angiography; TOF, time of flight.

amblyopia, astigmatism, strabismus, and visual field cuts, as well as impaired feeding because of involvement of the lips or mouth; and decreased mobility because of complicated involvement of the extremities. IHs involving the liver associated with high-output congestive heart failure and severe hypothyroidism require immediate intervention.

Propranolol has become the first-line treatment for IH and the preferred treatment for high-risk IH (**Fig. 6**).[28–30] The American Academy of Pediatrics has published

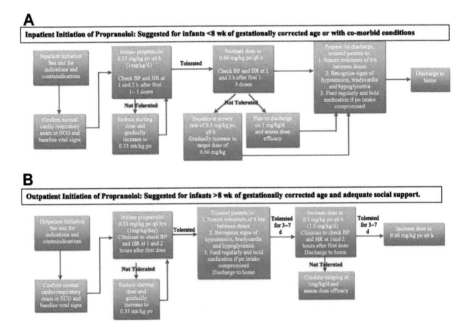

Fig. 6. (*A*) Summary of recommended dose initiation for inpatient scenario. (*B*) Summary of recommended dose initiation for outpatient scenario. BP, blood pressure; ECG, electrocardiogram; HR, heart rate. (*From* Drolet et al. Pediatrics 2013;131:128-140; with permission ©2013 by American Academy of Pediatrics.)

clinical practice guidelines.[27,28] An early therapeutic intervention was noted to be critical for complicated IHs to prevent medical complications and permanent disfigurement. The timing of intervention was noted to be best in the first 1 to 3 months of life. The guidelines specify hemangioma specialists because those practitioners have expertise in the management and care of hemangiomas, as well as knowledge of the risk stratification and treatment options. These providers include experts in the fields of dermatology, hematology and oncology, pediatrics, plastic surgery, general surgery, otolaryngology, and ophthalmology.[27] Propranolol is a nonselective beta-blocker. The potential mechanisms of action include vasoconstriction and/or decreased expression of VEGF and basic fibroblast growth factor, leading to apoptosis.[31,32] The dosing used is generally 1 mg/kg/d to 3 mg/kg/d, divided into 2 or 3 doses. The starting dose varies depending on risk factors and the location of initiation. Outpatients and inpatients are initially started at a dose of 0.5 mg/kg/d to 1 mg/kg/d and increased over time.[28,33,34] Initially, dosing of 3 times per day is recommended for infants younger than 5 weeks of age and for patients with PHACE syndrome.[28,35]

Patient monitoring varies depending on individual practice. However, oral propranolol peaks at 1 to 3 hours after administration and most centers measure heart rate and blood pressure 1 and 2 hours after each dose with initiation, and then when the dose is increased by at least 0.5 mg/kg/d. Parent and patient education includes instruction on when to hold the medication, signs of hypoglycemia, the necessity of feeding through the night, and when to call the physician with issues, such as illnesses that may interfere with oral intake or lead to dehydration or respiratory problems. Propranolol is contraindicated in infants with cardiogenic shock, sinus bradycardia, hypotension, second- to third-degree atrioventricular block, heart failure, history of airway responsiveness (eg, asthma and poor ventilation), aortic stenosis, and allergic reaction to propranolol. Common side effects of propranolol include gastrointestinal discomfort, sleep disorders, agitation, and body temperature fluctuations. Other β-blockers have also been used to treat IHs, including atenolol, nadolol, and acebutolol.[30,36] There are no consensus guidelines for the length of therapy with propranolol. In a prospective, multi-institutional study that assessed the efficacy and safety of propranolol in high-risk patients, the propranolol was administered for a minimum of 6 months, up to a maximum of age 12 months.

Before the widespread use of propranolol for IH treatment, glucocorticoids were the first-line therapeutic drugs for IH, and still have certain value for the treatment of refractory and complicated IHs. The use of topical β-blockers has also been effective; these agents are used mainly for the treatment of small, localized, superficial hemangiomas as an alternative to observation. Topical β-blockers include propranolol gel and timolol eye drops. The topical timolol that is used is the ophthalmic gel-forming solution 0.5%; 1 drop is applied to the hemangioma 2 times per day until a stable response is achieved. There have been studies using timolol maleate ophthalmic solution to treat IHs, involving more than 1000 patients.[37,38] Puttgen and colleagues[38] completed a multicenter retrospective cohort study at 9 centers to study 731 patients with IH who received topical timolol. This study suggested that timolol was a well-tolerated and safe treatment for IH, especially for superficial IH, with a good therapeutic efficacy. Surgical interventions are usually delayed unless an IH causes serious risks to the airway or orbit, or the IH ulcerates. Late surgery (ie, at age 3–5 years) may be needed for residual skin changes. Laser therapy is another modality and most suitable for superficial, naturally regressed, and residual IHs after drug treatment(s).[39,40]

CONGENITAL HEMANGIOMA

Congenital hemangiomas (CH) are rare vascular tumors that proliferate in utero and are fully present at birth; these hemangiomas may regress early, such as the rapidly involuting CHs (RICHs), whereas noninvoluting CHs (NICHs) do not regress. These lesions can occur both in the skin and in visceral organs such as the liver. Partially involuting CHs do not completely involute.

Pathogenesis and Natural History

The incidence of CH is rare (0.3%) with a male to female ratio of 1:1. Head and extremity lesions account for the majority of cases and are usually solitary lesions.[41–43] CH are negative for GLUT1, which is distinctly different from the IH that generally display GLUT1 positivity.[41] RICHs typically begin to regress a few days to a few weeks after birth (**Fig. 7**), and in most cases show complete regression in 6 to 14 months. In rare instances, involution may occur in utero, leaving areas of skin redundancy with dermal or subcutaneous atrophy, textural and color changes, and persistent telangiectasias or scattered veins. In a smaller proportion of patients with RICH, involution may be rapid but incomplete which leaves a vascular plaque with coarse telangiectasia on the surface and a peripheral bluish white border resembling a NICH (as discussed elsewhere in this article). Other local sequelae include permanent alopecia, superficial scarring, and milia formation.

NICHs display a slight preponderance of males to females (3:2); most lesions are solitary, with the majority of lesions in the head and neck, trunk, or limbs. Appearances are usually plaque-like or bossed, with a pink to purple color with prominent coarse telangiectasia on the surface. NICH, as the name implies, do not involute. They remain unchanged except for proportional growth and appearance of increased draining veins in the periphery of the lesion.[42] A partially involuting CH is a clinical subtype of CH that begins as a RICH with rapid involution during the first year of life, but fails to completely involute and persists as a NICH-like lesion with the residual tumor having the clinical, ultrasound, and histologic features of NICH.[43]

Clinical Presentation

CHs usually present as a raised violaceous soft tissue mass with prominent peripheral veins, or a soft tissue mass with overlying prominent, coarse telangiectasias admixed with blanched skin, including a halo of blanched skin at the periphery of the tumor. Ulceration, scarring, and atrophy are uncommon, but can occur during the involution period. The lesions are typically warm and may have areas of induration with well-circumscribed borders. They can also occur in the visceral organs, most commonly in the liver. Transient coagulopathy can occur, with thrombocytopenia and

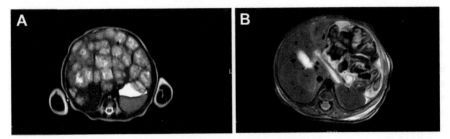

Fig. 7. Hepatic hemangioma. (*A*) Diffuse IH of the liver. (*B*) CH.

hypofibrinogenemia. Supportive treatment is recommended. High-output heart failure from arteriovenous shunting and cardiac overload has been seen with large CHs (>7 cm).

Management

The clinical diagnosis of CH is made in a newborn presenting with a fully grown soft tissue mass with overlying telangiectasias and peripheral vasoconstriction. The observation of rapid involution starting a few days to weeks after birth is usually sufficient to differentiate a RICH from a NICH. Imaging studies such ultrasound examination, MRI, or MR arteriography may be needed when the diagnosis is unclear. Ultrasound examination in both RICH and NICH shows a predominantly heterogeneous sonographic structure, with diffuse vascularity, high vessel density, and, occasionally, calcifications. Routine renal ultrasound examination increasingly detects CH, and Doppler examination can reveal high-flow vascular lesions. MRI of both RICH and NICH show heterogeneous enhancement, hyperintensity on T2-weighted sequences, flow voids, and the absence of peripheral edema.[44] Biopsy should be performed if the diagnosis is uncertain or if there is a clinical suspicion of malignant tumor.

RICHs are self-resolving and for the majority of the lesions; treatment is usually not necessary and is supportive in nature. Periodic clinical examinations are performed until complete involution has taken place. NICHs and partially involuting CHs do not resolve but, similar to RICHs, therapy may not be necessary if the lesion remains asymptomatic and does not bother the patient. Surgical excision may be necessary if deemed feasible. No medical treatment has been proven to be effective, because the lesions are not proliferative. Because RICH lesions spontaneously involute over time, their response to medical therapy is difficult to assess.

TUFTED ANGIOMA AND KAPOSIFORM HEMANGIOENDOTHELIOMA
Epidemiology

Tufted angiomas (TAs) (**Fig. 8**A) are rare locally aggressive vascular tumors of infants and young children (>50% occur in the first year of life) and are more common in males. To date, no genetic markers for TAs have been identified. Histopathology reveals multiple, discrete lobules of tightly packed capillaries (tufts) scattered in the dermis or the subcutis in a so-called cannonball pattern and fibrosis of surrounding dermis; the tufts are surrounded by cleft-like, semilunar empty vascular spaces and lymphatic differentiation is seen with thin-walled lymphatic spaces throughout. Immunohistochemistry of TAs is negative for GLUT1 but positive for CD31, CD34, VEGFR-3, D2-40, and proxy1.[45,46]

KHE (**Fig. 8**B) is a rare, locally aggressive vascular tumor that typically presents in infancy or early childhood. KHEs can be infiltrative, locally destructive, life-threatening tumors that are associated with the Kasabach–Merritt phenomenon (KMP), which includes thrombocytopenia and hypofibrinogenemia, with a significant risk of bleeding and an associated mortality rate as high as 20% to 30%.[47,48] There are no national registries documenting numbers of patients with KHE, but extrapolating data at the 2 largest vascular anomaly centers in the United States, the prevalence is 0.91 in 100,000 children. KHE has an equal sex predilection, but more recently a slight male predominance has been indicated by 2 large retrospective studies.[48,49] Approximately 50% of cutaneous lesions are visible or detectable at birth.[48] The etiology of KHE remains largely unknown and mutations in KHE tumor are sporadic rather than germline. Somatic translocations between chromosomes 13 (13q14) and 16 (16p13.3) have been identified in 10% of metaphase cells in KHE lesions; a somatic

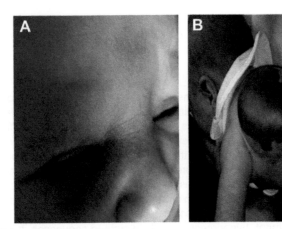

Fig. 8. (A) TA. (B). KHE.

activating GNA14 c.614 A > T (p.Gln205Leu) mutation was found in one-third of the KHE specimens and in one-fourth of the TA specimens. Somatic mutations in GNAQ and its paralogues (eg, GNA11 and GNA14) have also been identified in many other vascular tumors, vascular malformations, and solid tumors.[50–52] *GNAQ* family encodes Gα subunits that form a heterotrimer with Gβ and Gγ subunits and bind G-protein–coupled receptors. G-protein–coupled receptors are involved in many aspects of tumor and vascular biology as well as platelet aggregation, glucose secretion, and inflammation are among the physiologic processes affected by G-protein–coupled receptors[53]

Clinical Presentation

TAs present as infiltrated, firm, patches, plaques, or nodules with a dusky red to violaceous hue and ill-defined borders (**Fig. 9**A). Subcutaneous masses are seen rarely and may be inflammatory and painful. Hypertrichosis and hyperhidrosis present in the affected area. The most commonly locations are the extremities, abdomen and genitalia. TAs can follow a variable clinical course from chronic progression to spontaneous regression. In children, 3 distinct clinical patterns have been described: TA without complications, TA with the KMP and TA with coagulopathy and no thrombocytopenia.[54–56]

KHE can present as cutaneous lesions with various appearances or as deep masses without cutaneous signs. The clinical features also differ substantially between patients with KMP and patients without KMP. In the majority of patients, KHE is a single

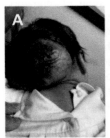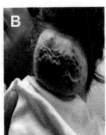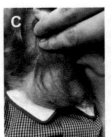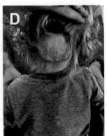

Fig. 9. CH.

soft tissue mass with cutaneous findings that range from an erythematous papule, plaque, or nodule to an indurated, purple, and firm tumor (**Fig. 9**B). In infants with KMP, the lesions are purpuric, warm or hot to the touch, swollen, and very painful. Most patients experience progressive lesion enlargement and/or symptom progression. There is more concern if the lesion extends into the deep tissue and vital organs, and if there is associated KMP.

Both TA and KHE can have associated KMP, which is defined as profound thrombocytopenia with associated consumptive coagulopathy with prolongation of the prothrombin time and partial thromboplastin time, as well as and hypofibrinogenemia. KMP has an estimated incidence of 42% to 71% in patients with TA and patients with KHE.[47] The thrombocytopenia is usually severe, with a median platelet count of 21 × 10^9/L at the initial presentation. KHE lesions with KMP display progressive engorgement and purpura. KMP can lead to significant pain and secondary bleeding. KHEs seem to be congenital, because the majority of cases are diagnosed in the newborn and infancy period. The risk of KMP is highest for congenital KHEs with a large size (especially >8 cm in diameter).[47,49] Anatomic location may also be a predictor of KMP. Clinically, intrathoracic KHEs are frequently associated with KMP.[47–49] The frequency of KMP in retroperitoneal KHEs is also high (**Fig. 9**C, D).

Management

Diagnosis may be made by tissue biopsy confirmed by histopathologic staining. It is also important to obtain laboratory evaluation including a complete blood count with platelet count, D-dimer, fibrinogen, prothrombin time, partial thromboplastin time, and international normalized ratio. Liver and renal function tests should be performed in acutely ill patients. MRI with gadolinium may be useful to determine the extent of involvement. Treatment must be individualized, based on the size, location, presence of symptoms such as tenderness or functional compromise, and the presence or absence of thrombocytopenia and coagulopathy. For patients without the KMP who have small or localized tumors, surgical excision is the treatment of choice. For nonresectable TAs, observation for spontaneous regression may be an option for lesions that are asymptomatic and not causing functional compromise and are not disfiguring. Infants with KMP require treatment for coagulopathy and hemostasis support. Surgical excision is the treatment of choice for small, localized tumors. For large, nonresectable tumors, chemotherapy with intravenous vincristine and systemic corticosteroids or/and oral sirolimus with or without systemic corticosteroids may be used.[57–59] Vincristine 0.05 mg/kg is given intravenously once weekly; oral prednisolone 2 mg/kg is given daily. Sirolimus is typically given orally at the dose of 0.8 mg/m^2 per dose, with close monitoring of blood levels and supportive care.[60–62] Consultation with a hematologist–oncologist who is part of a vascular anomaly multidisciplinary team is highly recommended.

ANGIOSARCOMA

Angiosarcoma is a rare, aggressive, vascular tumor that can arise in any part of the body but is more common in soft tissues, and accounts for 2% of sarcomas. Angiosarcoma has an estimated incidence of 2 cases per 1 million people; in the United States, each year it affects approximately 600 people who are typically aged 60 to 70 years.[63] Angiosarcomas are extremely rare in children, but cases have been reported in neonates and toddlers, with presentation of multiple cutaneous lesions and liver lesions, some of which are GLUT1 positive.[64–67] Angiosarcomas are positive for GLUT1 in 20% of cases. Most angiosarcomas involve the skin and superficial soft tissue, although the liver, spleen, and lung can be affected; bone is rarely affected.

Pathology

Angiosarcomas are largely aneuploid tumors. The rare cases of angiosarcoma that arise from benign lesions such as hemangiomas have a distinct pathway that is poorly understood. The histopathologic diagnosis can at times be difficult to make secondary to heterogeneous areas of varied atypia. The common feature is an irregular network of channels in a dissective pattern along dermal collagen bundles. There is varied cellular shape, size, mitosis, endothelial multilayering, and papillary formation. Epithelioid cells can also be present. Necrosis and hemorrhage are common. Tumors stain for factor VIII, CD31, and CD34. Some liver lesions can mimic IHs and have focal GLUT1 positivity. The nomenclature for these liver lesions has been difficult and confusing with use of terminology from 1971 (eg, type I hemangioendothelioma, IH; type II hemangioendothelioma, low-grade angiosarcoma; type III hemangioendothelioma, high-grade angiosarcoma).[65]

Management

Localized disease may be cured by aggressive surgery; complete surgical excision is crucial for angiosarcomas. Localized disease, especially cutaneous angiosarcoma, may also be treated with radiation therapy; most of these reported cases are in adults.[68] Multimodal treatment with surgery, systemic chemotherapy, and radiation therapy is used for metastatic disease, although it is rarely curative.[69] Disease control is the objective in metastatic angiosarcoma, with published progression-free survival rates between 3 to 7 months and a median overall survival rate of 14 to 18 months[70,71] In both adults and children, the 5-year overall survival rates of between 20% and 35% are reported.[71]

SUMMARY

Vascular tumors presenting in the newborn period represent a spectrum of disorders from a simple birthmark to life-threatening entities. An accurate diagnosis is crucial for appropriate evaluation and management, and often requires a multidisciplinary approach with a range of specialists. Recognition of clinical history, presentation, and examination is paramount to establish an appropriate diagnosis to most appropriately evaluate and manage the patients. Many neonatal vascular anomalies require no or minimal intervention, whereas others require a multidisciplinary approach with multimodal intervention. Understanding these nuances and complexities is essential for the most comprehensive care and optimal clinical outcomes with recommendation that patients be seen and referred by a dedicated pediatric vascular anomaly program.

DISCLOSURE

Dr D. Adams is a consultant for Venthura and Novartis.

REFERENCES

1. International society for the study of vascular anomalies (ISSVA) – updated classification. Available at: http://www.issva.org.
2. Goelz R, Poets CF. Incidence and treatment of infantile hemangioma in preterm infants. Arch Dis Child Fetal Neonatal Ed 2015;100:F85–91.

3. Blei F, Walter J, Orlow SJ, et al. Familial segregation of hemangiomas and vascular malformations as an autosomal dominant trait. Arch Dermatol 1998; 134(6):718–22.

4. Castrén E, Salminen P, Vikkula M, et al. Inheritance patterns of infantile hemangioma. Pediatrics 2016;138:1–7.

5. Boye E, Yu Y, Paranya G, et al. Clonality and altered behavior of endothelial cells from hemangiomas. J Clin Invest 2001;107:745–52.

6. Walter JW, North PE, Waner M, et al. Somatic mutation of vascular endothelial growth factor receptors in juvenile hemangioma. Genes Chromosomes Cancer 2002;33:295–303.

7. Chen T, Eichenfield L, Sheila FF, et al. Infantile hemangiomas: an update on pathogenesis and therapy. Pediatrics 2013;131(Number 1):99–108.

8. Yu Y, Flint AF, Mulliken JB, et al. Endothelial progenitor cells in infantile hemangioma. Blood 2004;103(4):1373–5.

9. Boscolo E, Mulliken JB, Bischoff J. Pericytes from infantile hemangioma display proangiogenic properties and dysregulated angiopoietin-1. Arterioscler Thromb Vasc Biol 2013;33(3):501–9.

10. Leon-Villapalos J, Wolfe K, Kangesu L. GLUT-1: an extra diagnostic tool to differentiate between haemangiomas and vascular malformations. Br J Plast Surg 2005;58:348.

11. North PE, Waner M, Mizeracki A, et al. GLUT1: a newly discovered immunohistochemical marker for juvenile hemangiomas. Hum Pathol 2000;31:11.

12. Colonna V, Resta L, Napoli A, et al. Placental hypoxia and neonatal haemangioma: clinical and histological observations. Br J Dermatol 2010;162(1):208–9.

13. de Jong S, Itinteang T, Withers AH, et al. Does hypoxia play a role in infantile hemangioma? Arch Dermatol Res 2016;308(4):219–27.

14. Ritter MR, Dorrell MI, Edmonds J, et al. Insulin-like growth factor 2 and potential regulators of hemangioma growth and involution identified by large-scale expression analysis. Proc Natl Acad Sci U S A 2002;99(11):7455–60.

15. Barnés CM, Huang S, Kaipainen A, et al. Evidence by molecular profiling for a placental origin of infantile hemangioma. Proc Natl Acad Sci U S A 2005; 102(52):19097–102.

16. Chang LC, Haggstrom AN, Drolet BA, et al. Growth characteristics of infantile hemangiomas: implications for management. Pediatrics 2008;122:360–7.

17. Christison-Lagay ER, Burrows PE, Alomari A, et al. Hepatic hemangiomas: subtype classification and development of a clinical practice algorithm and registry. J Pediatr Surg 2007;42:62–7.

18. Kulungowski AM, Alomari AI, Chawla A, et al. Lessons from a liver hemangioma registry: subtype classification. J Pediatr Surg 2012;47:165–70.

19. Yeh I, Bruckner AL, Sanchez R, et al. Diffuse infantile hepatic hemangiomas: a report of four cases successfully managed with medical therapy. Pediatr Dermatol 2011;28:267–75.

20. Xue L, Sun C, Xu DP, et al. Clinical outcomes of infants with periorbital hemangiomas treated with oral propranolol. J Oral Maxillofac Surg 2016;74(11):2193–9.

21. Metry D, Heyer G, Hess G, et al. Consensus statement on diagnostic criteria for PHACE syndrome. Pediatrics 2009;124(Number 5):1447–56.

22. Girard C, Bigorre M, Guillot B, et al. PELVIS syndrome. Arch Dermatol 2006;142: 884–8.

23. Stockman A, Boralevi F, Taïeb A, et al. SACRAL syndrome: spinal dysraphism, anogenital, cutaneous, renal and urologic anomalies, associated with an angioma of lumbosacral localization. Dermatology 2007;214:40–5.

24. Iacobas I, Burrows PE, Frieden IJ, et al. LUMBAR: association between cutaneous infantile hemangiomas of the lower body and regional congenital anomalies. J Pediatr 2010;157:795–801.

25. Horii KA, Drolet BA, Frieden IJ, et al. Hemangioma investigator group. Prospective study of the frequency of hepatic hemangiomas in infants with multiple cutaneous infantile hemangiomas. Pediatr Dermatol 2011;28(3):245–53. Epub 2011 Apr 26.

26. Huang SA, Tu HM, Harney JW, et al. Severe hypothyroidism caused by type 3 iodothyronine deiodinase in infantile hemangiomas. N Engl J Med 2000;343:185–9.

27. Krowchuk Daniel P, Ilona J, Mancini Anthony J, et al. Subcommittee on the management of infantile hemangiomas clinical practice guideline for the management of infantile hemangiomas. Pediatrics 2019;143(1):1–28.

28. Drolet B, Frommelt P, Sarah LC, et al. Initiation and use of propranolol for infantile hemangioma: report of a consensus conference. Pediatrics 2013;131:128–40.

29. Leute-Lebreze C, Voisard JJ, Nicholas M. Oral propranolol for infantile hemangioma. N Engl J Med 2015;373(3):284–5.

30. Chinnadurai S, Fonnesbeck C, Kristen MS, et al. Pharmacologic interventions for infantile hemangioma: a meta-analysis. Pediatrics 2016;137(Number 2):1–12.

31. Sharifpanah F, Saliu F, Bekhite MM, et al. β-Adrenergic receptor antagonists inhibit vasculogenesis of embryonic stem cells by downregulation of nitric oxide generation and interference with VEGF signalling. Cell Tissue Res 2014;358(2): 443–52.

32. Ma X, Zhao T, Ouyang T, et al. Propranolol enhanced adipogenesis instead of induction of apoptosis of hemangiomas stem cells. Int J Clin Exp Pathol 2014;7(7): 3809–17.

33. Solman L, Glover M, Beattie PE, et al. Oral propranolol in the treatment of proliferating infantile haemangiomas: British Society for Paediatric Dermatology consensus guidelines. Br J Dermatol 2018;179(3):582–9.

34. Hoeger PH, Harper JI, Baselga E, et al. Treatment of infantile haemangiomas: recommendations of a European expert group. Eur J Pediatr 2015;174(7): 855–65.

35. Garzon MC, Epstein LG, Heyer GL, et al. PHACE syndrome: consensus-derived diagnosis and care recommendations. J Pediatr 2016;178:24–33.e2.

36. Randhawa HK, Sibbald C, Garcia Romero M, et al. Oral nadolol for the treatment of infantile hemangiomas: a single-institution retrospective cohort study. Pediatr Dermatol 2015;32(No. 5):690–5.

37. Püttgen K, Lucky A, Adams D, et al. Topical timolol maleate treatment of infantile hemangiomas. Pediatrics 2016;138:1–9.

38. Chakkittakandiyil A, Phillips R, Frieden IJ, et al. Timolol maleate 0.5% or 0.1% gel-forming solution for infantile hemangiomas: a retrospective, multicenter, cohort study. Pediatr Dermatol 2012;29(1):28–31.

39. Witman PM, Wagner AM, Scherer K, et al. Complications following pulsed dye laser treatment of superficial hemangiomas. Lasers Surg Med 2006;38:116–23.

40. Reddy KK, Blei F, Brauer JA, et al. Retrospective study of the treatment of infantile hemangiomas using a combination of propranolol and pulsed dye laser. Dermatol Surg 2013;39:923–33.

41. Berenguer B, Mulliken J, Enjolras O, et al. Rapidly involuting congenital hemangioma: clinical and histopathologic features. Pediatr Dev Pathol 2003;6:495–510.

42. Krol A, MacArthur CJ. Congenital hemangiomas: rapidly involuting and noninvoluting congenital hemangiomas. Arch Facial Plast Surg 2005;7(5):307–11.

43. Mulliken John B, Enjolras Odile. Congenital hemangiomas and infantile hemangioma: missing links. J Am Acad Dermatol 2004;50(6):875–82.
44. Gorincour G, Kokta V, Rypens F, et al. Imaging characteristics of two subtypes of congenital hemangiomas: rapidly involuting congenital hemangiomas and non-involuting congenital hemangiomas. Pediatr Radiol 2005;35:1178.
45. Arai E, Kuramochi A, Tsuchida T, et al. Usefulness of D2-40 immunohistochemistry for differentiation between kaposiform hemangioendothelioma and tufted angioma. J Cutan Pathol 2006;33:492–7.
46. Le Huu AR, Jokinen CH, Rubin BP, et al. Expression of prox1, lymphatic endothelial nuclear transcription factor, in Kaposiform hemangioendothelioma and tufted angioma. Am J Surg Pathol 2010;34:1563–73.
47. Croteau SE, Liang MG, Kozakewich HP, et al. Kaposiform hemangioendothelioma: atypical features and risks of Kasabach-Merritt phenomenon in 107 referrals. J Pediatr 2013;162(1):142–7.
48. Ji Y, Yang K, Peng S, et al. Kaposiform haemangioendothelioma: clinical features, complications and risk factors for Kasabach-Merritt phenomenon. Br J Dermatol 2018;179(2):457–63.
49. Mahajan P, Margolin J, Iacobas I. Kasabach-Merritt phenomenon: classic presentation and management options. Clin Med Insights Blood Disord 2017;10:1–5.
50. Bean GR, Joseph NM, Folpe AL, et al. RecurrentGNA14 mutations in anastomosing haemangiomas. Histopathology 2018;73(2):354–7.
51. Ayturk UM, Couto JA, Hann S, et al. Somatic activating mutations in GNAQ and GNA11 are associated with congenital Hemangioma. Am J Hum Genet 2016; 98(6):1271.
52. Joseph NM, Brunt EM, Marginean C, et al. Frequent GNAQ and GNA14 mutations in hepatic small vessel neoplasm. Am J Surg Pathol 2018;42(9):1201–7.
53. Kimple AJ, Bosch DE, Giguere PM, et al. Regulators of G-protein signaling and their Galpha substrates: promises and challenges in their use as drug discovery targets. Pharmacol Rev 2011;63(3):728–49.
54. Osio A, Fraitag S, Hadj-Rabia S, et al. Clinical spectrum of tufted angiomas in childhood: a report of 13 cases and a review of the literature. Arch Dermatol 2010;146:758–63.
55. Okada E, Tamura A, Ishikawa O, et al. Tufted angioma (angioblastoma): case report and review of 41 cases in the Japanese literature. Clin Exp Dermatol 2000;25:627–30.
56. Herron MD, Coffin CM, Vanderhooft SL, et al. Variability of the clinical morphology. Pediatr Dermatol 2002;19:394–401.
57. Drolet BA, Trenor CC 3rd, Brandão LR, et al. Consensus-derived practice standards plan for complicated kaposiform hemangioendothelioma. J Pediatr 2013; 163:285–91.
58. Zhou SY, Li HB, Mao YM, et al. Successful treatment of Kasabach–Merritt syndrome with transarterial embolization and corticosteroids. J Pediatr Surg 2013; 48:673–6.
59. Chiu YE, Drolet BA, Blei F, et al. Variable response to propranolol treatment of kaposiform hemangioendothelioma, tufted angioma, and Kasabach–Merritt phenomenon. Pediatr Blood Cancer 2012;59:934–8.
60. Blatt J, Stavas J, Moats-Staats B, et al. Treatment of childhood Kaposi-form hemangioendothelioma with sirolimus. Pediatr Blood Cancer 2010;55:1396–8.
61. Hammill AM, Wentzel MS, Gupta A, et al. Sirolimus for the treatment of complicated vascular anomalies in children. Pediatr Blood Cancer 2011;57(6):1018–24.

62. Adams DM, Trenor CC, Hammill AM, et al. Efficacy and safety of sirolimus in the treatment of complicated vascular anomalies. Pediatrics 2016;137(2):1–10.

63. Cioffi A, Reichert S, Antonescu CR, et al. Angiosarcomas and other sarcomas of endothelial origin. Hematol Oncol Clin North Am 2013;27(5):975–88.

64. Jeng MR, Fuh B, Blatt J, et al. Malignant transformation of infantile hemangioma to angiosarcoma: response to chemotherapy with bevacizumab. Pediatr Blood Cancer 2014;61(11):2115–7.

65. Dehner LP, Ishak KG. Vascular tumors of the liver in infants and children. A study of 30 cases and review of the literature. Arch Pathol 1971;92(2):101–11.

66. Ferrari A, Casanova M, Bisogno G, et al. Malignant vascular tumors in children and adolescents: a report from the Italian and German soft tissue sarcoma cooperative group. Med Pediatr Oncol 2002;39(2):109–14.

67. Deyrup AT, Miettinen M, North PE, et al. Pediatric cutaneous angiosarcomas: a clinicopathologic study of 10 cases. Am J Surg Pathol 2011;35(1):70–5.

68. Sanada T, Nakayama H, Irisawa R, et al. Clinical outcome and dose volume evaluation in patients who undergo brachytherapy for angiosarcoma of the scalp and face. Mol Clin Oncol 2017;6(3):334–40.

69. Dickson MA, D'Adamo DR, Keohan ML, et al. Phase II trial of gemcitabine and docetaxel with bevacizumab in soft tissue sarcoma. Sarcoma 2015;2015:532478.

70. Ravi V, Patel S. Vascular sarcomas. Curr Oncol Rep 2013;15(4):347–55.

71. Grassia KL, Peterman CM, Iacobas I, et al. Clinical case series of pediatric hepatic angiosarcoma. Pediatr Blood Cancer 2017;64(11). https://doi.org/10.1002/pbc.26627.

Late Effects in Survivors of Neonatal Cancer

Sanyukta K. Janardan, MD[a,b], Karen E. Effinger, MD, MS[a,b],*

KEYWORDS

- Neonatal cancer survivor • Late effects • Long-term outcomes

KEY POINTS

- Survivors of neonatal malignancies may have increased risk for cancer treatment–related late effects because of their developing organ systems.
- Risk for late effects depends on treatment exposures.
- Radiation is often avoided in neonates because of its impact on growth and development.
- Evidence-based late effects surveillance recommendations published by the Children's Oncology Group serve as a reference for practitioners to monitor for late effects.

INTRODUCTION

Childhood cancer is rare, with an estimated yearly incidence of 210 per million children younger than 20 years in the United States; neonatal cancers comprise 2% of all childhood cancers.[1,2] Common neonatal cancers include leukemias, central nervous system (CNS) tumors, germ cell tumors, sarcomas, and other embryonal tumors (eg, neuroblastoma, mesoblastic nephroma, retinoblastoma, hepatoblastoma). Treatment modalities are diagnosis dependent and may include surgery, chemotherapy, radiation, and/or hematopoietic stem cell transplantation (HSCT). As treatments for childhood cancer improve, more infants are surviving their primary cancer diagnoses, with current 5-year survival rates of greater than 75%.[2] However, survivors of neonatal malignancies are at risk for chronic medical conditions from their cancer or its therapies, termed late effects. In this article, the authors focus on late effects of common treatments for neonatal malignancies; however, it bears noting that because studies in these survivors are quite limited, exposure-based risks are primarily extrapolated from studies of survivors of infant or childhood cancers.

a Division of Hematology/Oncology/BMT, Department of Pediatrics, Emory University, Atlanta, GA, USA; b Aflac Cancer and Blood Disorders Center, Children's Healthcare of Atlanta, 2015 Uppergate Drive, 4th Floor, Atlanta, GA 30322, USA
* Corresponding author. Aflac Cancer and Blood Disorders Center, Children's Healthcare of Atlanta, 2015 Uppergate Drive, Fourth Floor, Atlanta, GA 30322.
E-mail address: karen.effinger@emory.edu

Clin Perinatol 48 (2021) 199–214
https://doi.org/10.1016/j.clp.2020.11.009
0095-5108/21/© 2020 Elsevier Inc. All rights reserved.
perinatology.theclinics.com

LATE EFFECTS

Because of improvements in therapy, there are currently approximately 465,000 childhood cancer survivors living in the United States; yet, research has shown that these survivors have an increasing risk of morbidity and early mortality as they age.[2,3] By age 45, survivors have an estimated 95.5% cumulative prevalence of any chronic health condition and 80.5% cumulative prevalence of a serious or life-threatening condition.[4] The prevalence of late effects in neonatal cancer survivors, specifically, is unknown because of limited studies. However, because neonates' organs are immature and rapidly developing, their bodies are thought to be more vulnerable to the toxic acute and late effects of cancer treatments. These toxicities include medical late effects (eg, cardiovascular disease and growth disturbances), psychosocial late effects (eg, anxiety and depression), and neurocognitive late effects (eg, speech delay and low IQ).[5,6] An analysis of 33 neonatal cancer survivors treated between 1990 and 2018 revealed that only 18% developed late effects.[7] However, the length of follow-up and methods for capturing late effects were not described, and it is likely that this is an underestimate of the long-term health burden in these survivors. In a review of neonatal cancers treated in Denmark between 1943 and 1985, 2 of 19 five-year survivors (11%) developed a subsequent malignant neoplasm. One of these malignancies was probably related to a genetic predisposition and the other was in a radiation field.[8]

Although there is limited research specifically focused on neonates, there are several studies that have evaluated late effects in pediatric cancer survivors diagnosed at a young age. For example, research has shown that 26% to 60% of survivors of sacrococcygeal teratomas, which are typically diagnosed in the neonatal period, develop gastrointestinal late effects, and 41% to 66% suffer from urinary late effects.[9–12] Approximately 75% of infant leukemia survivors report at least 1 late effect, with growth, dental, and learning disturbances the most common.[6,13] However, in a series of 4 neonatal leukemia survivors, all of the survivors had growth impairment.[14] Studies of infant brain tumor survivors have reported neurocognitive and neurologic dysfunction in 70% to 83% of survivors as well as visual and endocrine late effects.[15,16] Although late effects are common in infant brain tumor and leukemia survivors, in a study of stage 4S neuroblastoma survivors, only 5 of 25 survivors (20%) developed chronic conditions.[17]

TREATMENT EXPOSURES

The specific type and severity of late effects that may develop in survivors depend on treatment exposures and intensity, which are related to diagnosis. **Table 1** summarizes common neonatal malignancies and their typical treatment exposures. **Table 2** summarizes organ systems affected by common treatments for neonatal malignancies.

Surgery

Surgical resection is an important component in the treatment of many neonatal malignancies in order to prevent the toxicities associated with chemotherapy, radiation, and HSCT. However, given the small size of neonates, surgery in this population poses unique challenges with regard to the morbidity of a major surgery and its impact on functional outcomes.

Neurosurgery

CNS tumors in the neonatal population are challenging to treat because of the morbidity associated with radiation therapy; however, surgical resection of these

Table 1
Common neonatal malignancies and associated treatment exposures[a]

Diagnosis	Treatment Modality/Exposure
Non-CNS solid tumors	
Sacrococcygeal teratoma	Surgery ± chemotherapy (bleomycin, cisplatin, etoposide)[b]
Neuroblastoma	Surgery ± chemotherapy (carboplatin, cyclophosphamide, doxorubicin, etoposide) ± radiation[c]
Sarcomas	Surgery ± chemotherapy (dactinomycin, vincristine ± cyclophosphamide, doxorubicin, ifosfamide, etoposide, NTRK inhibitors) ± radiation
Mesoblastic nephroma	Nephrectomy[d]
Wilms tumor	Nephrectomy ± chemotherapy (dactinomycin, vincristine ± doxorubicin) ± radiation
Rhabdoid tumor of kidney	Nephrectomy, chemotherapy (carboplatin, cyclophosphamide, doxorubicin, etoposide, vincristine), radiation
Hepatoblastoma	Chemotherapy (carboplatin, cisplatin, doxorubicin, etoposide, 5-fluorouracil, vincristine), surgery
Retinoblastoma	Laser surgery/cryotherapy/enucleation ± chemotherapy (carboplatin ± etoposide, vincristine) ± brachytherapy[e]
Leukemia	
Acute lymphoblastic leukemia	Chemotherapy (asparaginase, cytarabine,[f] cyclophosphamide, daunorubicin, dexamethasone, etoposide, mercaptopurine, methotrexate,[f] prednisone, thioguanine, vincristine) ± HSCT[g] ± radiation (cranial, testicular)[h]
Acute myeloid leukemia	Chemotherapy (asparaginase, cytarabine,[f] daunorubicin, etoposide, gemtuzumab ozogamicin,[i] mitoxantrone) ± HSCT[g]
CNS tumors	
Teratomas	Surgery
Astrocytoma	Surgery ± chemotherapy (carboplatin, cisplatin, etoposide, temozolomide, vinblastine, vincristine)
Medulloblastoma	Surgery, chemotherapy (carboplatin, cisplatin, cyclophosphamide, etoposide, methotrexate, vincristine) ± HSCT[j]
Choroid-plexus tumors	Surgery ± chemotherapy (carboplatin, cisplatin, etoposide, ifosfamide, vincristine) ± HSCT[j]

Abbreviation: NTRK, nonreceptor tyrosine kinase.

[a] Common treatment exposures listed; actual treatment is risk based and may vary.

[b] Chemotherapy is often not needed. Pelvic radiation may be required in relapsed or refractory disease.

[c] High-risk or relapsed disease may require additional chemotherapeutic agents (including retinoids and monoclonal antibodies) and autologous HSCT.

[d] Chemotherapy is sometimes required, especially for the cellular variant.

[e] Brachytherapy is preferred over external beam radiation therapy; however, external beam radiation may be necessary. Metastatic disease requires additional chemotherapeutic agents and autologous HSCT.

[f] Cytarabine and methotrexate are delivered via both intrathecal and intravenous routes. Methotrexate is also given orally.

[g] Based on disease response and cytogenetics. HSCT may include total body irradiation.

[h] Radiation is avoided as much as possible until age 3 y.

[i] Gemtuzumab ozogamicin is used for CD33+ acute myeloid leukemia.

[j] HSCT is used to avoid radiation as much as possible until age 3 y.

Table 2
Neonatal cancer treatments and organ systems with potential late effects

Cancer Treatment	Organ Systems with Potential Late Effects													
	SMN	Learning[a]	Neuro	MSK	Endo	Ocular	Auditory	Dental	Pulm	Cardiac	GI	Hepatic	GU[b]	Gonadal[c]
Surgery														
Neurosurgery, cranial		X	X		X	X	X							X
Neurosurgery, spinal			X								X		X	X
Enucleation				X		X								
Nephrectomy				X									X	
Abdominopelvic											X		X	X
Chemotherapy														
Anthracyclines[d]	X							X		X				
Bleomycin								X	X					
Traditional alkylators[e]	X					X[j]		X	X[j]				X[k]	X
Heavy metals[f]	X		X				X	X					X	X
Vinca alkaloids[g]			X					X						
Epipodophyllotoxin[h]	X							X						
Antimetabolites[i]		X[l]		X[m]				X				X		
Corticosteroids				X	X	X		X						
Radiation														
Cranial	X	X	X	X	X	X	X	X						
Spinal[n]	X		X	X	X			X		X	X		X	X
Neck	X				X			X						
Chest	X			X					X	X				
Abdominopelvic	X			X	X						X	X	X	X
Hematopoietic stem cell transplantation[o]														
Allogeneic/autologous	X	X	X	X	X	X	X	X	X	X	X	X	X	X

Abbreviations: Endo, endocrine; GI, gastrointestinal; GU, genitourinary; MSK, musculoskeletal; Neuro, neurologic; Pulm, pulmonary; SMN, subsequent malignant neoplasm.

[a] Learning includes treatment with a direct impact on neurocognitive function and not indirect influences seen in those with visual or auditory impairment.

[b] Includes renal toxicities.

[c] Includes central and direct gonadotoxicity as well as sexual dysfunction.

[d] Common anthracyclines used in neonatal cancers include daunorubicin, doxorubicin, mitoxantrone.

[e] Common traditional alkylators used in neonatal cancers include cyclophosphamide, ifosfamide, temozolomide. Busulfan is used in HSCT.

[f] Heavy metals include carboplatin and cisplatin.

[g] Vinca alkaloids include vincristine and vinblastine.

[h] Common epipodophyllotoxins include etoposide.

[i] Common antimetabolites used in neonatal cancers include cytarabine, mercaptopurine, methotrexate, thioguanine.

[j] Busulfan can cause cataracts and pulmonary dysfunction.

[k] Cyclophosphamide can cause urinary tract toxicity, and ifosfamide can cause renal toxicity.

[l] High-dose intravenous cytarabine and methotrexate as well as intrathecal methotrexate are associated with neurocognitive dysfunction.

[m] Methotrexate can cause decreased bone mineral density.

[n] Late effects associated with spinal irradiation depends on extent of spinal involvement.

[o] Late effects associated with HSCT depends on conditioning regimen and development of graft-versus-host disease.

tumors also carries risk for substantial late effects, including neurologic deficits, neurocognitive impairment, and endocrinopathies. In a study of patients younger than 6 months of age who underwent surgical resection for CNS tumors, all 8 survivors (median follow-up = 0.9 years) had neurologic deficits, ranging from motor difficulties in standing and crawling to seizures and hemiparesis.[18] Neurocognitive impairments, such as learning difficulties and developmental delay, were seen in 4 (50%) and aggressive behavior was seen in one (13%).[18] Precocious puberty was also reported in 1 patient, likely secondary to tumor location, because surgery in the suprasellar region can lead to pituitary dysfunction.[18]

Spinal involvement or surgical resection of paraspinal tumors can also be associated with significant neurologic sequelae.[19,20] Because of the need for a sacral approach and coccyx resection, sacrococcygeal teratoma survivors can develop neurologic impairments, including lower-extremity weakness, gait changes, and abnormal ambulatory muscle movements.[19–21] Similarly, neuroblastoma can arise in the paraspinal region, leading to nerve injuries, including hemiparesis. Nearly all neuroblastoma patients with epidural compression at birth have long-term sequelae unless they are detected prenatally and delivered prematurely.[22]

Enucleation

Enucleation may be required for local control in retinoblastoma and subsequently leads to at least partial vision impairment. Ross and colleagues[23] investigated the risk of developmental delay in children aged 6 to 40 months with retinoblastoma. They found that within the subpopulation of children with unilateral retinoblastoma (n = 21, 20 with enucleation), 7 of the survivors (33%) required visuomotor training, which they postulated may be due to vision impairments from enucleation. In addition, enucleation leads to abnormal orbital growth, which can cause facial deformities, especially if a prosthesis is not used.[24]

Nephrectomy

Nephrectomy is commonly used in the treatment of renal tumors, such as mesoblastic nephroma, Wilms tumor, and rhabdoid tumor of the kidney. Survivors who undergo a nephrectomy are at risk for hypertension, renal dysfunction, and renal failure. For example, a study of 3016 adult survivors of childhood cancer found that survivors who underwent nephrectomy were 1.68 times more likely to have hypertension as compared with the general population.[25] The risk of hypertension is important to consider when caring for these survivors given the serious consequences of untreated hypertension on the remaining kidney and heart. In adult survivors of childhood cancer, those with hypertension had 5.6 times higher risk for cardiac-specific mortality compared with survivors without hypertension.[26]

The development of renal dysfunction and/or failure is multifactorial in survivors, and nephrectomy can be a contributing factor to decreased glomerular filtration rate.[27] In addition, underlying genetic disorders, which are often associated with renal tumors in neonates, may increase the risk of renal failure after a unilateral nephrectomy. In a cohort of 15 unilateral Wilms tumor survivors with renal failure, two-thirds had Denys-Drash syndrome.[28] Although surgical interventions are limited as much as possible in patients with bilateral Wilms tumor, in a cohort of 39 patients with bilateral Wilms tumor, 24 patients (61.5%) progressed to renal failure iatrogenically because of the need for bilateral nephrectomies.[28]

Abdominopelvic resections

Abdominopelvic resections and/or laparotomies are often used in the resection of sacrococcygeal teratoma and neuroblastoma and can cause gastrointestinal and genitourinary late effects, especially in tumors with intraspinal extension.[9,12,20,29] Constipation is seen in most sacrococcygeal teratoma survivors, and fecal and bladder incontinence can occur.[9] Moreover, the intrapelvic surgery required for some of these tumors places survivors at risk of both pelvic floor and sexual dysfunction. It is also important to note that any survivor who has undergone major abdominal surgery is at risk for adhesions and bowel obstruction.

Chemotherapy

Chemotherapy serves as the backbone of many neonatal cancer treatment regimens that cannot be cured by surgery alone. Each chemotherapy drug has the potential to cause specific late effects regardless of the age at exposure; however, variable drug metabolism in neonates, including differences in renal blood flow, unpredictable rates of hepatic metabolism, and changes in plasma protein binding capacity can cause increased organ toxicity as young organ systems mature. Chemotherapy, in general, is associated with interruptions in dental development that can cause multiple dental anomalies, including hypodontia, root malformation, and enamel hypoplasia, especially when the exposure occurs before permanent dentition development.[30,31] Several chemotherapies, specifically alkylating agents, anthracyclines, and epipodophyllotoxins, place survivors at an increased risk of secondary leukemias with poor prognoses.[32–34]

Antitumor antibiotics

Antitumor antibiotics, like anthracyclines and bleomycin, cause DNA-strand breakage. The major late effect associated with anthracyclines is cardiotoxicity, which is the leading cause of non-cancer-related mortality in childhood cancer survivors.[35] Exposure to anthracyclines, including doxorubicin, daunorubicin, and mitoxantrone, can lead to cardiac late effects ranging from reduced cardiac contractility and left ventricular wall thinning to heart failure requiring heart transplantation. Anthracyclines may also impair cardiac muscle growth, which uniquely affects younger hearts that are still developing.[36] Risk for cardiotoxicity is correlated with exposure dose; however, it has also been shown that younger age at anthracycline exposure may increase risk.[36,37] For example, in a cohort of 120 childhood cancer survivors who received anthracycline therapy, those who were younger at diagnosis were more susceptible to cardiotoxicity, including left ventricular wall thinning and increased left ventricular afterload.[38]

Bleomycin has been associated with pulmonary late effects, specifically pulmonary fibrosis and obstructive as well as restrictive defects.[39,40] In a cohort of 80 childhood cancer survivors, children younger than 8 years at diagnosis were more likely to have abnormal pulmonary function testing as compared with older children. The investigators postulated that this may be due to disruption in alveolar development, which would make neonates particularly vulnerable to the pulmonary effects of this drug.[39]

Alkylating agents

Alkylating agents, which add alkyl groups to DNA and RNA in order to cause strand breakage and cell death, include traditional alkylating agents (eg, cyclophosphamide, ifosfamide, and temozolomide) as well as heavy metals like cisplatin and carboplatin. One of the most significant side effects of alkylating chemotherapy is gonadotoxicity, which is dose dependent. In female patients, higher doses of alkylating agents are associated with pubertal delay, premature ovarian failure, and infertility, but this risk is decreased in female patients who are prepubertal at the time of exposure.[41–44] In male patients, reduced quality and quantity of sperm can be seen secondary to alkylating agents at lower doses than associated with female gonadotoxicity; however, testosterone production is often preserved.[41,42] Unlike in female patients, the risk of gonadotoxicity in male patients is not impacted by pubertal status.[42]

Other notable late effects of alkylating chemotherapy include nephrotoxicity, ototoxicity, and dental anomalies. Nephrotoxicity can occur secondary to both heavy metals and ifosfamide.[45] Ifosfamide has been shown to have age-specific nephrotoxicity with more severe proximal tubular damage seen in children aged 5 years or younger as compared with older children. Proximal tubular damage not only impacts kidney function but also has the potential to cause hypophosphatemic rickets.[46] Ototoxicity is most commonly caused by platinum-based heavy metal chemotherapy, particularly cisplatin, and is more common in patients treated before age 5 years.[47] Importantly, in many common neonatal cancers, such as sacrococcygeal teratoma, neuroblastoma, CNS tumors, hepatoblastoma, and retinoblastoma, platinum-based chemotherapy is a crucial component of the treatment regimen if chemotherapy is recommended.[47] The resulting sensorineural hearing loss, which can develop both during and after treatment, is irreversible and has the potential to have far-reaching effects on early language development. Finally, although dental anomalies can develop secondary to chemotherapy in general, the use of alkylating chemotherapy has been specifically shown to cause dental anomalies in a dose-dependent fashion in children younger than 5 years of age.[31]

Plant alkaloids

Plant alkaloids disrupt cell division and include drugs such as vincristine and etoposide. Vincristine, a vinca alkaloid, is notable for causing cranial and peripheral neuropathies that can contribute to motor difficulties and reduced quality of life both during and after treatment. Cases of vincristine-related vocal cord paralysis and severe peripheral neuropathy leading to flaccid paralysis requiring intubation have been reported in infants undergoing cancer treatment.[48,49] Data regarding age-specific toxicity of vincristine are mixed.[50] To the authors' knowledge, no studies have specifically looked at the impact of vincristine on the incomplete and ongoing myelinization of the neonatal nervous system. Etoposide, the most common epipodophyllotoxin, has been implicated in the development of treatment-related acute myeloid leukemia. In the Childhood Cancer Survivor Study (CCSS), a multi-institutional, retrospective study of 13,581 five-year survivors of childhood cancer, an independent, statistically significant relationship between epipodophyllotoxins and secondary leukemias was identified.[33]

Antimetabolites

Antimetabolites, which are commonly used to treat leukemia, include cytarabine, methotrexate, mercaptopurine, and thioguanine. Cytarabine and methotrexate have both been shown to be associated with neurocognitive deficits in childhood cancer survivors. High doses of methotrexate can cross the blood-brain barrier, which is critical to the treatment of CNS leukemia; however, it can also damage cerebral white matter. The incomplete myelinization of the neonatal blood-brain barrier can potentially increase neonates' susceptibility to these toxic effects.[51] Buizer and colleagues[52] found that children with leukemia treated with higher methotrexate doses had more difficulties with functional attention. Survivors of non-CNS cancers who have received high-dose intravenous cytarabine, intravenous plus intrathecal cytarabine, or intravenous plus intrathecal methotrexate have also self-reported difficulties with emotional regulation.[53] In addition to neurocognitive and emotional late effects, methotrexate can increase bone resorption and impair bone matrix calcification, which may lead to decreased bone mineral density.[54] Methotrexate, mercaptopurine, and thioguanine are also associated with hepatotoxicity. Methotrexate has the potential to cause liver fibrosis, whereas mercaptopurine and thioguanine have been associated with the development of portal hypertension.[55,56]

Corticosteroids

Corticosteroids are used in the treatment of acute lymphoblastic leukemia and graft-versus-host disease after HSCT as well as to decrease edema associated with CNS tumors. The primary late effects from prolonged steroid use in childhood cancer survivors include decreased bone mineral density, growth impairments, and cataracts. Multiple studies have shown that high doses of corticosteroids, such as prednisone and dexamethasone, lead to osteopenia.[57,58] Although bone mass increases until approximately 30 years of age, the amount of childhood bone mass acquisition is important, as it can help determine the extent of bone loss later in life.[58] Short stature from corticosteroids can be due to reduced activity of chondrocytes at growth plates and reduced endogenous growth hormone release.[54] Prednisone, specifically, has also been implicated in the development of cataracts. In a cohort of patients within the CCSS, survivors treated with prednisone had 2.3 times higher risk of developing cataracts.[59]

Radiation

Radiation therapy has been demonstrated to have significant late effects in survivors of childhood cancer, including endocrinopathies, musculoskeletal deformities, neurocognitive impairments, and subsequent malignancies. These late effects are especially important to account for when using radiation in neonates, as their major organ systems are rapidly developing and, thus, are especially susceptible to injury.[60] Many common neonatal tumors, including CNS tumors, neuroblastoma, Wilms tumor, retinoblastoma, and leukemias, may include radiation as a component of the treatment plan; however, it is avoided as much as possible in neonates. In particular, neurocognitive deficits and bone and soft tissue hypoplasia can be significant in young patients after radiation exposure. Monitoring for subsequent neoplasms is particularly important in survivors who were exposed to radiation. Nonmelanomatous skin cancer is a common radiation-induced subsequent malignancy, with 90% of lesions in childhood cancer survivors found within a radiation field.[61]

Cranial radiation

Because of its toxicity on the developing brain leading to a longitudinal severe decline in IQ, the use of cranial radiation is now limited in young children.[62,63] In fact, it is rarely used before age 3 years in patients with CNS tumors because of the high treatment doses required; however, in some cases it may be needed for relapsed or refractory CNS tumors, neonatal leukemia, or head/neck solid tumors. The neurocognitive implications of radiation on the developing brain extend beyond decline in IQ and can impact academic achievement.[63–65] Silverman and colleagues[65] found that in 11 survivors of infant leukemia treated with cranial radiation (age at diagnosis 23 days to 11 months), 9 (82%) had varying degrees of neurocognitive impairment, with 2 of the 9 requiring multiple special education services and 1 who developed a seizure disorder. In addition to neurocognitive sequelae, cranial radiation can lead to pituitary dysfunction, including growth hormone deficiency, central diabetes insipidus, central hypothyroidism, and central hypogonadism through interruption of the hypothalamic-pituitary-adrenal axis.[5,66] Chemaitilly and colleagues[67] reported that in a cohort of adult childhood cancer survivors who had hypothalamus/pituitary radiation exposure as part of their cancer treatment, 50% had at least 1 anterior pituitary hormone deficiency and 11% had multiple pituitary hormone deficiencies. Radiation also causes growth disturbances in the bones and surrounding soft tissues. Retinoblastoma survivors who receive radiation are at risk of developing facial abnormalities, specifically bony orbital changes.[68,69] Radiation to the jaw has been shown to be independently associated with dental anomalies secondary to soft tissue atrophy, calcification abnormalities, and disruption of tooth and root growth as well as radiation-induced xerostomia, which can propagate the development of cavities.[31] Furthermore, radiation can impact sensory organs with increased risk for cataracts and hearing loss, which is exacerbated when radiation is combined with or precedes platinum-based chemotherapy.[47,59,70,71] Finally, those who have had cranial radiation exposure are at risk for the development of secondary intracranial malignancies, including astrocytoma, glioblastoma, and meningioma.[72–74]

Neck and chest radiation

Neck and chest radiation is sometimes used, depending on tumor location, in neuroblastoma and soft tissue sarcomas. Survivors of radiation to these fields are also at risk of secondary malignancies, including thyroid and breast carcinomas.[33,75] In addition, neck radiation is associated with primary hypothyroidism.[66] Radiation to the chest can cause cardiotoxicity, including cardiomyopathy, early coronary artery disease, and valvular abnormalities, and can result in pulmonary insufficiency.[6,20,35,60]

Abdominopelvic radiation

Abdominopelvic radiation is sometimes required for the treatment of Wilms tumor, neuroblastoma, and relapsed/refractory sacrococcygeal teratomas. Survivors exposed to abdominal radiation may develop scoliosis because of differential growth resulting from tissue hypoplasia.[20] In addition, radiation damage to the vertebral growth plates can result in poor spinal and linear growth.[20,76] Patients who undergo radiation to the abdominopelvic region are also at risk for gastrointestinal upset, hepatotoxicity, nephrotoxicity, cystitis, hypogonadism, and sexual dysfunction. Finally, abdominopelvic radiation can place childhood cancer survivors at an increased risk of colorectal cancer that approaches that of those with hereditary colorectal cancer predisposition syndromes.[77]

Hematopoietic Stem Cell Transplantation

HSCT is sometimes required for high-risk, refractory, or relapsed leukemia, neuroblastoma, or retinoblastoma. It is also used in neonatal CNS tumors to avoid radiation. HSCT preparative conditioning regimens involve a combination of high-dose chemotherapy and, at times, total body irradiation. Survivors of HSCT are at high risk for late effects of treatment because of the intensity of the preparative regimen and as a result of possible graft-versus-host disease. Several studies have shown that infant leukemia survivors who underwent HSCT are at increased risk for short stature, including those who do not receive radiation.[6,78] Compared with infant leukemia survivors treated with chemotherapy alone, those who received a HSCT had increased risk of hypothyroidism, pulmonary dysfunction, neurocognitive deficits, and cataracts.[6,13,78]

In addition, survivors of HSCT are at high risk for infertility because of exposure to high-dose alkylating agents and/or total body irradiation.[44]

DISCUSSION

Evidence-based late effects surveillance recommendations have been published by the Children's Oncology Group.[79] These recommendations are organized by treatment exposure and serve as a reference for both general physicians and oncologists in order to monitor late effects. The goal of surveillance is early detection and treatment to lessen morbidity. There has also been an increasing focus on the development and utilization of multidisciplinary cancer survivorship clinics. The complex and sometimes chronic nature of childhood cancer survivors' toxicities emphasizes the importance of this coordinated, comprehensive care in both identification and treatment of late effects as well as education of survivors about their exposure-based risks. A study of a regional childhood cancer survivor clinic found 98 new treatment-related late effects through risk-based surveillance in 34% of patients who presented for their first survivorship clinic visit.[80]

SUMMARY

Childhood cancer survivors are at risk for a wide range of late effects related to their therapy; however, neonatal survivors may have increased risk because of the age at which they undergo these treatments. When choosing appropriate treatments for neonates with malignancies, one must consider not only the treatment that will allow the best chance at a cure but also the associated morbidities that accompany each treatment regimen. In addition, it is important to consider underlying factors that may put the neonate at an increased risk for late effects. For example, premature neonates have organs that are even more immature and likely more susceptible to late effects than full-term neonates, and neonates with a family history of cancer may have an underlying predisposition syndrome that will further increase their risk of subsequent treatment-related malignancies.[60,75] An awareness of the potential late effects for which survivors are at risk is important so that appropriate surveillance can be undertaken and signs and symptoms of these late effects can be recognized. Well-rounded, comprehensive care of neonates with cancer is necessary to ensure the current and future health and well-being of this uniquely vulnerable patient population.

CLINICAL CARE POINTS

- Treatment of neonatal cancers, including surgery, chemotherapy, radiation, and HSCT, places survivors at long-term risk for morbidity and early mortality.[4]
- Neurosurgery (cranial and spinal) can lead to long-term neurologic and developmental deficits.[18–20]
- Depending on the type and dose, chemotherapy can have a wide range of late effects, impacting various organ systems, including dental, sensory, cardiac, reproductive, and cognitive.[4]
- Radiation is avoided as much as possible in neonates because of the devastating long-term growth and developmental sequelae associated with early exposure.[60]
- Evidence-based late effects surveillance recommendations published by the Children's Oncology Group serve as a reference for practitioners to monitor for late effects.[79]

Best Practices

What is the current practice for mitigating the late effects of cancer treatment in survivors of neonatal cancers?

Best Practice/Guideline/Care Path Objectives

- Survivors of neonatal cancer are at increased risk of late effects from their cancer treatments given the immaturity and ongoing development of their organ systems.
- Late effects for which neonates are at risk are treatment dependent and include neurocognitive impairment, altered growth, ototoxicity, dental anomalies, cardiotoxicity, nephrotoxicity, infertility, decreased bone mineral density, and subsequent neoplasms.
- Surgical resection of tumors in neonates has high morbidity and the potential to cause functional deficits.
- Variable drug metabolism in neonates makes chemotherapy administration challenging and increases the risk of drug toxicities.
- All efforts are made to avoid radiation in neonates and infants because of its severe impact on cognition and growth.
- Survivors of neonatal cancer require coordinated, comprehensive multidisciplinary care for risk-based late effects surveillance and treatment to improve their well-being and long-term outcomes.

What changes in current practice are likely to improve outcomes?

- Evaluation for underlying genetic syndromes at diagnosis can help guide selection of safe treatment options
- Regular monitoring for late effects based on exposure-based guidelines
- Referral to a comprehensive survivorship clinic after therapy completion to aid in late effect monitoring

Is there a Clinical Algorithm?

See Table 2 and Children's Oncology Group Long-Term Follow-up Guidelines[79]

Major Recommendations

- Avoidance of cranial radiation in young children whenever possible to minimize significant neurocognitive impairment
- Maintain awareness of unique and developing neonatal physiology in the setting of variable chemotherapy metabolism and potential for toxicities
- To reduce the morbidity of a large surgical resection, chemotherapy can be used as an adjuvant therapy before resection
- Survivors of neonatal cancer should be followed annually in a comprehensive survivorship clinic within 1 to 2 years of completing therapy

References/Source(s):[4,51,60,79]

DISCLOSURE

The authors have no conflicts of interest and no external funding.

REFERENCES

1. Alfaar AS, Hassan WM, Bakry MS, et al. Neonates with cancer and causes of death; lessons from 615 cases in the SEER databases. Cancer Med 2017;6(7): 1817–26.
2. Howlader N, Noone AM, Krapcho M, et al, editors. SEER cancer statistics review, 1975-2017. Bethesda (MD): National Cancer Institute; 2020. Available at: https://seer.cancer.gov/csr/1975_2017/. based on November 2019 SEER data submission, posted to the SEER web site.

3. Armstrong GT, Kawashima T, Leisenring W, et al. Aging and risk of severe, disabling, life-threatening, and fatal events in the Childhood Cancer Survivor Study. J Clin Oncol 2014;32(12):1218–27.

4. Hudson MM, Ness KK, Gurney JG, et al. Clinical ascertainment of health outcomes among adults treated for childhood cancer. JAMA 2013;309(22):2371–81.

5. Gerber NU, Zehnder D, Zuzak TJ, et al. Outcome in children with brain tumours diagnosed in the first year of life: long-term complications and quality of life. Arch Dis Child 2008;93(7):582–9.

6. Leung W, Hudson M, Zhu Y, et al. Late effects in survivors of infant leukemia. Leukemia 2000;14(7):1185–90.

7. Geurten C, Geurten M, Rigo V, et al. Neonatal cancer epidemiology and outcome: a retrospective study. J Pediatr Hematol Oncol 2020;42(5):e286–92.

8. Birch K, Jacobsen T, Olsen JH, et al. Neonatal cancer in Denmark 1943-1985. Pediatr Hematol Oncol 1992;9(3):209–16.

9. Draper H, Chitayat D, Ein SH, et al. Long-term functional results following resection of neonatal sacrococcygeal teratoma. Pediatr Surg Int 2009;25(3):243–6.

10. Gabra HO, Jesudason EC, McDowell HP, et al. Sacrococcygeal teratoma–a 25-year experience in a UK regional center. J Pediatr Surg 2006;41(9):1513–6.

11. Güler S, Demirkaya M, Balkan E, et al. Late effects in patients with sacrococcygeal teratoma: a single center series. Pediatr Hematol Oncol 2018;35(3):208–17.

12. Shalaby MS, Walker G, O'Toole S, et al. The long-term outcome of patients diagnosed with sacrococcygeal teratoma in childhood. A study of a national cohort. Arch Dis Child 2014;99(11):1009–13.

13. Gandemer V, Bonneau J, Oudin C, et al. Late effects in survivors of infantile acute leukemia: a study of the L.E.A program. Blood Cancer J 2017;7(1):e518.

14. Ishii E, Oda M, Kinugawa N, et al. Features and outcome of neonatal leukemia in Japan: experience of the Japan infant leukemia study group. Pediatr Blood Cancer 2006;47(3):268–72.

15. Nomura Y, Yasumoto S, Yanai F, et al. Survival and late effects on development of patients with infantile brain tumor. Pediatr Int 2009;51(3):337–41.

16. Pillai S, Metrie M, Dunham C, et al. Intracranial tumors in infants: long-term functional outcome, survival, and its predictors. Childs Nerv Syst 2012;28(4):547–55.

17. Levitt GA, Platt KA, De Byrne R, et al. 4S neuroblastoma: the long-term outcome. Pediatr Blood Cancer 2004;43(2):120–5.

18. Lang SS, Beslow LA, Gabel B, et al. Surgical treatment of brain tumors in infants younger than six months of age and review of the literature. World Neurosurg 2012;78(1–2):137–44.

19. Malone PS, Spitz L, Kiely EM, et al. The functional sequelae of sacrococcygeal teratoma. J Pediatr Surg 1990;25(6):679–80.

20. Pintér AB, Hock A, Kajtár P, et al. Long-term follow-up of cancer in neonates and infants: a national survey of 142 patients. Pediatr Surg Intl 2003;19(4):233–9.

21. Zaccara A, Iacobelli BD, Adorisio O, et al. Gait analysis in patients operated on for sacrococcygeal teratoma. J Pediatr Surg 2004;39(6):947–52 [discussion: 947–52].

22. Gigliotti AR, De Ioris MA, De Grandis E, et al. Congenital neuroblastoma with symptoms of epidural compression at birth. Pediatr Hematol Oncol 2016;33(2):94–101.

23. Ross G, Lipper EG, Abramson D, et al. The development of young children with retinoblastoma. Arch Pediatr Adolesc Med 2001;155(1):80–3.

24. Chojniak MM, Chojniak R, Testa ML, et al. Abnormal orbital growth in children submitted to enucleation for retinoblastoma treatment. J Pediatr Hematol Oncol 2012;34(3):e102–5.

25. Gibson TM, Li Z, Green DM, et al. Blood pressure status in adult survivors of childhood cancer: a report from the St. Jude Lifetime Cohort Study. Cancer Epidemiol Biomarkers Prev 2017;26(12):1705–13.

26. Armstrong GT, Oeffinger KC, Chen Y, et al. Modifiable risk factors and major cardiac events among adult survivors of childhood cancer. J Clin Oncol 2013;31(29): 3673–80.

27. Kooijmans EC, Bökenkamp A, Tjahjadi NS, et al. Early and late adverse renal effects after potentially nephrotoxic treatment for childhood cancer. Cochrane Database Syst Rev 2019;(3):CD008944.

28. Ritchey ML, Green DM, Thomas PRM, et al. Renal failure in Wilms' tumor patients: a report from the National Wilms' Tumor Study Group. Med Pediatr Oncol 1996; 26(2):75–80.

29. Schmidt B, Haberlik A, Uray E, et al. Sacrococcygeal teratoma: clinical course and prognosis with a special view to long-term functional results. Pediatr Surg Intl 1999;15(8):573–6.

30. Effinger KE, Migliorati CA, Hudson MM, et al. Oral and dental late effects in survivors of childhood cancer: a Children's Oncology Group report. Support Care Cancer 2014;22(7):2009–19.

31. Kaste SC, Goodman P, Leisenring W, et al. Impact of radiation and chemotherapy on risk of dental abnormalities: a report from the Childhood Cancer Survivor Study. Cancer 2009;115(24):5817–27.

32. Le Deley MC, Leblanc T, Shamsaldin A, et al. Risk of secondary leukemia after a solid tumor in childhood according to the dose of epipodophyllotoxins and anthracyclines: a case-control study by the Société Française d'Oncologie Pédiatrique. J Clin Oncol 2003;21(6):1074–81.

33. Neglia JP, Friedman DL, Yasui Y, et al. Second malignant neoplasms in five-year survivors of childhood cancer: Childhood Cancer Survivor Study. J Natl Cancer Inst 2001;93(8):618–29.

34. Sandler ES, Friedman DJ, Mustafa MM, et al. Treatment of children with epipodophyllotoxin-induced secondary acute myeloid leukemia. Cancer 1997; 79(5):1049–54.

35. Armstrong GT, Ross JD. Late cardiotoxicity in aging adult survivors of childhood cancer. Prog Pediatr Cardiol 2014;36(1–2):19–26.

36. Lipshultz SE, Colan SD, Gelber RD, et al. Late cardiac effects of doxorubicin therapy for acute lymphoblastic leukemia in childhood. N Engl J Med 1991;324(12):808–15.

37. Trachtenberg BH, Landy DC, Franco VI, et al. Anthracycline-associated cardiotoxicity in survivors of childhood cancer. Pediatr Cardiol 2011;32(3):342–53.

38. Lipshultz SE, Lipsitz SR, Mone SM, et al. Female sex and higher drug dose as risk factors for late cardiotoxic effects of doxorubicin therapy for childhood cancer. N Engl J Med 1995;332(26):1738–43.

39. De A, Guryev I, LaRiviere A, et al. Pulmonary function abnormalities in childhood cancer survivors treated with bleomycin. Pediatr Blood Cancer 2014;61(9): 1679–84.

40. Zorzi AP, Yang CL, Dell S, et al. Bleomycin-associated lung toxicity in childhood cancer survivors. J Pediatr Hematol Oncol 2015;37(8):e447–52.

41. Green DM, Sklar CA, Boice JD Jr, et al. Ovarian failure and reproductive outcomes after childhood cancer treatment: results from the Childhood Cancer Survivor Study. J Clin Oncol 2009;27(14):2374–81.

42. Hudson MM. Reproductive outcomes for survivors of childhood cancer. Obstet Gynecol 2010;116(5):1171–83.

43. Jenkins A. Late effects of chemotherapy for childhood cancer. Paediatrics Child Health 2013;23(12):545–9.

44. Sklar CA, Mertens AC, Mitby P, et al. Premature menopause in survivors of childhood cancer: a report from the Childhood Cancer Survivor Study. J Natl Cancer Inst 2006;98(13):890–6.

45. Dekkers IA, Blijdorp K, Cransberg K, et al. Long-term nephrotoxicity in adult survivors of childhood cancer. Clin J Am Soc Nephrol 2013;8(6):922–9.

46. Skinner R, Pearson AD, Price L, et al. The influence of age on nephrotoxicity following chemotherapy in children. Br J Cancer Suppl 1992;18:S30–5.

47. Grewal S, Merchant T, Reymond R, et al. Auditory late effects of childhood cancer therapy: a report from the Children's Oncology Group. Pediatrics 2010;125(4):e938–50.

48. Anghelescu DL, De Armendi AJ, Thompson JW, et al. Vincristine-induced vocal cord paralysis in an infant. Paediatr Anaesth 2002;12(2):168–70.

49. Baker SK, Lipson DM. Vincristine-induced peripheral neuropathy in a neonate with congenital acute lymphoblastic leukemia. J Pediatr Hematol Oncol 2010; 32(3):e114–7.

50. van de Velde ME, Kaspers GL, Abbink FCH, et al. Vincristine-induced peripheral neuropathy in children with cancer: a systematic review. Crit Rev Oncol Hematol 2017;114:114–30.

51. Siegel SE, Moran RG. Problems in the chemotherapy of cancer in the neonate. Am J Pediatr Hematol Oncol 1981;3(3):287–96.

52. Buizer AI, de Sonneville LM, van den Heuvel-Eibrink MM, et al. Chemotherapy and attentional dysfunction in survivors of childhood acute lymphoblastic leukemia: effect of treatment intensity. Pediatr Blood Cancer 2005;45(3):281–90.

53. Kadan-Lottick NS, Zeltzer LK, Liu Q, et al. Neurocognitive functioning in adult survivors of childhood non-central nervous system cancers. J Natl Cancer Inst 2010; 102(12):881–93.

54. van Leeuwen BL, Kamps WA, Jansen HW, et al. The effect of chemotherapy on the growing skeleton. Cancer Treat Rev 2000;26(5):363–76.

55. Castellino S, Muir A, Shah A, et al. Hepato-biliary late effects in survivors of childhood and adolescent cancer: a report from the Children's Oncology Group. Pediatr Blood Cancer 2010;54(5):663–9.

56. McIntosh S, Davidson DL, O'Brien RT, et al. Methotrexate hepatotoxicity in children with leukemia. J Pediatr 1977;90(6):1019–21.

57. Kadan-Lottick NS, Dinu I, Wasilewski-Masker K, et al. Osteonecrosis in adult survivors of childhood cancer: a report from the Childhood Cancer Survivor Study. J Clin Oncol 2008;26(18):3038–45.

58. Wilson CL, Ness KK. Bone mineral density deficits and fractures in survivors of childhood cancer. Curr Osteoporos Rep 2013;11(4):329–37.

59. Whelan KF, Stratton K, Kawashima T, et al. Ocular late effects in childhood and adolescent cancer survivors: a report from the Childhood Cancer Survivor Study. Pediatr Blood Cancer 2010;54(1):103–9.

60. Littman P, D'Angio GJ. Radiation therapy in the neonate. Am J Pediatr Hematol Oncol 1981;3(3):279–85.

61. Perkins JL, Liu Y, Mitby PA, et al. Nonmelanoma skin cancer in survivors of childhood and adolescent cancer: a report from the Childhood Cancer Survivor Study. J Clin Oncol 2005;23(16):3733–41.

62. Bishop AJ, McDonald MW, Chang AL, et al. Infant brain tumors: incidence, survival, and the role of radiation based on Surveillance, Epidemiology, and End Results (SEER) Data. Int J Radiat Oncol Biol Phys 2012;82(1):341–7.

63. Mulhern RK, Merchant TE, Gajjar A, et al. Late neurocognitive sequelae in survivors of brain tumours in childhood. Lancet Oncol 2004;5(7):399–408.

64. Ferster A, Bertrand Y, Benoit Y, et al. Improved survival for acute lymphoblastic leukaemia in infancy: the experience of EORTC-Childhood Leukaemia Cooperative Group. B J Haematol 1994;86(2):284–90.

65. Silverman LB, McLean TW, Gelber RD, et al. Intensified therapy for infants with acute lymphoblastic leukemia: results from the Dana-Farber Cancer Institute Consortium. Cancer 1997;80(12):2285–95.

66. Rose SR, Horne VE, Howell J, et al. Late endocrine effects of childhood cancer. Nat Rev Endocrinol 2016;12(6):319–36.

67. Chemaitilly W, Li Z, Huang S, et al. Anterior hypopituitarism in adult survivors of childhood cancers treated with cranial radiotherapy: a report from the St Jude Lifetime Cohort study. J Clin Oncol 2015;33(5):492–500.

68. Halperin EC. Neonatal neoplasms. Int J Radiat Oncol Biol Phys 2000;47(1):171–8.

69. Kaste SC, Chen G, Fontanesi J, et al. Orbital development in long-term survivors of retinoblastoma. J Clin Oncol 1997;15(3):1183–9.

70. Alloin AL, Barlogis V, Auquier P, et al. Prevalence and risk factors of cataract after chemotherapy with or without central nervous system irradiation for childhood acute lymphoblastic leukaemia: an LEA study. Br J Haematol 2014;164(1):94–100.

71. Crom DB, Wilimas JA, Green AA, et al. Malignancy in the neonate. Med Pediatr Oncol 1989;17(2):101–4.

72. Chester AN, Tan CH, Muthurajah V, et al. Concurrent pituicytoma, meningioma, and cavernomas after cranial irradiation for childhood acute lymphoblastic leukemia. World Neurosurg 2020;136:28–31.

73. Magdum SA. Neonatal brain tumours - a review. Early Hum Dev 2010;86(10):627–31.

74. Yamanaka R, Hayano A. Secondary glioma following acute lymphocytic leukemia: therapeutic implications. Neurosurg Rev 2017;40(4):549–57.

75. Campbell AN, Chan HS, O'Brien A, et al. Malignant tumours in the neonate. Arch Dis Child 1987;62(1):19–23.

76. Gale GB, D'Angio GJ, Uri A, et al. Cancer in neonates: the experience at the Children's Hospital of Philadelphia. Pediatrics 1982;70(3):409–13.

77. Reulen RC, Frobisher C, Winter DL, et al. Long-term risks of subsequent primary neoplasms among survivors of childhood cancer. JAMA 2011;305(22):2311–9.

78. Tomizawa D, Koh K, Sato T, et al. Outcome of risk-based therapy for infant acute lymphoblastic leukemia with or without an MLL gene rearrangement, with emphasis on late effects: a final report of two consecutive studies, MLL96 and MLL98, of the Japan Infant Leukemia Study Group. Leukemia 2007;21(11):2258–63.

79. Children's Oncology Group. Long-term follow-up guidelines for survivors of childhood adolescent and young adult cancer, version 5.0. Monrovia (CA): Children's Oncology Group; 2018. Available at: www.survivorshipguidelines.org.

80. Staba Hogan M-J, Ma X, Kadan-Lottick NS. New health conditions identified at a regional childhood cancer survivor clinic visit. Pediatr Blood Cancer 2013;60(4):682–7.

Moving?

Make sure your subscription moves with you!

To notify us of your new address, find your **Clinics Account Number** (located on your mailing label above your name), and contact customer service at:

Email: journalscustomerservice-usa@elsevier.com

800-654-2452 (subscribers in the U.S. & Canada)
314-447-8871 (subscribers outside of the U.S. & Canada)

Fax number: 314-447-8029

Elsevier Health Sciences Division
Subscription Customer Service
3251 Riverport Lane
Maryland Heights, MO 63043

*To ensure uninterrupted delivery of your subscription, please notify us at least 4 weeks in advance of move.